Manual Medicine
Diagnostics

2nd edition

Manual Medicine
Diagnostics

Jiří Dvořák and Václav Dvořák

with contributions by:
H. Baumgartner, D. Dalley, T. Drobný, W. Gilliar, D. Grob,
N. Gschwend, U. Munzinger, W. Schneider, B. R. Simmen,
B. Tait, W. Trautmann, T. Tritschler

Translated and edited by
Wolfgang G. Gilliar and Philip E. Greenman

2nd, revised edition
467 illustrations

Foreword by M. M. Panjabi

1990
Georg Thieme Verlag   Thieme Medical Publishers, Inc.
Stuttgart · New York   New York

Editors and Co-Workers:

Jiří Dvořák, M.D., Head of Dept. of Neurology, Spine Unit, Wilhelm Schulthess Hospital; Chairman of the Educational Program of the Swiss Medical Association of Manual Medicine, 8008 Zurich, Switzerland

Václav Dvořák, M.D., Internal and Musculoskeletal Medicine in General Practice, 7402 Bonaduz, Switzerland

Hubert Baumgartner, M.D., Head of the Department of Rheumatology, Spine Unit, Schulthess Hospital, Zurich, Switzerland

Don Dalley, M.D., Sports and Musculoskeletal Medicine, St. Albans Medical Center, Christchurch, New Zealand

Tomáš Drobný, M.D., Department of Orthopedic Surgery, Knee Unit, Schulthess Hospital, Zurich, Switzerland

Wolfgang Gilliar, D.O., Dept of Rehabilitation Medicine, Tufts University School of Medicine; Associate Director, Rehabilitation Medicine, Greenery Rehabilitation and Skilled Nursing Center, Boston, MA, USA

Dieter Grob, M.D., Head of the Department of Orthopedic Surgery, Spine Unit, Schulthess Hospital, Zurich, Switzerland

Norbert Gschwend, M.D., Professor and Chairman, Department of Orthopedic Surgery, Schulthess Hospital, Zurich, Switzerland

Urs Munzinger, M.D., Head of the Department of Orthopedic Surgery, Knee Unit, Schulthess Hospital, Zurich, Switzerland

Werner Schneider, M.D., Physical Medicine, Rehabilitation, spec. Rheumatology, Kreuzlingen, Switzerland

Beat R. Simmen, M.D., Head, Department of Orthopedic Surgery, Hand and Upper Extremity Unit, Schulthess Hospital, Zurich, Switzerland

Barrie Tait, M.D., Senior Lecturer, Department of Orthopedic Surgery and Musculoskeletal Medicine, Christchurch School of Medicine, Christchurch, New Zealand

Wolfgang Trautmann, R.P., Physiotherapy, 3063 Ittingen, Switzerland

Thomas Tritschler, R.P., Chairman, School of Physiotherapy, Kantonsspital, 8208 Schaffhausen, Switzerland

Library of Congress Cataloging-in-Publication Data

Dvořák, Jiří:
Manual medicine : diagnostics / Jiří Dvořák and Václav Dvořák. With the collab. of Tomás Drobný. Transl. and ed. by Wolfgang G. Gilliar and Philip E. Greenman. – 2., rev. ed. – Stuttgart ; New York : Thieme ; New York : Thieme Med. Publ., 1990
  Deutsche Ausg. u.d.T.: Dvořák, Jiří: Manuelle Medizin
NE: Dvořák, Václav:

This book is an authorized and revised translation from the 3rd German edition, published and copyrighted 1988 by Georg Thieme Verlag, Stuttgart, Germany.
Title of the German edition: Manuelle Medizin. Diagnostik.

1st German edition 1983   1st English edition 1984
2nd German edition 1985   1st Italian edition 1986
3rd German edition 1988   1st Japanese edition 1988
                               1st Spanish edition 1989

© 1990 Georg Thieme Verlag, Rüdigerstrasse 14,
D-7000 Stuttgart 30, Germany
Thieme Medical Publishers, Inc.,
381 Park Avenue South, New York, N.Y. 10016
Typesetting by Druckhaus Götz KG,
D-7140 Ludwigsburg (System 5, Linotron 202)
Printed in Germany by K. Grammlich,
D-7401 Pliezhausen
ISBN 3-13-660002-9 (GTV, Stuttgart)
ISBN 0-86577-306-8 (TMP, New York)   1 2 3 4 5 6

Foreword

Although my work is centered in biomechanics, I often find myself in need of more specific information to further my understanding of a particular certain research matter. For example, knowing the precise anatomic relationships between the back muscles and the spinal column plays a strategic part in developing a biomechanical understanding of the spine. *Manual Medicine: Diagnostics* has been a most valuable source of information here. Most standard anatomic texts lack the clear, instructive manner of this text, which presents the material of diagnostic manual medicine in an easily accessible style and arrangement. Clearly, the book was designed with both the clinician and the research scientist in mind.

Even if it becomes difficult for the clinician to grasp the importance of biomechanics, its inclusion in the methodology of the book is vital. The authors see the relationship of this discipline to their own to be one which aids the clinician in analyzing the pathophysiology of joint disturbances, both organic and functional. Many of the research papers produced by biomechanics laboratories clarify some hitherto unknown functions of the spine: information which attests to the need for biomechanical principles in elucidating a clinical diagnosis.

The new edition of *Manual Medicine: Diagnostics* tries to present a clinical examination according to biomechanical knowledge and principles. For each examination, the region of interest is clearly identified by a drawing, while a set of photographs depicts and describes the examination procedure. Superimposed graphics are combined with the photographic images to indicate the points of applied pressure as well as the direction of the linear and rotary forces as they are applied. Finally, the accompanying text elaborates possible pathological findings to complete the presentation of the examination.

More than simply a convenient and beneficial way of combining the intimately related fields of biomechanics and manual medicine diagnostics, Dr. Dvorak's method becomes both the substance and the structure of the text. In the second edition, careful improvements elucidate this process. Photographs in which subjects display the muscles in question have been added to accompany the anatomical drawings, and these draw on the author's knowledge of clinical medicine and biomechanical principles. In a chapter on radiologic diagnosis, new to the second edition, each clinical radiograph is accompanied by a photograph of a corresponding skeletal section.

I extend my thanks to the authors for their contribution to developing a methodology that correlates clinical manual medicine diagnostics with biomechanics. The new book presents the material in a precise, accessible manner, with many innovative graphic supplements, so that it may provide clinicians and research scientists with a complete understanding of their work, and for this I congratulate them.

Manohar M. Panjabi, Ph.D.
Professor
Department of Orthopedics and Rehabilitation;
Director
Biomechanics Research
Yale University School of Medicine
New Haven, Connecticut

Preface

The ratio of physicians practicing manual medicine in Switzerland is 1 : 9000 per head of population. 97% of the members of the Swiss Society of Manual Medicine are board-certified specialists — largely rheumatologists, internists and general practitioners. A recent survey by the Swiss Medical Association showed that 79% of all general practitioners and specialists refer their patients with functional disorders of the spine to physicians with a thorough grounding in manual medicine, or to board-certified chiropractors. According to the data of the Swiss Institute for Medical Statistics, 4 million medical consultations for disorders of the spine take place every year. 15% of these (some 600000) involve manual medicine. These numbers reflect the important role that manual medicine plays within the Swiss Medical Association.

Recent prospective and well-controlled studies have proved the validity of manual treatment in dealing with low back pain, both in the acute and in the chronic stages. Although the question of cost-effectiveness still remains unanswered, one may assume that manual medicine is not one of the more expensive therapeutic modalities.

The importance of, and responsibilities connected with, education in manual diagnostics and treatment are obvious from the above-mentioned figures. In this second edition, we have again tried to present the field of manual medicine in language which is understandable, and to base our approach on the results of clinical biomechanics as well as applied anatomy and neurophysiology.

Our close collaboration with M. M. Panjabi, Ph. D., from Yale Medical School, not only helped us to understand the complex mechanisms of segmental spinal motion, but also stimulated us to undertake our own research, combining basic science with the practical experience of everyday clinical practice.

The interdisciplinary approach we employ at the Schulthess Hospital in Zurich has helped us to determine the limitations of manual therapy, especially in relation to degenerative disorders. The chapter on clinical examination of the peripheral joints was written by our colleagues who are experts in the fields of orthopedic surgery and rheumatology. Input connected with sports and musculoskeletal medicine was provided by Dr. B. Tait and Dr. D. Dalley from New Zealand. The thesis written by Dr. T. Rudolph provided useful material for the chapter on the sacroiliac joint.

As editors, we would like to thank all our co-workers for their valuable contributions in expanding the scope of manual diagnostics. Special thanks go to our translator, erstwhile co-worker, and friend, Dr. W. Gilliar, who forms a link between European manual medicine and American osteopathic medicine.

The continuing support of the Bertelsmann Foundation, and the personal involvement of Mr. and Mrs. R. Mohn, are key factors in merging international experience in the field of manual medicine.

We are also indebted to Mr. A. Lütscher and Mrs. V. Zwicker from our Department of Medical Documentation, and to Mrs. J. Reichert for her secretarial skills in revising and typing the manuscripts.

We are grateful to Dr. Bremkamp and Mr. A. Menge from Thieme Publishers for giving us the opportunity to present a second edition. Support for the field of manual medicine from such prestigious publishers is an exciting and stimulating factor in helping to bridge the gap between classical academic medicine and this so-called "new method."

Zurich and Bonaduz   *Jiři Dvořák, M.D.*
August, 1990   *Václav Dvořák, M.D.*

Foreword to the 1st Edition

Articular neurology is the branch of neurology that is concerned with the morphology, physiology, pathology, and clinical features of the innervation of the joints of the body (including those in the vertebral column), but until about 15 years ago this discipline did not exist as an organized body of knowledge, since it had never been studied systematically in the laboratory or the clinic. Happily, articular neurology has now been developed to the point where it forms one of the basic sciences of orthopedic medicine and surgery, as well as of clinical neurology.

The observations reported in this monograph represent an important clinical application of some of what is now known of articular reflexology in a diagnostic context, and as such should prove to be of considerable significance to practitioners of manual medicine and physical therapy, as well as of orthopedics, rheumatology, and neurology. For too long, manual medicine has existed as an empirical art rather than as a clinical science, but this monograph — based as it is on some of the scientific data currently available in the field of articular neurology — should go some way toward remedying this state of affairs. It therefore gives me considerable pleasure to contribute this foreword to a work that I hope will serve as a stimulus to clinicians in a variety of disciplines, as well as to practitioners of manual medicine.

London   *Prof. Dr. B. D. Wyke, M.D., B.S.*
Director of the Neurological Unit,
Royal College of Surgeons of England

Foreword to the 1st Edition

The undersigned has neither received a formal education in manual therapy, nor does he practice such (this sentence is not a pleonasm!). Furthermore, he is neither disappointed by his own field or frustrated because of other reasons. When he recommended that this book should appear at all, this was not due to personal or complex psychological motives, nor an innate trust in this form of medicine itself.

The reasons are, on the contrary, quite rational. As a recent poll by the Swiss Medical Society for Manual Medicine indicated, approximately 300 000 manipulations are performed by physicians in Switzerland every year. About 100 chiropractors manipulate nearly 800 000 times per year. This amounts to a total of some 1.1 million manipulations in Switzerland every year. We neurologists especially, however, tend to see the undesirable side-effects and complications of manual medicine. Is this therefore not enough reason in itself to recommend a thorough explanation of one of the techniques and its fundamentals? Further, the author of this foreword has been privileged to have had numerous personal contacts with nonmedical chiropractors and physicians practicing manual medicine who have demonstrated a responsible and ethically irreproachable attitude, in-depth training and convincing therapeutic success. This alone would be a good reason for a representative of formal, organized medicine to support a publication which advocates manual therapy.

On the other hand, one experiences in diverse discussions, as always in this field, that one school of thought is set against another, when irrational and unverifiable elements with confusing terminology come into play; actually, therapeutic acts begin to assume the form of pure magic! The beneficial effects of this therapy became simply a "last resort," albeit obligatory, alternative for treatment due to the ubiquitous prejudicial consensus of opinion concerning this form of medicine. Patient demands, however, or official control, forced many therapists into a sterile confinement and restricted them in every case which presented itself into using this single approach in a one-sided intractability. A further reason in this respect for publishing one of these methods of treatment was the need for a clear and unambiguous statement of principles, claims and limitations.

This leads to the fourth and probably the most important reason for this publication: even though manual therapy has developed empirically, as indeed today's medicine has originally developed, it might nevertheless fulfill some of, the patients' expectations by a direct, "close-hand" approach which corresponds to their wishes for a "magical" panacea. With its own intrinsic procedures, manual therapy can further be viewed as a challenge to the technical and impersonal aspects of modern medicine. All this, however, is not a reason to not subject manual medicine to scientific methodology. In this context, the term "scientific" implies:

- building on existing foundations, identifying the tangible phenomena, and
- making these comprehensible and learnable.

Many representatives of this type of treatment and other "alternatives" to formal medicine have largely evaded any meaningful discussion of their particular field of activity, when brought to task. Usually, they shelter behind a mass of esoteric terminology and avoid a rational promulgation of their fundamentals, preventing them from being studied.

The physicians Jiří Dvořák, who has a comprehensive knowledge of general medicine as well as a training in neurology, Václav Dvořák, trained in internal medicine, and Tomáš Drobný, with a surgical and orthopedic specialist training behind him, have all worked as students under the auspices of the internal specialist Max Sutter as well as pursuing their own interest in manual medicine. They were thus presented with the opportunity not only to demonstrate their reproducible successes in therapeutics, but also had the courage to establish the scientific basis of the principles pertaining thereto, and lay these open to discussion. They have done this knowing that the last word in this matter has not yet been reached. They would like their interpretation of the mechanisms of manual medicine to be scrutinized, challenged and perhaps corrected. To this end it is essential that the subject be candidly laid bare. Only in this respect is the chance presented for the material to become useful and valid in the long term. To this effect, this book is scientific.

Bern   *Mark Mumenthaler*

Contents

Contents

Contents

Contents

Contents

1 Biomechanics and Functional Examination of the Spine

An understanding of the biomechanics of the spinal column is indispensable, not only for examination procedures, but also for the evaluation of radiographs and therapy. In this chapter, therefore, emphasis is placed on the biomechanics based on the fundamental work by White and Panjabi (1978a and b). Described are only those methods of examination that, in addition to rheumatological, orthopedic, and neurological procedures, have proven to be useful.

1.1 General Biomechanic Principles

1.1.1 The Axial System

Any movement in space can be defined within the framework of a three-dimensional coordinate system. Derived from general principles in the field of mechanics, this system has also found general acceptance and application in biochemanics, allowing precise definition of movement of the body and body parts in space.

The fundamental determinants of the three-dimensional coordinate system are represented by three axes. By convention, the human body in its neutral, anatomic position is placed into space, with the anteroposterior view being the standard examination view (Fig. 1.**1**). The point of intersection (O-point) of the three axes is hypothetically placed between the sacral horns. By convention, a set of three reference arrows is arranged such that they point into the positive direction, whereas arrows pointing into the opposite direction are, again by convention, designated as negative.

The primary axes in this three-dimensional coordinate system are as follows (Figs. 1.**1**, 1.**2**):

- The transverse (horizontal) x-axis. The direction to the left from the center point is designated as +x, whereas the direction to the right is designated as −x
- The vertical y-axis, which is perpendicular to the x-axis. The superior direction is designated as +y, while the inferior direction is designated as −y
- The sagittal z-axis, which is perpendicular to the x-axis in the horizontal plane. The anterior direction is designated as +z, whereas the posterior direction is designated as −z

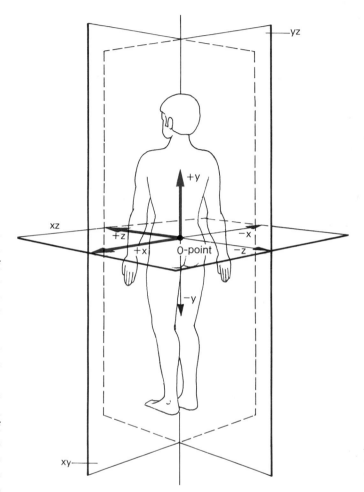

Fig. 1.**1** Three-dimensional coordinate system

yz Sagittal plane
xz Horizontal plane
xy Frontal plane

Combining two of the three axes allows definition of the three major planes in this coordinate system. The *sagittal plane* is formed by the y- and z-axes, the *horizontal plane* by the x- and z-axes, and the *frontal plane* by the x- and y-axes (Fig. 1.**1**). It is then possible to analyze each individual motion component in reference to these axes and planes, or according to the rotation around a certain axis in a specific plane.

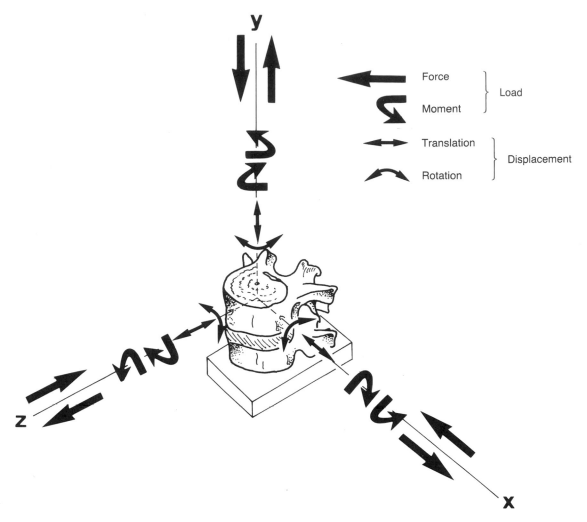

Fig. 1.2 A three-dimensional coordinate system has been placed at the center of the upper vertebral body of a vertebral unit (motion segment). A total of 12 load components, linear and rotatory, can act on theses axes; the application of any one of the load components (linear or rotatory) produces displacement of the upper vertebra with respect to the lower vertebra. This displacement consists of translation and rotation (after White and Panjabi, 1978a)

Clockwise rotation is designated as positive $(+)$ direction, whereas counter-clock-wise rotation is designated as negative $(-)$ direction.

Six major movement possibilities (degrees of freedom) can thus occur at the spine (Figs. 1.2, 1.3):

- Flexion
  $(+\varnothing x)$ describes the positive direction around the x-axis in the sagittal plane
- Extension
  $(-\varnothing x)$ describes the negative rotation around the x-axis in the sagittal plane
- Sidebending (lateral bending)
  to the right $(+\varnothing z)$, positive rotation around the z-axis in the frontal plane

- Sidebending (lateral bending)
  to the left $(-\varnothing z)$, negative rotation around the z-axis in the frontal plane
- Axial rotation
  $(+\varnothing y)$, positive rotation to the left around the y-axis in the horizontal plane
- Axial rotation
  $(-\varnothing y)$, negative rotation to the right around the y-axis in the horizontal plane

Using this convention, it is possible to break down the more complex movements into individual uniformly defined movement components. Thus, any movement can be viewed as undergoing a specific rotational movement around a certain axis (the posi-

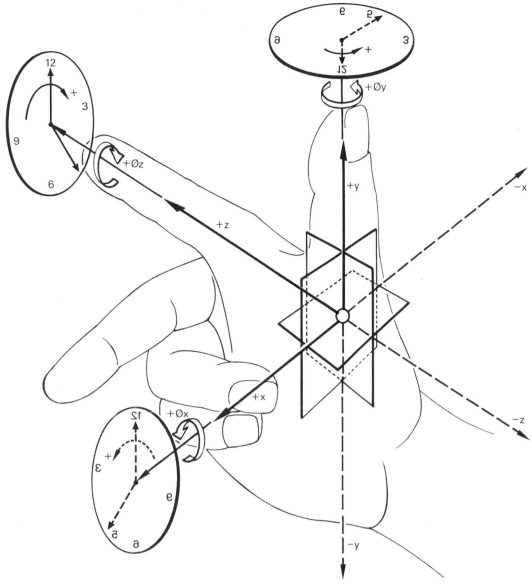

Fig. 1.3   Three finger model applied to the three-dimensional coordinate system

tive component of the previously defined three major axes). Clockwise rotation is designated as $+\varnothing$, in contrast to the counter-clockwise rotation, which is designated as $-\varnothing$ (Fig. 1.2). Thus, rotation denoted as $+\varnothing z$ corresponds to sidebending movement to the right, while $-\varnothing z$ corresponds to sidebending to the left. Flexion motion corresponds to $+\varnothing x$ and extension to $-\varnothing x$. Axial rotation to the left is identical to $+\varnothing y$, whereas rotation to the right corresponds to $-\varnothing y$.

Specifically, when interpreting either gross movement of the spine or specific segmental movement,

the following rules (conventions) should be kept in mind:

– Movement, or rotation, around a particular axis is defined in relationship to the superior and anterior aspect of the vertebral body in question (Fig. 1.4); in practice, axial rotation of the vertebra to the left ($+\varnothing y$) describes the fact that the anterior aspect of the vertebral body moves towards the left.
– Description of motion between two adjacent vertebrae (the two partners of a spinal segment) is such that motion of the superior vertebra is defined in relationship to its inferior partner

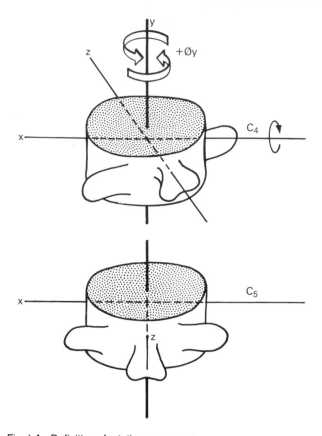

Fig. 1.4   Definition of rotation movement

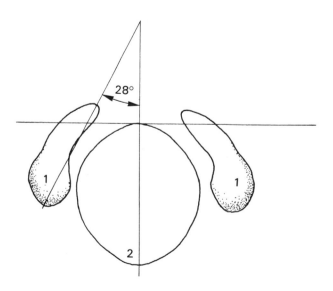

Fig. 1.5   Sagittal angle of the joint axes for the occipital condyles (after Ingelmark, 1947). 1: occipital condyles; 2: foramen magnum

Even though individual physiologic movement components can, in theory, be analyzed (i. e., using the mathematical-model), it must always be remembered that the vertebral column is both anatomically and functionally a very complex system having to fulfill the dual requirements for stability and motion. Movement in the different spinal segments can be viewed as a combination of translatory and rotatory movements around a particular axis defined by the three-dimensional coordinate system (refer to Fig. 1.3).

Axial rotation ($\pm\emptyset y$) and sidebending ($\pm\emptyset z$) in a spinal segment are coupled to each other; this has become known as *coupling patterns* (Lysell, 1969; White and Panjabi, 1978; Stooboy, 1967). The individual coupling of movements is governed by the anatomy of the different vertebrae and their joint surfaces, in addition to a complex ligamentous apparatus; they are also governed by the function of the paraspinal muscles. The physiologic curvature of the spine in the sagittal plane is of further contributing significance.

1.2   Biomechanics of the Upper Cervical Spinal Joints (C0-C1-C2)

1.2.1   Atlanto-Occipital Joint (C0-C1)

The articulation between the skull and the atlas is formed by two paired structures, each pair consisting of the occipital condyle and the superior facets of the atlas. The articulating surfaces are oval, sometimes showing a beanlike configuration. The upper surface of the condyles is convex, and the surface of the superior facets of the atlas is concave. The sagittal axial angle of the joints is 50° to 60° for the adult (Ingelmark, 1947; Bernhard, 1976) (Fig. 1.5).

The frontal axial angle of the joints (Fig. 1.6) results from lines drawn parallel to the articulating surfaces of the condyles. On the average, it is 124,2° (Stoff, 1976). This axial angle is increased in the event of condylar hypoplasia and basilar impression.

Von Lanz and Wachsmuth (1979) describe the joint between the skull and the atlas as a modified spherical articulation, with mobility around two axes according to the anatomical arrangement. The left and right joints acting in conjunction allow movement around the larger transverse axis and the smaller sagittal axis.

Flexion and extension movements take place around the transverse axis, whereas lateral bending is around the sagittal axis (Fig. 1.7).

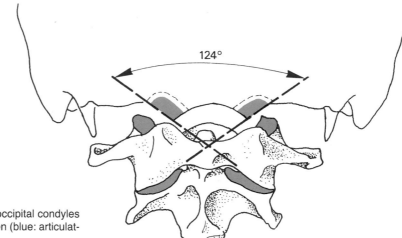

Fig. 1.**6**   Frontal angle of the joint axes for the occipital condyles (after Stoff, 1976) is 124° for men, 127° for women (blue: articulating surface)

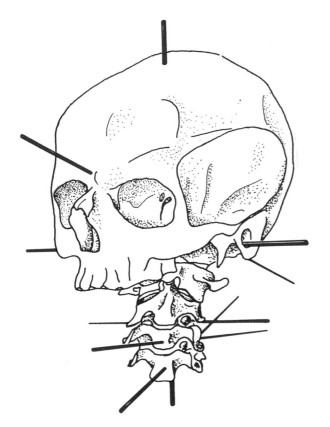

Fig. 1.**7**   Axes of motion of the occipital-atlanto-axial and cervical joints (after Knese, 1947/50)

1.2.1.1 Function of the Upper Cervical Joints (C0-C1)

Rotation takes place around the transverse axis, measuring an average of twenty-four degrees. It is limited by the bony and surrounding soft tissue structures (Panjabi, Dvořák et al. 1988) (Table 1.**1**).

Rotation at this level has been specifically termed inclination and reclination motion, analogous to forward flexion and extension, respectively.

Cervical spine flexion takes place in two phases (Dul 1982; Arlen 1977; Gutmann 1981). During the first phase, only a positive rotation around the x-axis in the C0-C1 spinal segment has been observed. This forward movement of the head in relation to the atlas measures approximately 8° and has also been assigned a specific term, that is, the "nodding" (nutation) motion. The spinal segments below this point remain in the neutral position. It is not until the second phase that rotation $(+\emptyset x)$ takes place in the other cervical spinal segments: C1-C2 (tilted forward); C2-C3 to C6-C7 (flexion). In respect to C7, the axis rotates 45 degrees. Furthermore, during this second phase a positional change occurs in the C0-C1 segment at the same time that the head rotates backward (in relation to the atlas). This relative negative rotation of the head in reference to the atlas and the axis (i. e., backward rotation) prevents an exaggerated cervical spine kyphosis and possible associated changes in the spinal canal.

Table 1.**1**   Restriction of the range of motion of the occipital-atlanto-axial joints about the transverse axis

Flexion	Extension
Nuchal ligament	Bony limitation
Posterior longitudinal ligament	Anterior muscles of the back
Longitudinal fasciculus of the cruciform ligament	
Tectorial membrane	Alar ligaments
Posterior muscles of the back	Anterior longitudinal ligament

5

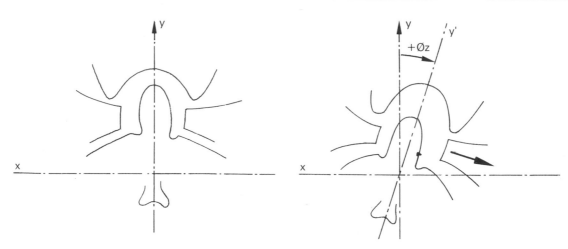

Fig. 1.**8**   Gliding movement of the atlas with sidebending to the right

Sidebending, also known as lateral bending, takes place around the sagittal axis and measures approximately 5° to one side (Panjabi, Dvořák et al., 1988; Penning 1978). It is greatest when the head is slightly flexed. Sidebending movement usually does not occur when the head is in extension, due to the action of the alar ligaments.

With sidebending, Gutmann (1981) reports a transverse gliding movement of the atlas between the condyles and the body of the axis (in the atlanto-occipital an atlantoaxial joints). The gliding movement is in the same direction as the gross sidebending movement (Fig. 1.**8**).

Reports in the literature dealing with the biomechanics of sidebending movement have been contradictory. Pure cervical spine sidebending movement without simultaneous rotation of the head is a complex movement. In addition to segmental tilting, there is always forced coupled rotation in the same direction as in sidebending in the C2-C7 vertebrae. Starting superiorly, the degree of this forced rotational movement decreases while moving inferiorly along the cervical spine. Werne (1957) and Fielding (1957) report that with maximal sidebending the axis actually rotates to a greater degree than during maximal rotation of the head and cervical spine. Lewit's (1987) findings vary from those reported by the former two authors, while Gutmann (1987) and Kamieth (1987) emphasize that there is virtually no atlas rotation with pure sidebending movement.

Various mechanisms have been proposed to explain the cause of this forced rotation. Most authors agree that it is due to the unique anatomic arrangement of the joints and their articulations in the cervical spine.

Werne (1957) suggests that the forced rotation of the axis is the result of the eccentric insertion of the alar ligaments. Jirout (1973) postulates that, in addition to the influence of the articular processes, the muscles in the head and neck region with their insertions at the spinous processes play a specific role in achieving forced rotation during the second phase.

In the atlantoaxial joint, in addition to axial rotation, there ist displacement of the atlas in the same direction as sidebending (in the frontal plane). This becomes apparent on the anteroposterior view of X-rays where the dens of the axis is located asymmetrically, on either side of the center between the two lateral masses. The offset is termed positive when the surface of the atlas projects beyond the surface of the axis, and negative when the surface of the axis projects beyond that of the atlas. Furthermore, the appearance and degree of offset is dependent upon those changes stemming from the rotation of the axis itself. According to Gutmann (1986) and Lewit (1986), it is the wedgelike anatomic arrangement of the atlas that causes it to be displaced towards the side of lateral bending.

Reports about lateral atlas displacement have also been inconsistent. Keim (1986) was able to demonstrate this deplacement with maximal sidebending in all 25 of cases studied. In contrast, out of a group of 30 subjects, Lewit (1986) found only four cases of paradoxical displacement, that is, where the atlas was displaced towards the side opposite to that of lateral bending. In both of these studies, the sidebending movement was actively performed by the subjects. Jirout (1986) found that atlantoaxial changes are more pronounced when there is passive, rather than

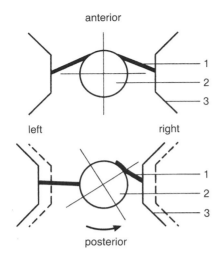

Fig. 1.9 Atlas displacement with sidebending; hypothetical mechanism. Coupled rotation of the axis causes the anterior portion of the right alar ligament to be wrapped around the dens, thus bringing the right-sided lateral mass of the atlas closer to the dens. The anterior portion of the left alar ligament does not become tight until its insertion has been rotated into the posterior position (after Werne)

1 Alar ligament
2 Dens of the axis
3 Atlas (lateral mass)

active, sidebending. Kamieth (1986) postulates that the displacement is a function of the degree of axis rotation.

The author has postulated that lateral atlas displacement is affected by the anterior portion of the alar ligament, which wraps itself around the dens. This presumes that the forced rotation of the axis is primary to that of the lateral displacement of the atlas, and that the course of the alar ligaments is as reported by Ludwig (1957), (Fig. 1.9).

In all 30 adolescents studied by the author, the gliding movement of the atlas was found to occur in the same direction as sidebending. This gliding movement was more pronounced in patients with proven atlantoaxial instability secondary to rheumatoid arthritis. The distance between the dens of the axis and the lateral mass of the atlas was used for measurement (Reich and Dvořák 1986).

Reports about the *rotation movement* in the atlantoaxial joint differ as well. Fielding (1957, 1978), White and Panjabi (1978a and b), and Penning (1968) reported that rotation in this joint is nonexistent, whereas Depreux and Mestdagh (1974) described approximately 5° of motion, with values being significantly higher in cases of atlantoaxial fusion. Gutmann (1981) reports that when the head is being

turned, the atlas undergoes a rotation movement (±∅y) in relation to the axis. The lateral portion of the fibrous joint capsule associated with the facet joints in the upper cervical spine is taut, providing specific control of rotation and sidebending (in conjunction with other limiting anatomic factors, such as joint inclination and arrangement). Caviezel (1976) clinically examines the "passive endpoint rotation" of the atlas by using the springing test.

Using functional computed tomogram (CT) scans of the upper cervical spine in fresh cadavers, rotation between the occiput and atlas were clearly demonstrated (Dvořák and Panjabi, 1986). The mean values were 4.5° and 5.9° for rotation to the right and to the left, respectively. In healthy adults as well, rotation between the occiput and the atlas was clearly demonstrated on functional CT scans, with the average value being 4°(Dvořák and Hayek, 1987). The recent in vitro study by Panjabi, Dvořák et al. (1988) analyzing the three-dimensional movements of the upper cervical spine using stereophotogrammetry confirmed the atlanto-occipital rotation of 7° to one side. Table 1.2 summarizes the mean values of motion at the atlanto-occipital joint.

Table 1.2 Range of motion at the C0−C1 joint (Panjabi et al., 1988)

	Flexion/ extension (total)	Lateral bending (one side)	Axial rotation (one side)
Fick (1904)	50	30−40	0
Poirier and Charpy (1926)	50	14−40	0
Werne (1957)	13	8	0
Penning (1978)	30	10	0
Dvořák et al (1985)	—	—	5.2
Clark et al (1986)	22.7	—	4.8
Dvořák et al (1987)	—	—	4.0
Penning and Wilmink (1987)	—	—	1.0
Panjabi et al (1988)	3.5/21.0	5.5	7.2

1.2.2 Atlantoaxial Joint (C1-C2)

The atlantoaxial joint with its dominant rotatory movement, is also important. Motion takes place in four articular spaces, one of which is designated the bursa atlantodentalis; this is the space between the transverse ligament of the atlas and the dens of the axis.

The middle atlantoaxial joint is located between the dens of the axis and the posterior surface of the anterior arch of the atlas. The two articular spaces of

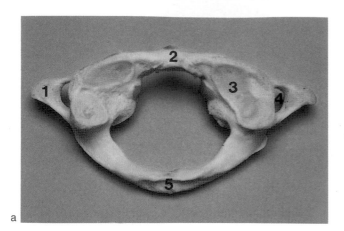

a

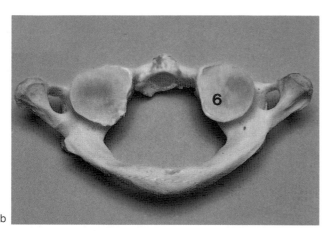

b

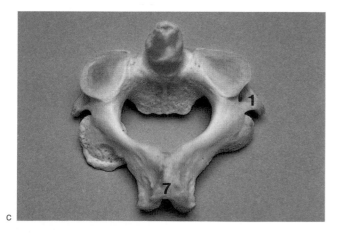

c

Fig. 1.**10a** Atlas, superior view; the superior joint surfaces are oval, sometimes with double formation (left)
b Atlas, view from inferior; round joint surfaces
c Axis, superior view; the joint surfaces point inferiorly (meniscoid)

1 Transverse process
2 Anterior tubercle
3 Superior articular facet of the atlas
4 Transverse foramen
5 Posterior tubercle
6 Inferior articular facet of the atlas
7 Spinous process

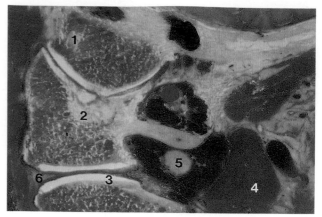

Fig. 1.**11** Sagittal section of the upper cervical spine

1 Occipital condyle   4 Vertebral artery
2 Atlas   5 Great occipital nerve
3 Axis   6 Meniscoid

the lateral atlantoaxial joint are of primary importance (Fig. 1.**10**). The joint surfaces are usually round, but sometimes triangular, and covered with cartilage of 1.4 to 3.2 mm thickness. The articular surfaces of the axis are convex, and those of the atlas are relatively flat, causing an anterior and posterior gap of 2 to 5 mm (Knese, 1947/50) (Fig. 1.**11**). The joint capsule is wide and flabby, and from the medial wall a cuneiform synovial fold reaches into the articular space (meniscoid).

1.2.2.1 Function of the Atlantoaxial Joint

Flexion/extension: The bony structures of the articular surfaces, along with the securing ligamentous apparatus, allow minimal movement around the transverse axis of not more than 21° (Panjabi et al., 1988) (Fig. 1.**7**). In the lateral X-ray, the effectiveness of the ligaments can be determined by the distance between the back of the anterior arch of the atlas and the dens of the axis. As this distance increases, so does insufficiency.

Sidebending: An average of 13° sidebending between C1 and C2 is only possible with simultaneous rotation around the axis. This is described as forced rotation and is probably the result of the physiologic function of the alar ligaments. Lewit (1970) and Jirout (1973) report dislocation of the atlas in the direction of the bending when lateral bending is forced.

Rotation: The head and atlas rotate simultaneously on the axis around the dens. The rotational axis passing through the dens of the axis is determined by the transverse ligament of the atlas (Fig. 1.**7**). Average rotation in the young, healthy adult has been

Table 1.**3**   Range of motion at C1−C2 joint

	Flexion/ extension (total)	Lateral bending (one side)	Axial rotation (one side)
Fick (1904)	0	0	60
Poirier and Charpy (1926)	11	—	30−80
Werne (1957)	10	0	47
Penning (1978)	30	10	70
Dvořák et al (1985)	—	—	32.2
Clark et al (1986)	10	—	14.5
Dvořák et al (1987)	—	—	43.1
Penning and Wilmink (1987)	—	—	40.5
Panjabi et al (1988)	11.5/10.9	6.7	38.9

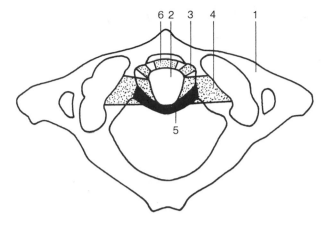

Fig. 1.**12** Schematic representation of the ligamentous apparatus at the craniocervical junction

1 Atlas
2 Dens of the axis
3 Atlantal portion of the alar ligament
4 Occipital portion of the alar ligament
5 Transverse ligament of the atlas
6 Anterior atlantodental ligament

determined to be 43° (SD = 6°), which amounts to approximately half of the cervical spine rotation (Dvořák and Hayek, 1987). Normal values for axial rotation in the upper cervical spine are listed in Table 1.**2**. Cinematographic studies by Fielding (1957, 1978) clearly demonstrate that, starting from the neutral position, rotation takes place in the atlantoaxial joints first. Once their motion is completed, the lower cervical spine segments begin to rotate. The limitation of the rotation is primarily effected by the alar ligaments (Fig. 1.**15**, 1.**16**).

Coupled movement: Motion between segments is primarily a coupling between that in the frontal plane ($\pm\varnothing z$) and the transverse plane ($\pm\varnothing y$). This may occur either in two or three dimensions. According to Gutmann (1981), axial rotation of the head ($\pm\varnothing y$) and atlas rotation in the opposite direction occur with sidebending, while C2 undergoes axial rotation toward the same side as in sidebending.

Translatory gliding: Minimal lateral translatory gliding of up to 2 to 3 mm takes place in the sagittal plane (z-axis) and transverse plane (x-axis) (Hohl, 1964). These two movements are always coupled to axial rotation movement. Axial rotation is accompanied by a vertical translatory gliding movement (y-axis). The review of the literature as related to the motion of the atlantoaxial joint are summarized in Table 1.**3**.

1.2.3   Ligaments of the Upper Cervical Spine

In this context, only those ligaments are described that appear important for the function of the atlantooccipital and atlantoaxial joints, such as the alar ligaments and the cruciform ligament of the atlas (Fig. 1.**12**).

1.2.3.1 Alar Ligaments

Ludwig (1952) describes the alar ligament as an irregular, quadrilateral pyramidlike trunk. The rectangular base lies against the superior two thirds of the lateral surface of the dens. The superior, posterior, and anterior surfaces connect the dens with the occipital condyle, and the inferior and lateral surfaces connect the dens with the lateral mass of the atlas (Fig. 1.**13**).

The orientation of the fibers in the sagittal plane is primarily a function of the height difference between the tip of the dens of the axis and the occipital condyles (Fig. 1.**13c**). The ligament that connects the dens of the axis and the anterior arch of the atlas is part of the alar ligament as well (Fig. 1.**14**). Occasionally, the presence of another ligamentous connection between the base of the dens of the axis and the anterior arch of the atlas has been observed that is, the so-called anterior atlanto-dental ligament (described by Barrow, 1841).

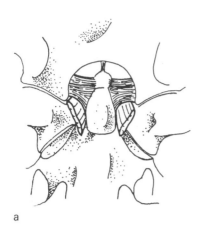

a

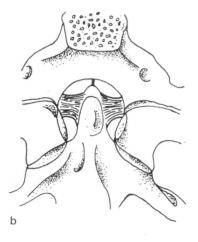

b

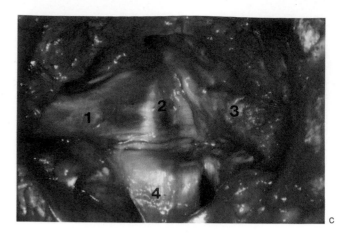

c

Fig. 1.13 The alar ligaments, seen **a** from superior and **b** from anterior (after Ludwig, 1952) **c** Anatomic specimen in the anteroposterior view

1 Left alar ligament
2 Dens of the axis
3 Right alar ligament
4 Longitudinal ligament

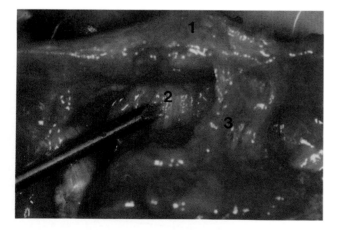

Fig. 1.14 Ligamentous interconnection between the dens of the axis and the atlas. View from superior onto the ligaments associated with the upper cervical spinal joints. The probe is on the anterior atlantodental ligament

1 Anterior arch of the atlas
2 Anterior atlantodental ligament
3 Alar ligament

Biomechanics of the Alar Ligaments

The mechanical properties of the alar ligaments depend primarily on three factors:

– Fiber orientation
– The proportion of collagenous versus elastic fibers
– The mechanical properties of the collagenous and elastic fibers

The collagenous fibers will be irreversibly stretched if subjected to a stretch beyond 6% to 8% of resting length, and will ultimately start to tear when stretched further (Abrahams, 1967). Elastic fibers, in contrast, can be stretched to 200% of their resting length, at which point they rupture abruptly. Within this context then, it can be said that, in essence, the collagenous fibers cannot be stretched.

The alar ligaments are almost entirely made up of collagenous fibers (Saldinger et al. 1989) (Fig. 1.15). At the attachments they run parallel, while at the center they tend to be interdigitated in a criss-cross

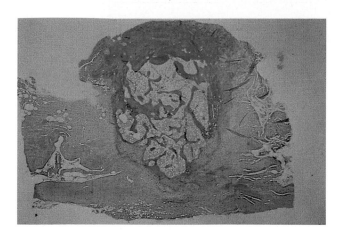

Fig. 1.**15** The alar ligaments are made up of collagenous fibers (Giemsa stain)

1 Dens axis
2 Left alar ligament
3 Right alar ligament

pattern (Dvořák and Schneider, 1987). It was determined by mechanical testing that, on the average, the alar ligaments rupture at 200 N.

Function of the Alar Ligaments

It is not difficult to deduce the function of the alar ligaments, especially when considering their course, which is governed by the attachment at the occipital condyles and the atlas. The primary role of the alar ligaments is to limit axial rotation in the upper cervical spine (C0-C1 and C1-C2 joints). Rotation to the right is limited by the left alar ligament, and vice versa. Rotation to one side causes the contralateral ligament to become more taut (Fig. 1.**16**). During sidebending to one side (equal to rotation around the z-axis), the occipital portion of the ligament on that side is relaxed. In contrast, the atlantal portion becomes tight and thus limits gliding of the atlas in

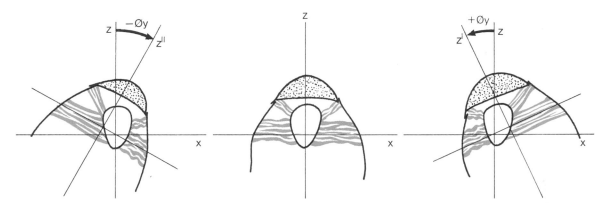

Fig. 1.**16** Function of the alar ligaments during rotation in the atlantoaxial joint (C1−C2)
z−z′ Rotation to the right, z−z″ Rotation to the left

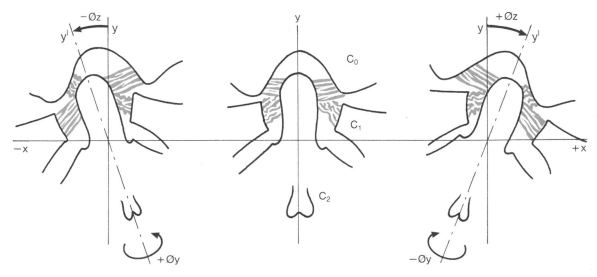

Fig. 1.**17** Function of the alar ligaments during sidebending in the atlantoaxial joint (C1−C2)

the ipsilateral direction as in sidebending. At the same time, the occipital portion of the opposite alar ligament becomes tighter, which limits gliding of the occipital condyles in the opposite direction (Fig. 1.**17**). The tight occipital portion of the alar ligament with its posterior and eccentric origin at the dens of the axis, together with the opposite atlantal portion and its anterior eccentric origin at the dens of the axis, induces forced rotation of the axis towards the same side as in sidebending. Clinically, the spinous process of the axis moves towards the opposite side, that is, in the direction of the convexity (Fig. 1.**17**). (Reich and Dvořák, 1985; Dvořák et al., 1987). Based on data from various experimental studies, it cannot be concluded that only the action of the alar ligaments causes forced rotation of the axis, especially since the anatomy of the joint itself, that is surface inclination, must be taken into account. Further studies are necessary to clarify the complex function of the ligaments.

Flexion in the upper cervical spine is primarily limited by the nuchal and posterior longitudinal ligaments, the tectorial membrane, the longitudinal fascicles of the cruciform ligament, and, finally, a taut alar ligament. Extension movement is primarily limited by the transverse-orientated alar ligaments.

The alar ligaments are subjected to the greatest tension forces and therefore are more likely to be irreversibly stretched or even ruptured. This could be especially true when the head is rotated maximally (rotation around the y-axis) followed by flexion and extension movements (rotation around the x-axis). A similar positional arrangements has frequently been observed in people involved in rear-end motor vehicle collisions. It can therefore be surmised that under similar circumstances it is the alar ligaments that are damaged, while the transverse ligament may remain essentially unaffected.

During *rotation* of the atlantoaxial joint, the ligament of the opposite side is stretched and "rolled up" around the dens of the axis; the ligament on the same ride relaxes. Thus, during rotation to the right, the left alar ligament is "rolled up", and the right ligament relaxes (Fig. 1.**16**).

During *sidebending,* the alar ligament of that same side relaxes, and the stretched ligament of the opposite side causes a forced rotation of the axis in the direction of the bending, due to the attachment to the dens of the axis (the spinous process of the axis moves contralaterally; Fig. 1.**17**). Thus, the strong alar ligaments are able to limit the rotation of the atlantoaxial joints.

1.2.3.2 The Cruciform Ligament of the Atlas

The cruciform ligament consists of the horizontal transverse ligament of the atlas and the vertical longitudinal fasciculi. The transverse ligament of the atlas arises from the medial surfaces of the lateral masses of the atlas, portions of the fibers being attached to the tip of the dens. The ligament consists primarily of collagen fibers that can be irreversibly stretched under strong tension (Kennedy et al., 1976). The central portion of the ligaments is 10 mm high, 2 mm thick, and covered by a thin layer of cartilage. The longitudinal fasciculi are weak and are present inconsistently. They merge with the atlanto-occipital membrane (Fig. 1.**18**).

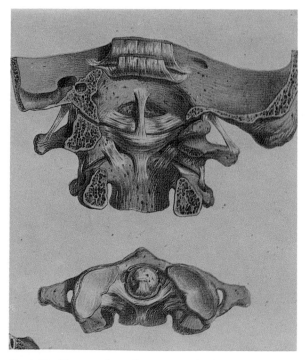

Fig. 1.**18** The cruciform ligament and other ligaments of the occipital-atlanto axial complex. Above: posterior view; below: superior view (from Arnold, 1845)

Biomechanics of the Transverse Ligament of the Atlas

The transverse ligament is primarily made up of collagenous fibers. The collagenous fiber bundles are oriented in parallel at the insertion only to form a criss-cross pattern at the center of the ligament, which is also the thickest portion. The portion facing the dens of the axis may have undergone fibrocartilagenous changes.

This ligament ruptures at approximately 350 N. Histologic examinations reveal that the primary site of rupture is at the bone-cartilage insertion interface (Dvořák et al., 1987).

Function of the Cruciform Ligament of the Atlas

The function of the cruciform ligament is to secure physiologic rotation between C1 and C2 and to protect the spinal cord form the dens of the axis.

Macalister (1893) found that the transverse ligament of the atlas tears at a load of 130 kg. Fielding et al. (1974) examined the tensile strength of the alar ligaments and the cruciform ligament of the atlas in 20 corpses. They found that the ligaments tear at a load of 400 N to 1800 N (average, 1100 N).

The transverse ligament of the atlas tears when stretched to a length beyond 4.8 to 7.6 mm. Overstretching will lead to tearing of the collagenous fibers, which can be seen on radiographs as an increase in the distance between the dens and the posterior surface of the anterior arch of the axis of more than 3 mm (more prominent in radiographs taken in the flexed position). With a distance of 7 mm, complete separation of the transverse ligament from the atlas is to be expected; with distances greater than 10 to 12 mm, tearing of the alar ligaments is to be expected.

The spatial relationship between the bony structures of the atlas, the dens of the axis, the spinal cord, and the free zone is designated as an anatomical constant. Generally, the rule of thirds by Steele (1968) has proved valuable (Fig. 1.**19**). One third of the space is occupied by the dens, one third by the spinal cord, and one third by a free space, the socalled safety zone of the spinal cord.

Considering the anatomical position of the cardiac and respiratory centers in the medulla oblongata, the double control is plausible in regard to the prevention of a dens dislocation via the alar ligaments and the transverse ligament of the axis. Huguenin (personal communication, 1980) points out the clinical symptomatology and the resulting changes seen on radiographs for the partial and complete tearing of the ligaments in the occipital-atlanto-axial joint region, both in functional tomograms and CT scans.

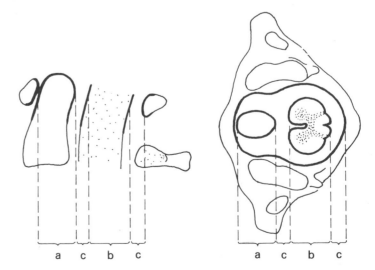

Fig. 1.**19** Steel's rule of thirds (1968): a = b = 2c = ⅓ (a + b + 2c). a: dens axis; b: spinal cord, c: safety zone

1.2.4 Radiologic Studies of the Upper Cervical Spine

Conventional anteroposterior and lateral radiographs provide only limited information about the function of the upper cervical spine. Normal relationships as seen in the upper cervical spine of a healthy adult are depicted in Figure 1.20. In contrast, the radiographs of a 67-year-old female patient with proven atlantoaxial instability secondary to rheumatoid arthritis is shown in Figure 1.21 (same views). Conventional X-rays do not provide information about axial rotation, which is the dominant movement of the upper cervical spine. Thus, functional CT scans may be considered as a supplement to the classic conventional X-ray studies (Dvořák and Panjabi, 1987; Dvořák and Hajek, 1987; Penning and Willming, 1987). The ligaments can be visualized in the sagittal cuts of the CT scans (Fig. 1.22).

In the functional CT studies of the upper cervical spine, the head is passively rotated to its extreme. This allows evaluation of the range of motion between the occiput and atlas, the atlas and axis, and the vertebrae below. The technique itself, as well as the interpretation of the results, require a good

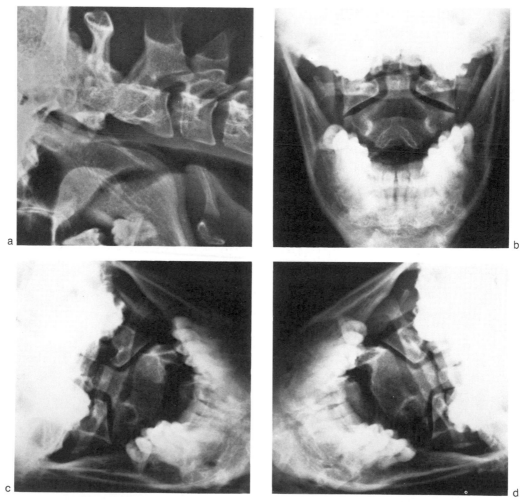

Fig. 1.20 Conventional radiographs in lateral and anteroposterior projections in a 23-year-old, healthy adult male (from Reich and Dvořák, 1986)

a Maximal flexion (flexion at the upper cervical joints)
b Neutral anteroposterior position
c Sidebending to the right
d Sidebending to the left

three-dimensional understanding and significant practice.

For the measurements, Penning (1987) has used identical bony landmarks and avoided the unclear situation by superimposing the next levels in order to determine the range of motion. By controlling the measurement errors, he has found the biggest difference in the upper cervical spine, trying to explain that by the lateral tilting of the occiput and atlas. Based upon the author's further development of this technique, this measurement error could be avoided by using the Arrange program of General Electric (GE). As landmarks for the occiput, the protuberantia occipitalis and the nasal septa for C1 and C2 and for the rest of the vertebrae below the traverse foramina are marked. For each segment it is possible to connect two points on a set of four images and obtain the exact rotatory angle, which is immediately calculated by the computer. This technique is especially helpful for the measurement of the atlas rotation, since the transverse foramina of this vertebra seldom appears on the same image due to lateral tilting (Dvořák 1988) (Fig. 1.**23**).

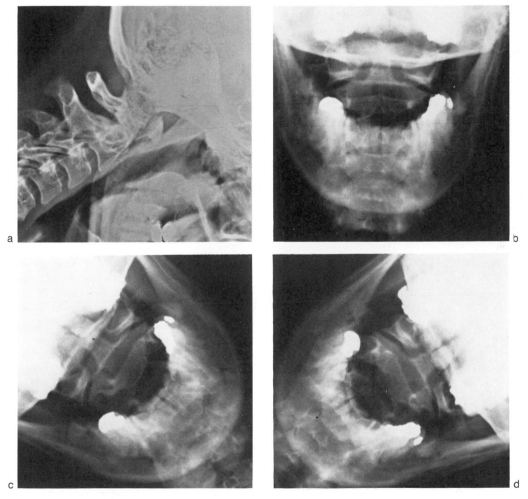

Fig. 1.**21**   67-year-old patient with chronic polyarthritis

a   Maximal flexion; in this lateral view, there is significant atlantoaxial instability

b   Neutral position in the anteroposterior projection

c, d   There is increased distance between the dens of the axis and the lateral mass of the atlas during sidebending to both the left and right (Reich and Dvořák, 1986)

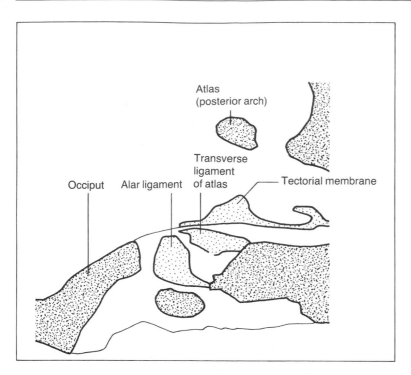

Atlas
(posterior arch)

Transverse
ligament
of atlas

Occiput   Alar ligament   Tectorial membrane

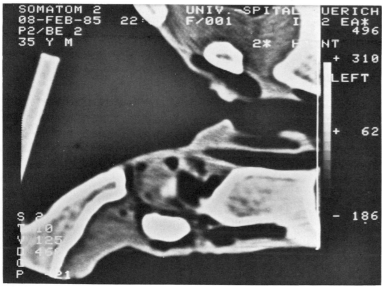

Fig. 1.22   CT scan: sagittal section at the
upper cervical spine (cadaver specimen)

Based on examinations of both healthy subjects and patients with soft tissue injuries, a set of values have been reported that indicate the possibility of hypermobility or hypomobility. These values are presented in Table 1.3. Figure 1.23 is an example of a normal functional CT scan in a healthy adult. The values presented in Figure 1.24 suggests that there is rotational instability to the right.

Fig. 1.23   Functional CTs of the upper cervical spine. Female, 39 ▶
years old, after severe soft-tissue injury of the cervical spine
(whiplash injury). *Rotation to the right* was measured as: occiput
86°, atlas 88°, axis 33° — C0 C1 −2° (paradoxical rotation),
C1–C2 55° (increased), C2–C7 33°. *Rotation to the left* was
measured as: occiput 86°, atlas 82°, axis 30° — C0–C1 4°,
C1–C2 52°, C2–C7 30°

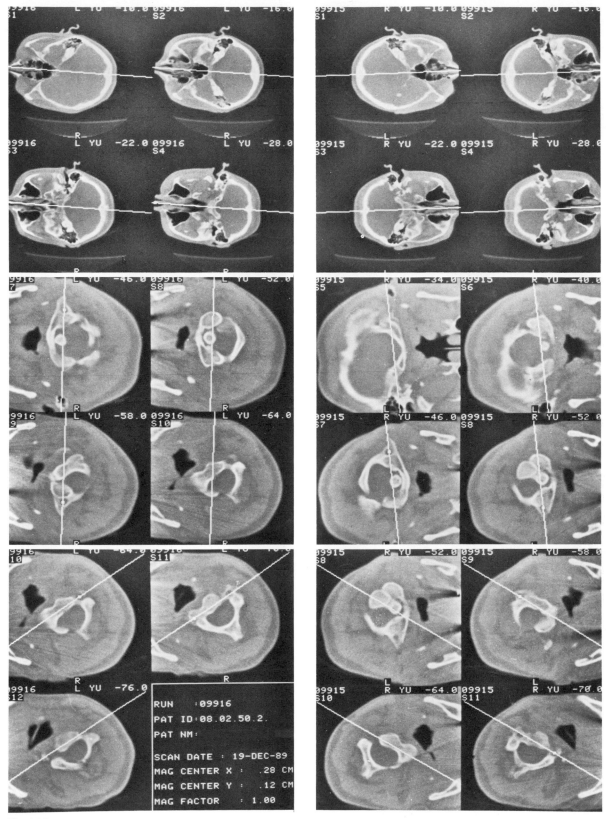

Fig. 1.23

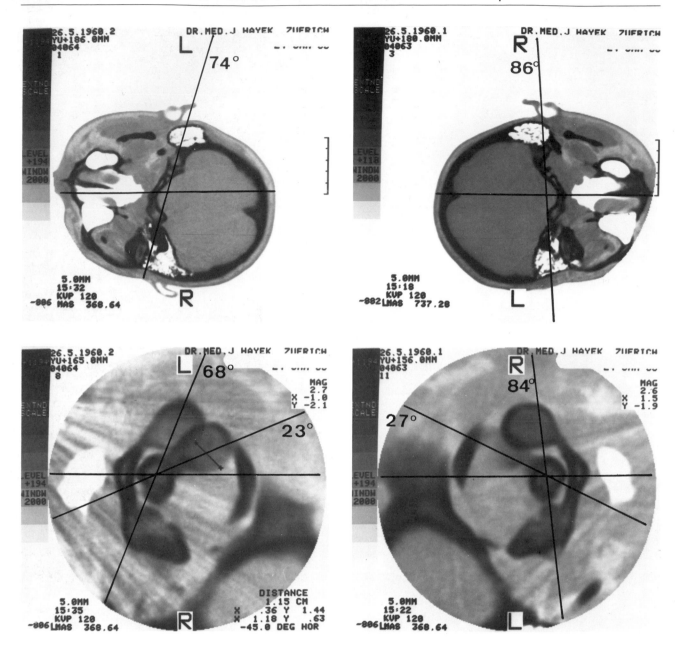

Fig. 1.**24** Functional CTs of the upper cervical spine of a 26-year-old patient with soft-tissue injuries to the cervical spine. Rotation of the axis and the spinal segments below measures 23° to the right and 27° to the left; rotation of the atlas in relationship to the axis measures 45° to the right and 57° to the left; rotation of the occiput measures 6° to the right and 2° to the left. The left-right difference of rotation at the C1–C2 joint measures 12° (suspicious for instability of rotation to the right at C1–C2)

1.3 Biomechanics of the Lower Cervical Spine (C3-C7)

The axis is a transitional vertebra between the upper and lower cervical spine. The greatest range of motion takes place in the mid-cervical spine region where the following motions are possible: flexion/extension, lateral bending (lateral flexion), and rotation (Table 1.**4**).

The inclination of the central and lower cervical spine facets is 45° to the horizontal plane. The lower segments are steeper than the upper segments (Figs. 1.**25**, 1.**26**).

The motions possible in an individual segment (vertebral unit) can be considered as the combined translatory-rotatory motion around the respective axis of the three-dimensional coordinate system.

For flexion and extension, Lysell (1969) describes a so-called top angle upon which the individual segments move. This so-called segmental arch is flat at C1, and almost semicircular at C7 (Fig. 1.**27**). The top angle is determined by the inclination of the individual facets and the condition of the intervertebral disk.

Flexion/extension motion ($\pm\emptyset x$) is greatest in the central portion of the cervical spine (Table 1.**4**), with the largest value at C5-C6 (approximately 17°). This phenomenon is often quoted as being one of the causes of cervical spondyloarthropathy in the midcervical spine.

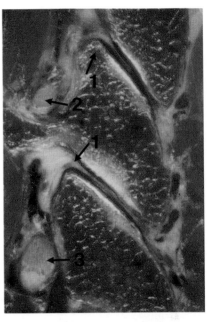

Fig. 1.**26** Sagittal section through the zygapophyseal joints at the lower cervical spine. The orientation of the articular process is approximately 45° (with permission from W. Rausching, Uppsala, Sweden)

1 Meniscoid   2 Spinal nerve   3 Ganglion

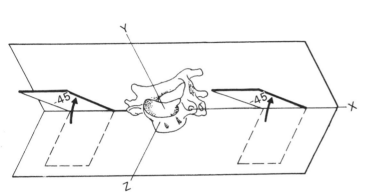

Fig. 1.**25** Facet joint inclinations and axes of motion for vertebra C4 (after White and Panjabi, 1978a)

Table 1.**4** Limits and representative values of range of rotation of the lower cervical spine (after White and Panjabi, 1978a)

Spinal segments	Flexion/extension (x-axis rotation)		Lateral bending (z-axis rotation)		Axial rotation (y-axis rotation)	
	Limits of ranges (degrees)	Representative angle (degrees)	Limits of ranges (degrees)	Representative angle (degrees)	Limits of ranges (degrees)	Representative angle (degrees)
C2–C3	5–23	8	11–20	10	6–28	9
C3–C4	7–38	13	9–15	11	10–28	11
C4–C5	8–39	12	0–16	11	10–26	12
C5–C6	4–34	17	0–16	8	8–34	10
C6–C7	1–29	16	0–17	7	6–15	9
C7–T1	4–17	9	0–17	4	5–13	8

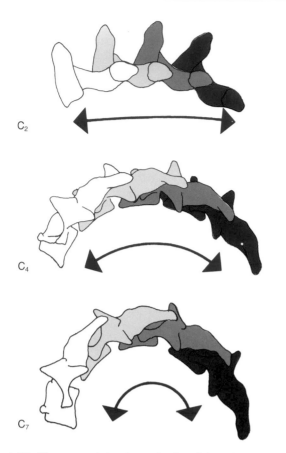

C₂

C₄

C₇

Fig. 1.**27** The segmental arches, after Lysell (1969) (from White and Panjabi, 1978b)

Translatory gliding movement takes place in the sagittal plane, and measures between 2.0 and 3.5 mm ($\pm$ z-axis) (White, 1975).

1.3.1 Coupling Patterns with Lateral Bending and Rotation

Lysell (1969) postulated and measured the coupling patterns for lateral flexion and rotation of the cervical spine. These coupling patterns are of clinical importance and are evaluated during the functional examination.

When the head is sidebent, the spinous processes move in the direction of the convexity, that is, in lateral bending to the left they move to the right. Motion about the z-axis is coupled to a rotation around the y-axis, and vice versa. At the second cervical vertebra, there are 2° of coupled axial rotation for every 3° of lateral bending. At the seventh cervical vertebra, there is 1° of coupled rotation for every 7.5° of lateral bending (White and Panjabi, 1978b) (Figs. 1.**28**, 1.**29**).

In the osteopathic literature, this coupling of movements is described as type-II movement (Ward and Sprafka, 1981; Fryette, 1954). In other words, with the vertebral column being either flexed or extended (in the sagittal plane), sidebending to one side is associated with rotation to the same (concave) side.

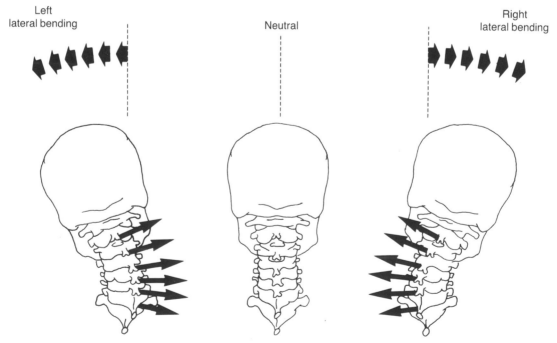

Left lateral bending   Neutral   Right lateral bending

Fig. 1.**28** Major cervical spine coupling patterns (after White and Panjabi, 1978b)

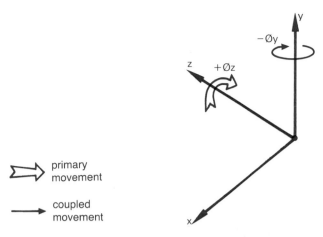

primary
movement

coupled
movement

Fig. 1.**29** Coupled movements in the cervical spine. $+\varnothing z$ is accompanied by $-\varnothing y$

1.4   Vertebral Artery

The vertebral artery must be mentioned in connection with the functional examination and biomechanics of the cervical spine. It enters the costotransverse foramen of C6, occasionally that of C5, and runs to the axis through the costovertebral

foramina of the individual vertebra. After a slight posterolateral curvature, it enters the costotransverse foramen of the atlas and upon exit forms a posterosuperiorly directed loop that punctures the atlanto-occipital membrane and the dura mater in the region of the foramen magnum at the occiput (Fig. 1.**30**).

It is known that extreme rotation of the head can cause neurological symptoms, such as dizziness, nausea, and tinnitus. These are often caused by a transient, decreased blood supply in the basilar region, since rotation of the head between 30° and 45° to one side causes the blood flow to be diminished in the opposite vertebral artery at the atlantoaxial junction (Fielding, 1957) (Fig. 1.**31**, 1.**32**).

Rotational instability in the upper cervical spine, both constitutional as well as acquired (i. e., trauma), may lead to a mechanical reduction of the blood supply. Furthermore, due to the close anatomic proximity of the vertebral artery with the margins of the C1 and C2 facet joints during rotation, mechanical irritation is much more likely and may lead to reflex spasms (Fig. 1.**32**). Of significance, in addition to rotational instability, are degenerative changes which

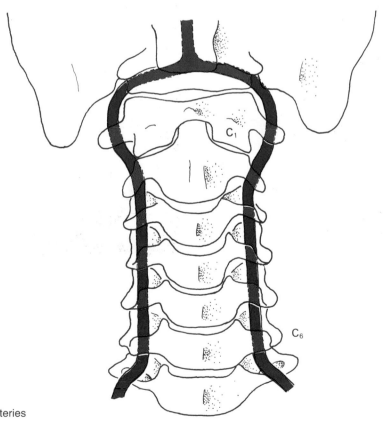

Fig. 1.**30**   The vertebral arteries

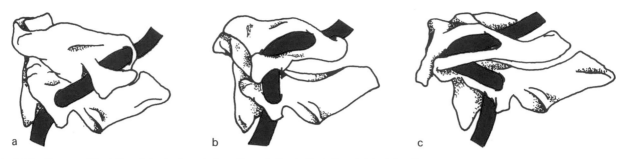

Fig. 1.**31**   Course of the left vertebral artery during atlas rotation to the left and right (after Fielding, 1957)

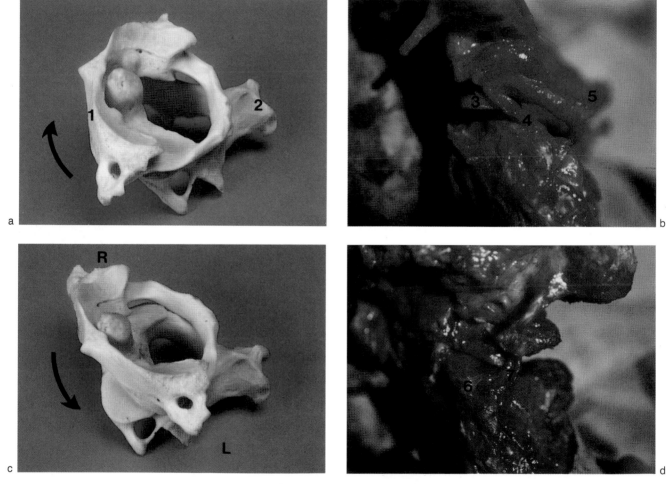

Fig. 1.**32**   Dissection specimens demonstrating changes in the vertebral artery with C1–C2 rotation to the right (**a**–**b**) and left (**c**–**d**)

1   Atlas
2   Axis
3   Left articular process of the atlas
4   Left vertebral artery
5   Posterior arch of the atlas
6   Articular process of the axis
7   Vertebral artery

may cause reflex spasms as well (Fig. 1.**33**). Figure 1.**34** demonstrates the close relationsship of the vertebral artery to the uncovertebral and zygapophyseal joints.

It is known that "high velocity thrust techniques" can cause vascular accidents (Dvořák and Orelli, 1982). In order to prevent accidents, it is necessary to employ provocative examination before thrust is applied (Memorandum of the German Society for Manual Medicine, 1979). It is sometimes necessary to include ultrasound examination of the vertebral artery.

Provocative test (extension and rotation of head): With the patient sitting the examiner conducts passive motion of the head to either side, starting from both the neutral and extended positions. The passive motions should be conducted slowly, and the patient

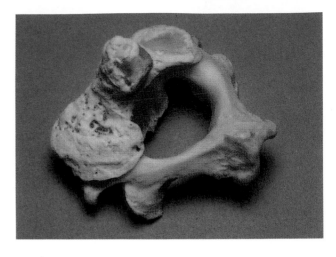

Fig. 1.**33** Prominent degenerative changes of the axis in a 64-year-old female patient

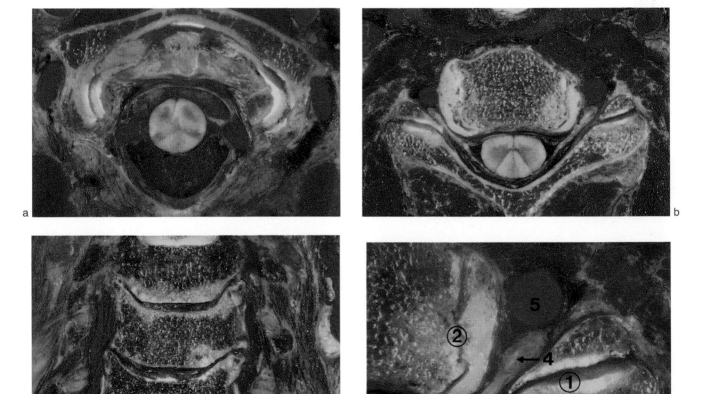

Fig. 1.**34** Vertebral artery at the level of the atlas (with permission from W. Rausching, Uppsala, Sweden)

a Midcervical spine
b Coronal section
c Close relationship to the uncovertebral joints
d Detail of the intervertebral canal

1 Zygapophyseal joint
2 Uncovertebral joint
3 Nerve root
4 Spinal ganglion
5 Vertebral artery

is asked to report any subjective symptoms (see also pp. 89 and 90 in the section "examination").

Kleijn Hanging Test: The patient is supine with the head beyond the examining table, being held by the examiner. From this hanging position, the head is passively rotated to both sides. While the examiner observes the patient's eye movements (nystagmus), the patient is again asked to report subjective symptoms.

Ultrasound examination: Noninvasive ultrasound examination of the carotid and vertebral arteries can be helpful when vertebral basilar insufficiency is suspected, with subclavian steal syndrome, with hypersensitive carotid sinus syndrome, and with possible increased risk of cerebral vascular disease. The ultrasound examination provides further information about the vertebral artery and its function in cervical spine motion. With an ultrasound probe of approximately 15 cm in length, which is inserted in the oropharynx, the vertebral arteries can be

detected at the C3–C4 level both on the left and right sides. The following criteria are diagnostically useful: direction of blood flow, differences between both vertebral arteries (diastolic phase and pulsation amplitude), reaction of the carotid upon compression and reaction upon head rotation, flexion and extension. Since it is physiologically normal for blood flow to decrease with rotation, it is important to verify early blood flow arrest in this examination (Adorjani, personal communications, 1980; Keller et al., 1976).

1.5 Biomechanics of the Thoracic Spine

The facets of the individual vertebrae show a twofold inclination, that is, inclination around the x-axis of 60° and around the y-axis of 20° (Fig. 1.**35**). These doubly inclined facets still allow rotation around all axes (flexion and extension, lateral bending, axial rotation) (Table 1.**5**).

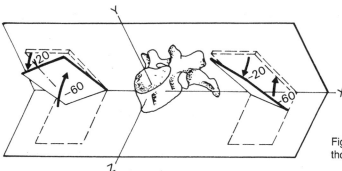

Fig. 1.**35** The facet joint inclinations and axes of motion of a thoracic vertebra (after White and Panjabi, 1978a)

Table 1.**5** Limits and representative values of range of rotation of the thoracic spine (after White and Panjabi, 1978a)

Spinal segment	Flexion/extension		Lateral bending		Axial rotation	
	Limits of ranges (degrees)	Representative angle (degrees)	Limits of ranges (degrees)	Representative angle (degrees)	Limits of ranges (degrees)	Representative angle (degrees)
T1–T2	3–5	4	5	6	14	9
T2–T3	3–5	4	5–7	6	4–12	8
T3–T4	2–5	4	3–7	6	5–11	8
T4–T5	2–5	4	5–6	6	4–11	8
T5–T6	3–5	4	5–6	6	5–11	8
T6–T7	2–7	5	6	6	4–11	8
T7–T8	3–8	6	3–8	6	4–11	8
T8–T9	3–8	6	4–7	6	6–7	7
T9–T10	3–8	6	4–7	6	3–5	4
T10–T11	4–14	9	3–10	7	2–3	2
T11–T12	6–20	12	4–13	9	2–3	2
T12–L1	6–20	12	5–10	8	2–3	2

Flexion/extension: range of motion in the upper segments of the thoracic spine is limited. Starting at the T7−T8 level, flexion and extension movement increases progressively in the more inferior segments.

Sidebending (lateral bending): occurs essentially to the same extent at all thoracic spinal segments.

Axial rotation: opposite to that encountered in the flexion and extension movement. The segments from T1 to T7−T8 can undergo significantly greater rotational motion than their lower counterparts (below T7−T8).

Coupled-movements: According to Panjabi et al. (1978), coupled movement in the thoracic spine is not unlike that in the cervical spine. Sidebending (lateral bending, $\pm\varnothing z$) to one side is accompanied by axial rotation to the same side ($+\varnothing y$) (Fig. 1.**36**).

Greenman (personal communications, 1983) and Mitchell et al. (1979) distinguish between two types of coupled movements:
− Type I: sidebending to one side ($\pm\varnothing z$) is accompanied by axial rotation ($\pm\varnothing y$) to the opposite side.
− Type II: sidebending to one side ($\pm\varnothing z$) is accompanied by axial rotation ($\pm\varnothing y$) to the same side.

According to the above criteria, and because there is usually a slight kyphotic curvature in the thoracic spine, flexion ($\pm\varnothing x$) in the thoracic spine is usually accompanied by coupled type-I movement.

It is well known that vertebral motion in the thoracic spine is minimal, especially when compared with movement in the remainder of the vertebral column. The range of motion between the individual vertebrae is limited due to the restrictive effect of the

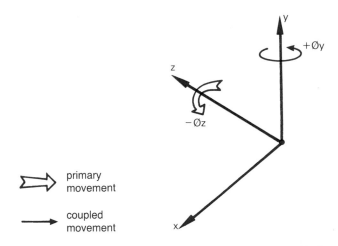

Fig. 1.**36** Coupled movement in the thoracic spine. $-\varnothing z$ is accompanied by $-\varnothing y$

longitudinal ligament, the anulus fibrosus, and the spatial arrangement of the spinous processes and their connections to the ribs.

1.6 Biomechanics of the Thorax and Ribs

The union of the thoracic spine with the ribs and consequently with the sternum significantly increases the rigidity and stability of the longest portion of the vertebral column. Strong ligaments stabilize the costovertebral and costotransverse joints (Fig. 1.**37**).

The relatively rigid union between the sternum and the thoracic spine by way of the ribs markedly increases the resistance of the spine against forces that cause rotation. An interesting experiment was conducted by Schulz, et al. (1974a). Loads were

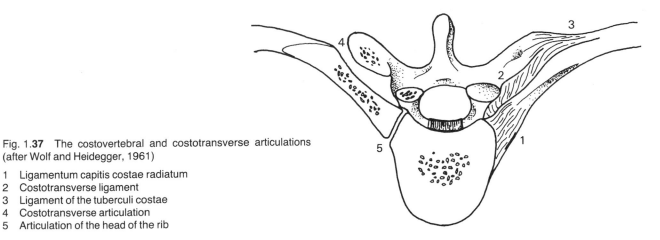

Fig. 1.**37** The costovertebral and costotransverse articulations (after Wolf and Heidegger, 1961)

1 Ligamentum capitis costae radiatum
2 Costotransverse ligament
3 Ligament of the tuberculi costae
4 Costotransverse articulation
5 Articulation of the head of the rib

applied to individual ribs from different directions and the mobility of the ribs was measured. It was noted that the second rib exhibited the greatest resistance when the force was applied from the posteroanterior direction. The lowest stiffness and resistance (highest flexibility) was exhibited by the tenth rib when loaded either from the superior or inferior direction. According to Panjabi, et al. (1978), the costovertebral joints play an important role in the stability and the segmental mobility of the thoracic spine. Their function, in addition to the stabilizing action of the whole thorax, is verified in a mathematical model by Andriacchi, et al. (1974).

Due to its connection with the ribs and sternum, the thoracic spine can tolerate a greater amount of loading forces when subjected to various physiologic movements, in particular the extension component. The thorax also enhances axial mechanical stabilization during anteroposterior compression.

1.7 Biomechanics of the Lumbar Spine

Motion in the region of the lumbar spine is possible around all three axes. Motion around the x-axis (flexion and extension) increases in the inferior direction, the maximum motion being in the vertebral unit L5–S1 (Table 1.**6**). Lateral bending and rotation around the z-axis are the most limited in the lumbosacral junction. According to Lumsden and Morris (1968), axial rotation is greatest in the lumbosacral junction. Compared with lateral bending and axial rotation, flexion and extension are large, which is easily explained by the arrangement of the facets (Fig. 1.**38**).

Coupled movements: sidebending ($\pm\varnothing z$) is strongly coupled to axial rotation ($\pm\varnothing y$) (Panjabi et al., 1978; Miles, 1961). In the lumbar spine, with its normal lordosis, sidebending to one side is accompanied by rotation to the opposite side (Fig. 1.**39**). The osteopathic literature further describes a more complex coupling of motion (Mitchell et al., 1979; Greenman, personal communications, 1983). When the lumbar spine is flexed ($\pm\varnothing x$) and sidebent to one side ($\pm\varnothing z$), there is coupled rotation ($\pm\varnothing y$) to the same side as sidebending (Fig. 1.**40**). Translatory gliding in the sagittal plane ($\pm y$-axis), a though rare, has been reported to occur with axial rotation (Rolander, 1966).

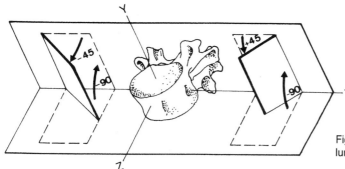

Fig. 1.**38** The facet joint inclinations and axes of motion of a lumbar vertebra (after White and Panjabi, 1978a

Table 1.**6** Representative values of the range of rotation of the lumbar spine (after White and Panjabi, 1978a)

Spinal segment	Flexion/extension (x-axis rotation)		Lateral bending (z-axis rotation)		Axial rotation (y-axis rotation)	
	Limits of ranges (degrees)	Representative angle (degrees)	Limits of ranges (degrees)	Representative angle (degrees)	Limits of ranges (degrees)	Representative angle (degrees)
L1–L2	9–16	12	3–8	6	1–3	2
L2–L3	11–18	14	3–9	6	1–3	2
L3–L4	12–18	15	5–10	8	1–3	2
L4–L5	14–21	17	5–7	6	1–3	2
L5–S1	18–22	20	2–3	3	3–6	5

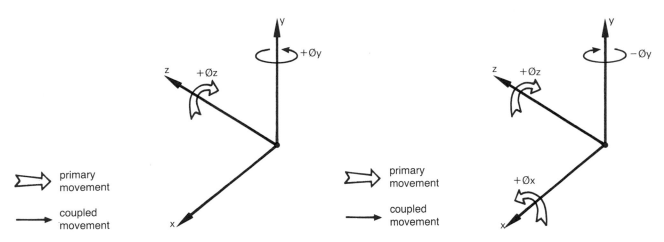

Fig. 1.39 Coupled movement in the lumbar spine. $+\emptyset z$ is accompanied by $+\emptyset y$

Fig. 1.40 Coupled movement in the lumbar spine. With $+\emptyset x$, there is $+\emptyset x$ primary movement accompanied by $-\emptyset y$

1.8 Biomechanics of the Pelvic Girdle

The functional unit of the pelvic girdle is comprised of the sacrum, both wings of the ilium, and the fifth lumbar vertebra, connected through the sacroiliac joints (SIJs) and the symphysis pubis. The SIJs are representatives of a diarthrosis, yet function as an amphiarthrosis where movement, even though minimal, is felt to be present. The SIJ takes on an auricular or a "C" shape, with the convex side facing anteriorly and inferiorly (Fig. 1.41). There is significant variation in regard to size, ranging from 5.3 cm to 8.0 cm in length and 1.8 to 4.1 cm in width (Schunke, 1938).

1.8.1 Macroscopic and microscopic Joint Anatomy

The SIJs, with their surfaces oriented vertically, are arranged such that they form a certain angle in respect to the sagittal plane (i. e., oblique orientation). In a horizontal plane through the center of the joint, the distance between either side of the SIJ is smaller anteriorly than posteriorly. The situation reverses at the inferior portion, where the distance between both sides of the joint is smaller posteriorly than anteriorly (Fig. 1.42).

Various differences have been observed at the two joint sides (sacral versus iliac side). The sacral cartilage is approximately 2 to 3 mm thick, whereas at the iliac side it measures 1.5 mm. Furthermore, the chemical composition of the joint cartilage is different at the two locations. The sacral cartilage is primarily made up of hyaline material, whereas the surface of the iliac cartilage is comprised of fibrous

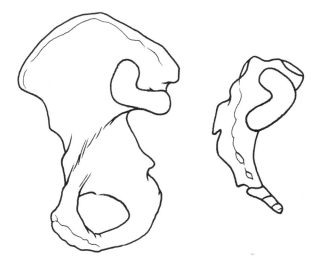

Fig. 1.41 Anatomic arrangement of the sacroiliac joint

material. Sacral cartilage contains large chondrocytes grouped in pairs which fill the lacunes. These lacunes are distributed evenly throughout the hyaline matrix of the cartilage. The ground matrix is homogeneous, with little fibrous tissue present except in areas of degenerative change (Bowen and Cassidy, 1981). In contrast, the ground matrix of the iliac cartilage is made up of thick bundles of collagenous fibers, The lacunes, surrounded by collagenous fibers, are filled with chondrocytes that tend to clump.

In order to understand the biomechanics of the SIJs, the histological changes that occur in these joint surfaces as a function of advancing age must be appreciated. Previous anatomic descriptions may

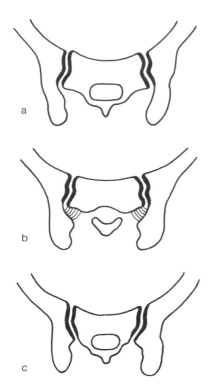

Fig. 1.42 Horizontal sections through the sacroiliac joints at various levels

a Superior
b Middle
c Inferior

have been inconsistent for the simple reason that the joints studied were not those of young, healthy adults. The "normal" anatomic description had often been inferred from studies involving older joints already affected by degenerative processes, for instance. Thus, it is important to arrange the description systematically according to different age groups.

First decade: In children, the cartilage of the sacrum is three to four times as thick as that of the ilium. On the iliac side, the bone and cartilage are interdigitated in a manner similar to that found in the cartilaginous growth plates of the vertebrae or the symphysis during the growth period. The joint capsule, even though already well developed at this age, still allows great mobility of the joint, with gliding movement possible in any direction.

Second decade: In the sacral cartilage of a 15-year-old, the divisions into cell-rich and cell-poor areas have become even more pronounced, particularly in the deeper layers. The columnar appearance of the

iliac cartilage remains unchanged. By the second decade, a cartilaginous joint space has developed behind the joint surface on each side. The joint space is perpendicular to the joint line. The pronounced changes observed in the cartilage of this joint space are more likely to be due to mechanical stress and damage to the growing cartilage than to growth processes themselves (Putschar 1931).

Third decade: Growth-related changes cease to occur on the sacral side before they cease on the iliac side. It is not until the third decade that the iliac surface assumes a convex shape and the sacral surface a concave shape. While the deeper layers remain histologically unchanged, the superficial joint surfaces show crevices with rough edges and erosions especially on the iliac side, more so than on the sacral side (Bowen and Cassidy, 1981).

Fourth decade: The capsule grows still thicker with a proportional increase of the fibrous material in the synovial layer. There is a decrease in the vasculature. The joint surface is microscopically irregular and discontinuous with flattened, longitudinal cells. At this age, the iliac cartilage reveals clumping of chondrocytes into bundles. In contrast, except for discrete rough edges at the borders, the sacral hyaline cartilage appears unchanged. Osteophytes have frequently developed at the margins, especially on the iliac side. The joint cavity contains flakelike clumps of yellow amorphous debris (Bowen and Cassidy, 1981). Despite the loss of elasticity at this age, overall joint mobility continues to be good.

Fifth decade: Degenerative processes become more prominent, with the joint surface being more irregular due to erosions. Eosinophils, and amorphous and exfoliated material have accumulated in the joint space. The iliac cartilage is more affected, with joint thickness being diminished in the presence of significant accumulation of chondrocytes. The ground matrix is infiltrated with fibrous material. Osteophytes at the sacroiliac joint have been observed in 85% of men and 50% of women in the fifth decade (Frigerio, 1974).

Sixth decade: Capsule and synovium continue to grow thicker and stiffer. In particular, the iliac portion has lost a significant share of its cartilaginous substance to the point of exposure of the subchondral bone. A thick layer of flaky amorphous debris covers both joint surfaces, and the iliac surface cannot be distinguished by its blue appearance (Bowen and Cassidy, 1981). The sacral portion is less involved, even though superficial erosions and fibrillation have been noted. Osteophytes at the joint margin, especially prominent superiorly and anteriorly, continue to broaden and interconnect the joint space. Motion in the SIJ becomes minimal or even entirely absent at this point. Partial or complete ankylosis at this age has been observed to occur in 60% of males, in contrast to 15% of females (Frigerio, 1974).

Seventh decade: Cartilage has undergone further atrophic changes on both sides. While the process may have progressed to erosions and fibrillatory changes at some locations, thus leading to only bone being present at that portion of the articular surface, some of the cartilage may show material primarily void of living cells, as well as signs of necrosis. The remainder of the cartilage reveals an increase in collagenous materials and clustering of chondrocytes. There is more amorphous material in the joint space, and fibrous degenerative changes have led to intra-articular fibrous interconnections. The joints may have undergone complete ankylosis in up to 70% of the cases (MacDonald, 1952). Calcifications at the capsular attachments have also been noted at both joints.

Eighth decade: At this age, the joints have ankylosed in the majority of the cases, with significant calcification at the periphery of the fibrous capsule. Subcapsular osteophytes are present in almost all of the joints, and the interdigitation between them is so pronounced that essentially any movement is prohibited. Diminished movement may be compounded by the presence of intra-articular fibrous connections (Bowen and Cassidy, 1981). Erosions and necrotic changes, exposure of the deeper layers, and fibrillatory changes are found to a significant degree in all joints, yet less so on the sacral side. Subchondral bone has become thin and atrophied (Fig. 1.**43**).

1.8.2 Ligaments associated with the SIJs

Of great importance, in addition to a tight joint capsule, are the ligaments associated with the SIJ. There are two major sets of ligaments, an anterior and posterior group. The anterior group is made up of the anterior sacroiliac ligament, whereas the posterior group is comprised of the long and short sacroiliac ligaments as well as the interosseous sacroiliac ligament.

The anterior sacroiliac ligament, which is essentially no more than the thickened portion of· the joint capsule, is thin and weak. During movement it is stretched obliquely (Duckworth, 1970); it receives its

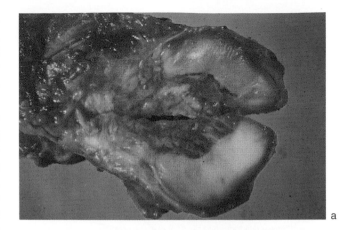

a

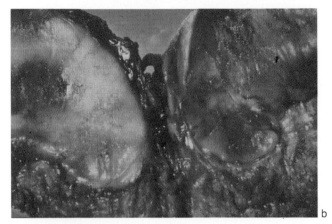

b

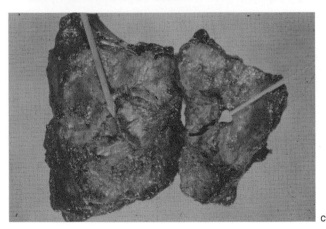

c

Fig. 1.**43** Degeneration of the sacroiliac joints (with permission from D. Cassidy, Saskatoon, Canada)

a First decade
b Fourth decade
c Seventh decade

sensory innervation from the ventral rami of the spinal nerves L2 and L3. The posterior ligaments, that is, the short, long, and interosseous sacroiliac ligaments, are much thicker and stronger. The long

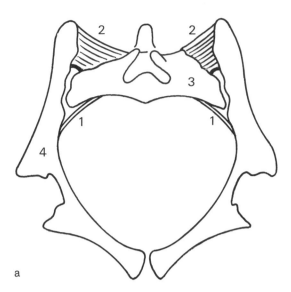

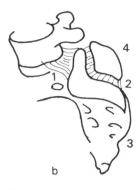

Fig. 1.**44**   The sacral suspension

a   Superior view (after Kapandji)   **b**   Medial view
1   Anterior sacroiliac ligament
2   Interosseous sacroiliac ligament
3   Sacrum
4   Ilium

and short sacroiliac ligaments are supplied by both the sensory portion of the ventral rami of spinal nerves L5-S2 and the dorsal rami of L1-L5 and S1-S3. The interosseous ligament receives its sensory supply from the dorsal rami of L5-S2.

According to Sutter (1972), the sacrum is suspended from the posterior prominence of the iliac tuberosity by the interosseous sacroiliac ligament. The position of the sacrum is secured not only by the safeguarding function of the sacroiliac ligaments (i. e., limiting motion) but also by the shape and congruity of the SIJs, which converge inferiorly. Forces that are directed towards the sacrum and the innominate bones are countered by forces originating in conjunction with the "clamp down mechanism" (anatomical arrangement with inferior convergence of the SIJ): This mechanism remains intact only as long as the short sacroiliac ligaments allow the mechanically important posterior closure between the sacrum and ilia. If these ligaments are too weak, the ilia can deviate laterally to some minor extent. When lateral movement of the ilia occurs, the upper pole of the sacrum is obligatorily pulled into a more posterior position, thus approximating the prominence of the iliac tuberosity. This mechanism is mediated by the strong interosseous sacroiliac ligament (Fig. 1.**44**).

1.8.3   Function of the SIJ

An excellent review of the literature concerning the SIJ has been presented in the medical thesis by Rudolf (1985). It is likely that no other joint in the human body has been subjected to more controversy

and hypothetical postulates regarding its function and pathology than the SIJ. This may be primarily due to two reasons: first, the significance of this joint, especially as far as movement is concerned, is undoubtedly less obvious than that of the hip or knee joint, for instance; second, it has been extremely difficult in the past to design the proper experiment and, let alone, make conclusive interpretation of studies investigating the mechanics of this joint. A final, all encompassing description of the physiology of the SIJ has not been presented thus far. A brief review of the literature reveals that Hippocrates and Vesalius believed the SIJ to be mobile. It is interesting to note that Hippocrates had already surmised a certain degree of mobility to occur at the SIJ during pregnancy. In the 19th century, those in the field of obstetics and gynecology became more interested in the function and mechanics of the pelvic girdle. Some authors report changes in measurements of the pelvic inlet that could only be explained on the basis of mobility at the SIJ. A decrease in diameter of the pelvic inlet was always found to be associated with an increase in the pelvic outlet. This led to the conclusion that the sacrum rotates around a horizontal axis. This rotational movement of the sacrum has been termed *nutation* ("nodding") movement in the literature. However, the anatomic placement of this axis varies depending on the individual author. Pitkin and Pheasant (1936) describe two types of rotation based on measuring the angle between a line that connects both superior iliac spines and lines constructed through the sacrum. In one type, the axis of rotation (Fig. 1.**45**, the point labeled *a*) is at the center of the SIJ (a tubercle between the superior and inferior

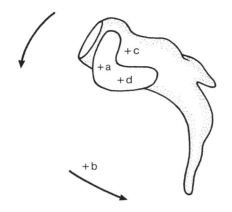

Fig. 1.**45** Different positions for axis of rotation allowing sacroiliac nutation („nodding") motion

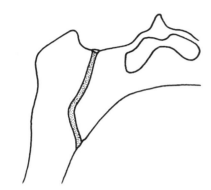

Fig. 1.**46** Sacrum: flat type (after Delmas)

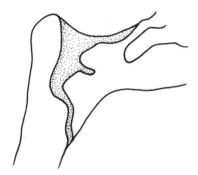

Fig. 1.**47** Sacrum: wide type (after Delmas)

As early as 1937, Lloyd pointed out the close relationship between stability and structural components of the SIJ. The somewhat rectangular shape of the sacrum is associated more with a vertical SIJ position, leading to relative instability. This concept was further developed by Delmas (1950) and later supported by Sandoz (1981).

According to these and other functional considerations, it is possible to differentiate between two prototypes:

– the so-called *flat* type: the joint surfaces between the sacrum and ilium are fairly congruent, and the retroarticular space is relatively small. The short and strong interosseous ligaments span the narrow joint. In this type, the balance between mobility and stability is unquestionably shifted in the direction of stability with less mobility possible. This configuration is more typical of the male pelvis (Fig. 1.**46**).

– the so-called *wide* type: the joint surfaces are less congruent, the retroarticular space being wider and the interosseous ligaments longer than in the flat type. This configuration allows greater mobility due to loss of stability. This type is found predominantly in women, often in association with an exaggerated lordosis (Fig. 1.**47**). Thus, in this type, there is a predisposition to instability.

The wide and flat prototypes occur in approximately 25% of the population, with the remaining 50% being of the mixed or intermediary type.

Weisl (1955), using controlled X-ray studies, abandoned the conventional concept of a fixed axis of rotation. Concluding from his controlled geometric measurements, he placed the axis of rotation approximately 10 cm below the promontorium. Here, it is not fixed but rather, can undergo up-and-down movement of up to 5 cm. This indicates that movement of the sacrum is not only rotatory around one stationary axis, but also follows a translatory path. Kapandji (1974) and Colachis (1963) came to similar conclusions. Both confirm that motion at the SIJ is a combination of rotation and gliding movement. Sutter (1977) postulates four axes of movement for the SIJ around which movement can take place either unilaterally or bilaterally (Fig. 1.**48**). Various other authors, applying modern diagnostic techniques such as CT and three-dimensional modeling, attempt to elucidate the three-dimensional biodynamic mechanisms in the SIJ (Frigerio, 1974; Egund et al., 1978; Reynolds and Hubbard, 1980).

portions of the joint surface). The second type is that in which the center of the axis is located at the symphysis pubis (Fig. 1.**45**, point labeled *b*). Duckworth (1970) refers to a nutation movement with the axis of rotation being at the site of the shortest and strongest portion of the interosseous ligament (Fig. 1.**45**, point labeled *c*). Beal (1982) reported that the axis of rotation is at the inferior portion of the SIJ (Fig. 1.**45**, point labeled *d*).

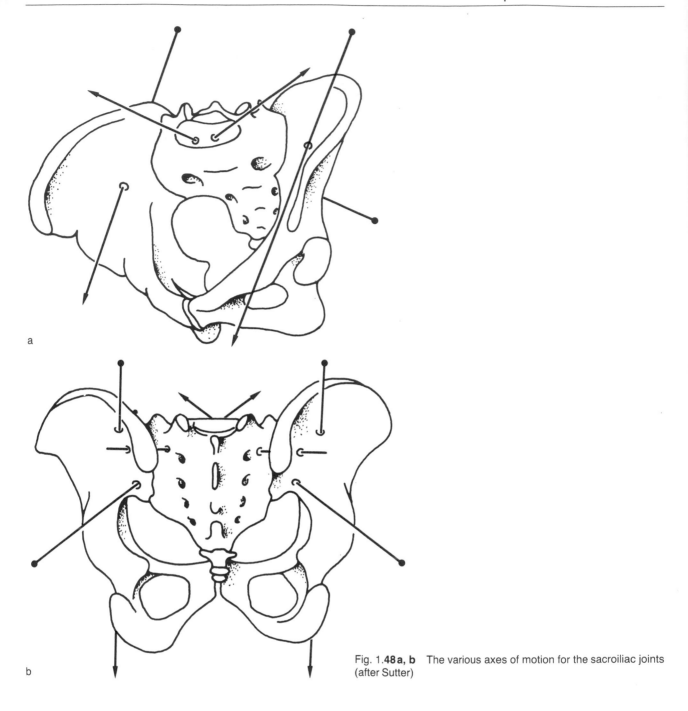

Fig. 1.**48a, b** The various axes of motion for the sacroiliac joints (after Sutter)

Even though these studies fulfill the requirements of modern research, adequate clinical studies are still lacking, especially in regard to sufficient patient numbers. Such investigations are needed to conclusively answer the question of SIJ movement, both qualitatively and quantitatively. Thus, the final answer regarding the physiology and biomechanics of SIJ movement remains a matter of interpretation, with many unanswered questions.

Lewit (1973) reports that the SIJ functions as an elastic buffer zone between the spine and the lower extremities. Sandoz (1981) suggests a similar concept. Movement at this joint should be understood as that causing compression of a specific region with simultaneous distraction of another, rather than that of mere joint gliding. The cushioning or buffering function of the SIJ should be viewed in the context of all the forces that are directed towards the pelvic

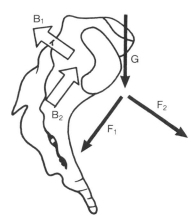

Fig. 1.**49** Loading force vector associated with trunk weight and its unit vectors (after Kapandji)

G   Body weight (gravity)
F1   Nutation
F2   Translatory force (displacement)
B1   Pulling force exhibited by the superior interosseous Ligament
B2   Pulling force exhibited by the inferior interosseous Ligament

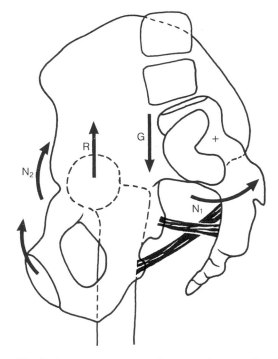

Fig. 1.**50** Body posture and its effects on the sacroiliac joint (after Kapandji)

G   Body weight (gravity)
R   Reaction of the ground
N1   Nutation motion of sacrum
N2   Counter-nutation by the innominate bone

girdle due to the human's assumption of an erect posture (Kapandji, 1974; Beal, 1982). The influence of the various forces involved is described below.

The vertical vector of the gravitational force caused by the body's (trunk's) weight is directed towards the superior surface of the sacrum, that is, S1 (Fig. 1.**49**). As a result of the anatomical arrangement of this joint, this vector (G) can be further separated into two unit components, indicating the two motion forces labeled F1 and F2 in Figure 1.**49**. F1 is the force causing nutation, a movement controlled by the sacrospinous and sacrotuberous ligaments, as well as a portion of the superior sacroiliac ligaments (force B1). Translatory displacement along the joint's longitudinal axis (F2 in Fig. 1.**49**), is counteracted by the inferior portion of the sacroiliac ligaments (force B2, Fig. 1.**49**). At the same time, the reaction of the ground (R), transmitted by the femur and applied to the hips, combines with the body weight (G) to form a rotatory couple. This causes the iliac bone to tilt posteriorly (N2; also known as "counter-nutation"), which is a rotation in direction opposite to that of sacral nutation (N1, Fig. 1.**50**).

The relationship of these forces applies to a person standing on one foot or taking a step during walking. The forces in that instance are applied to the SIJ on the side of the supporting stance (non-swing) leg (Beal, 1981; Kapandji, 1974). The reaction of the ground (R), transmitted by the supporting limb, elevates the corresponding hip and bony pelvis, whereas the contralateral hip tends to be pulled down by the

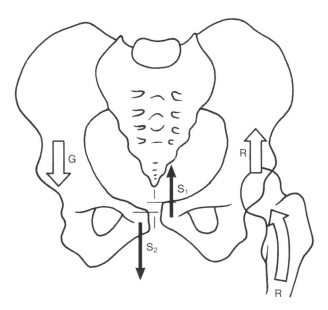

Fig. 1.**51** Shearing forces encountered at the symphysis during stance phase (standing on one leg) (Kapandji)

G   Body weight (gravity)
R   Reaction of the ground
S1, S2   Shearing forces

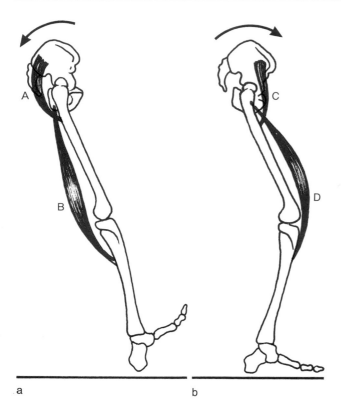

Fig. 1.**52a** Early stance phase **b** Swing phase (after Grice)

A Gluteus maximus muscle
B Biceps femoris, semitendinosis and semimembranosus muscles
C Iliopsoas muscle
D Quadriceps femoris muscle

the nutation movement of the sacrum and the counter-nutation of the ilium, occurs with every step. The force distribution described applies to the stance leg.

Additional forces are introduced with active muscle action: in early stance phase the major active muscle groups are the gluteus maximus and the hamstring muscles (Fig. 1.**52a**, labeled A and B, respectively). Due to the origin and insertion of these muscles, the posterior superior iliac spine (PSIS) is being pulled posteriorly, a movement correlating with that described above as "counter-nutation" (Fig. 1.**52a**). The other leg, now in swing phase, primarily activates the iliopsoas muscle and quadriceps femoris muscle (Fig. 1.**52b**, labeled C and D, respectively). The forces generated through this action cause the pelvis on that same side to rotate anteriorly (Fig. 1.**52b**). During the gait cycle, there is then a dynamic and alternating interplay of small movements involving both SIJs. Movement between the sacrum on one side and the ipsilateral ilium is such that the sacrum typically moves in a direction opposite to that of the ilium. Motion is more in an anterior and inferior direction on the stance side, and more posterior and superior on the swing side. This introduces a rotational component at the sacrum, which is transmitted to the lowest lumbar vertebra via the intervertebral disk. Due to the counter-nutation of the ilium and the recruited action of the iliolumbar ligament, this vertebra is actually rotated in the opposite direction (Illi, 1951). As a result, rotation at the lower lumbar spine during the gait cycle is held to a minimum when the SIJ functions normally.

Dejung (1985) describes the so-called sacroiliac syndrome or sacroiliac joint dysfunction in 58 patients predominately in the age range of 20 to 40 years. In many cases, the patient reported a history of low back pain, occasionally radiating to the buttocks but rarely to the knee. The radiation of the pain is usually on the same side as the side of joint restriction. The symptoms are often related by the patient to either a previous fall onto the sacrum or concurrent pregnancy. Mobility at the lumbosacral junction is remarkably decreased.

Joint motion restriction due to a somatic dysfunction in this area must be diagnostically differentiated from loss of motion due to antalgic posture secondary to a herniated disk. In the latter case, the surrounding muscles may reveal localized muscle "spasm" or a hard palpable band, in particular in the gluteus maximus, longissimus lumborum, adductor longus, iliopsoas, and piriformis muscles.

weight of the free limb. This leads to a shearing force at the symphysis pubis (Fig. 1.**51**). The description thus far takes into account only passive (static) forces and not the influence and action of the various muscle groups (Kapandji, 1974).

Under physiologic conditions, these ligaments exert such a strong force that they substantially limit gross movement, thus making objective measurement difficult. It should not be difficult, however, to imagine how the various forces correspondingly alternate and interplay during the walking cycle, repetitively causing a temporary and reversible pelvic torsion (Lewit, 1968). Grice points out that this elastic give-way of the joints at the pelvis, together with the tendency of the iliac to undergo concomitant flexion-extension movement, reduces to a minimum the torsional forces at the spine during walking. The force interplay described above (forces G and R) brings about alternating movement at the SIJ that, together with

2 Neurophysiology of the Joints and Muscles

2.1 Neuropathophysiology of the Apophyseal Joints

It is not the intention of this chapter to treat the different theories and hypotheses developed in relation to manual medicine. Little is actually known about those neurophysiologic processes that are initiated with manipulation or mobilization of the apophyseal joints and joints of the extremities.

In light of the increased interest in manual medicine among physicians, it became necessary to support and promote clinical and basic research.

An important step was undertaken in 1975 upon the recommendation of the National Institutes of Health. Upon the invitation of the National Institute of Neurological and Communicative Disorders and Stroke (Goldstein, 1975) a conference was held on the topic "The Research Status of Spinal Manipulative Therapy." References here are mainly to Sato's (1975) work on the somatosympathetic reflexes. Perl's (1975) work on pain and spinal and peripheral nerve factors, and White and Panjabi's work (1978b) on the biomechanics of the spine.

In 1978, a symposium was held in Pisa, Italy on "Reflex Control of Posture and Movement" (Granit and Pompeiano, 1979). Even though manual medicine was not discussed per se, this symposium offers a broad basis of the theoretical research in this field.

In 1982, Michigan State University held a symposium entitled "Empirical Approaches to the Validation of Manual Medicine" (Greenman and Buerger, 1984). Researchers and clinicians from the fields of biomechanics and neurophysiology discussed their basic and clinical research findings as related to the field of manual medicine.

Based on his basic experimental research with Freeman (1967), Wyke coined the expression "articular neurology". His work, published in 1967, 1975 (Wyke and Polacek), 1979, and 1980, and that of Jayson (1980) make use of this expression and – enable a better understanding of the neurophysiological processes involved in manual medicine. These will be subsequently described.

2.2 Articular Neurology

The following presentation is based mainly on the work of Wyke and coworkers.

This branch of neurology deals with the morphology, physiology, pathology, and the clinical aspects of the innervation of the joints of the entire skeleton. Here, concentration ist on the apophyseal joints.

Wyke's important contribution regarding articular neurology is the description of the structure and innervation pattern of the four receptor types, their distribution and charakteristic behavior, the evidence of their presence in all synovial joint capsules, and their effects on static and dynamic reflex controls of the striated musculature, under both normal and pathologic conditions.

2.2.1 Receptors of the Joint Capsule

It is well known that all synovial joints in the human body are supplied by the mechanoreceptors and nociceptive-free nerve endings (nociceptors). Their organization was visualized in neurohistologic studies (Wyke and Polacek, 1973 and 1975; Freeman and Wyke, 1967; Vrettos and Wyke, 1979) (Table 2.**1**).

Type-I Receptors (Mechanoreceptors)

This type of mechanoreceptor consists of multiple (three to eight), thinly encapsulated, globular corpuscles ($100\,\mu m \times 40\,\mu m$) that are found in the outer layer of the fibrous joint capsule. The thinly myelinated (6 to $9\,\mu m$) afferent nerve fibers connect these corpuscles with the corresponding articular branches of the dorsal rami of the spinal nerves.

Function:
- Slowly adapting receptors. They control tension of the outer layers of the joint capsule
- Transsynaptic inhibition of the centripetal flow of the activity of the nociceptive afferent receptors (type-IV nociceptors) or, in other words, inhibition of the impulses arising from pain receptors
- Tonic reflexogenic effects on the montoneurons of the neck, limb, jaw, and eye muscles (Wyke 1975, 1977; Molina et al., 1976; Biemond and DeJong, 1969; Igarashi et al., 1972; Hirosaka and Maeda, 1973; DeJong and Cochen 1977)

Table 2.1 Morphologic and functional characteristics of articular receptor symptoms (Wyke, 1979b; Freeman and Wyke, 1967)

Type	Morphology	Location	Parent Nerve Fibers	Behavioral Characteristics	Function
I	Thinly encapsulated globular corpuscles (100 µm × 40 µm) in clusters of 3–8	Fibrous capsulae of joint (superficial layers)	Small myelinated (6–9 µm)	Static and dynamic mechanoreceptors: low threshold, slowly adapting	Tonic reflexogenic effects on neck, limb, jaw, and eye muscles. Postural and kinesthetic sensation. Pain suppression
II	Thickly encapsulated conical corpuscles (280 µm × 100 µm) singly or in clusters of 2–4	Fibrous capsulae of joint (deeper layers). Articular fat pads	Medium myelinated (9–12 µm)	Dynamic mechanoreceptors: low threshold, rapidly adapting	a) Phasic reflexogenic effects on neck, limb, jaw, and eye muscles. b) Pain suppression
III	Fusiform corpuscles (600 µm × 100 µm) usually singly, also in clusters of 2–3	Ligaments, also in related tendons	Large myelinated (13–17 µm)	Mechanoreceptor: high threshold, very slowly adapting	
IV	Three-dimensional plexus of unmyelinated nerve fibers	Entire thickness of fibrous capsulae of joint. Walls of articular blood vessels. Articular fat pads	Very small myelinated (2–5 µm), and unmyelinated	Nociceptor (pain-provoking): high threshold, nonadapting	a) Tonic reflexogenic effects on neck, limb, jaw, and eye muscles. b) Evocation of pain. c) Respiratory and cardiovascular reflexogenic effects

Type-II Receptors (Mechanoreceptors)

The type-II receptors consist of oblong, conical, thickly encapsulated corpuscles (about 280 µm × 100 µm) that most often appear singly in the deeper layers of the fibrous joint capsule. These receptors are connected with the articular rami by way of the thickly myelinated nerve fibers.

Function:

– Rapidly adapting mechanoreceptors with a low threshold reacting to changes in tension of the fibrous joint capsule (less than 0.5 seconds).
– Phasic and reflexogenic effects on neck, limb, jaw, and eye muscles
– Transitory inhibition of the nociceptive activity of the joint capsule

Type-III Receptors (Mechanoreceptors)

Mechanoreceptors of the type-III category are the typical receptors of the ligaments and tendons inserting close to the joint capsule and are not found in the joint capsule itself. They do, however, play an important role in relation to the function of the joint. Morphologically, they consist of broad, fusiform corpuscles (600 µm × 100 µm) and usually appear singly.

Occasionally, they occur in clusters of one to three and are found at the end of the ligament or tendon.

Type-III receptors are innervated by large myelinated (13 to 17 µm) fibers and are connected with the articular branches. Their form resembles the ligamentous receptors of the Golgi's corpuscles, and it is assumed that they have the same function. Furthermore, it is believed that these slowly adapting receptors have an inhibitory reflexogenic effect on motoneurons (Freeman and Wyke, 1967).

Type-IV Receptors (Nociceptors)

Nociceptive fibers are sensitive to noxious changes in the tissue. The nociceptors are free, very thinly myelinated, or nonmyelinated plexiform nerve endings. They are ubiquitous in the fibrous portion of the joint capsule. This receptor system is activated by depolarization of the nerve fibers. For instance, depolarization occurs with constant pressure on the joint capsule (such as nonphysiological position and abrupt motions), with narrowing of the intervertebral disk, with fracture of the vertebral body, with dislocation of the apophyseal joints, or with chemical irritation (for example, potassium ions, lactic acid, 5-

hydroxytryptamine, and histamine), as well as with interstitial edema of the joint capsule in acute or chronic inflammatory processes.

Function:

– Tonic reflexogenic effects on neck, limb, jaw, and eye muscles
– Evocation of pain
– Respiratory and cardiovascular reflexogenic effects

2.2.2 Innervation of the Joint Capsule

The joint capsules are supplied by the dorsal rami of the spinal nerves. It should be emphasized that the articular rami of a nerve root are not only contributing to one segmental joint capsule, but that collateral rami lead to neighboring joints as well. Therefore the joint capsules are innervated pluri-segmentally

(Auteroche, 1983). The cross-section of the thoracic spine, for instance, shows the nerve supply of the joints, tendons, paravertebral musculature, and the periosteum (Fig. 2.1).

2.2.3 Central Interaction of the Mechanoreceptors and Nociceptive Impulses

Figure 2.2 shows, in a simplified manner, that the nociceptive and mechanoreceptive fibers enter the gray matter of the spinal cord through the dorsal root in the posterior horn. In the spinal cord, the nociceptive fibers divide into many collateral rami. Some of these rami run through the gray matter directly to the basal nuclei (basal spinal nucleus or lamina IV and V after Rexed). Furthermore, they run through the lateral spinothalamic tract (anterolateral) and reach

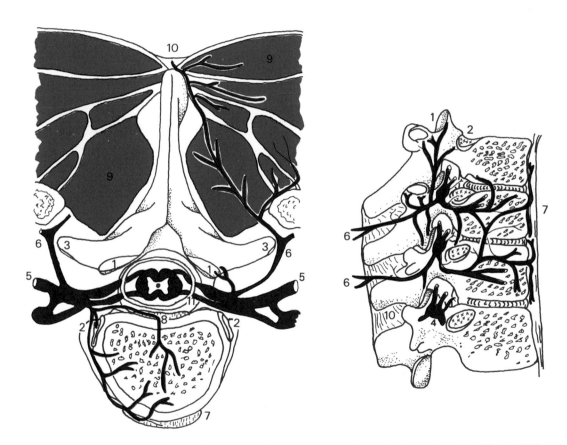

Fig. 2.1 The nerve supply of the joints, muscles, ligaments, and periosteum in the thoracic spine region (after Wyke, 1967)

1	Apophyseal joint	7	Anterior longitudinal ligament
2	Costovertebral joint	8	Posterior longitudinal ligament
3	Costotransverse joint	9	Paravertebral musculature
4	Spinal ganglion	10	Interspinous ligament
5	Ventral ramus of the spinal nerve	11	Ventral ramus of the spinal nerve
6	Dorsal ramus of the spinal nerve		

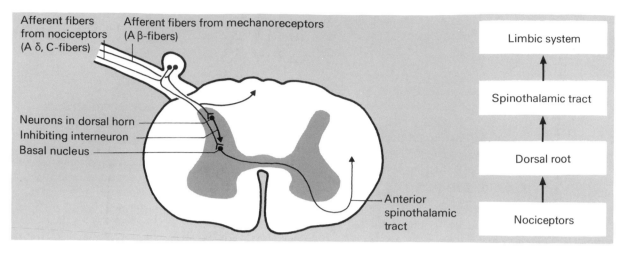

Fig. 2.**2**   Fibers of nociceptors and mechanoreceptors in the region of the posterior horns (after Wyke, 1979a)

the limbic system, where the actual perception of pain occurs. Pain cannot be subjectively perceived unless depolarization of the synapse has occurred at the level of the basal nuclei as a result of the nociceptive impulses.

The mechanoreceptive afferent fibers enter the posterior horn of the gray matter of the spinal cord through the dorsal root (Fig. 2.**2**). Important for this theory is that some of the many divided rami form synapses at the level of the apical spinal nucleus (or lamina II after Rexed). The apical spinal interneurons arising from this location conduct the activity of the mechanoreceptive afferent stimuli to the basal spinal nucleus and, at this level, are thus able to presynaptically inhibit the arriving pain-inducing nociceptor stimuli to a certain extent. Thus, they interrupt conduction to the spinothalamic tract and the limbic system (Wyke, 1979; Bonica and Albe-Fessard, 1980).

Experiments on adult cats demonstrate that a portion of the thinly myelinated afferent fibers ends in the substantia gelatinosa of the dorsal horns. By application of opiates to the substantia gelatinosa, the transmission of nociceptive impulses (initiated by peripheral stimulation of the nociceptors) could be blocked. Transmission of other sensory modalities, such as that of light touch, remain intact (Yoshimura and North, 1983). It is possible that opiates inhibit those cells of the substantia gelatinosa that function as interneurons in the transmission of pain. Electron-microscopic studies found an endogenous enkephalin in the substantia gelatinosa (Benett et al., 1982), which again would indicate that the interneurons have an inhibitory function. The encephalin may thus

serve as an inhibiting neurotransmitter. It also appears that strong stimulation of type-II-mechanoreceptors leads to a depotlike increase of the encephalins in the dorsal horns (Wyke, personal communications, 1983).

2.2.4   Mechanoreceptors and Nociceptive Reflexes

A significant contribution to the understanding and the basis for research of the clinically observed spondylogenic reflex syndrome (SRS) came from Wyke and co-workers. This experimental work is of such significance that it is described here in detail.

In anesthetized cats, the joint capsule and the articular nerve C3—C4 were microsurgically exposed. Using a probe and a stimulator, the joint capsule was irritated. A substantially lower voltage (2 V) was necessary to stimulate the mechanoreceptors than that necessary for the stimulation of the nociceptors (8 V). Wyke's results, reproduced here, very clearly show the reflexogenic relationship between the receptors of the fibrous joint capsule, the apophyseal joints, and the peripheral musculature (Figs. 2.**3**–2.**6**).

Akio Sato (1975) made similar observations in his investigation of the somatosympathetic reflexes. Based on clinical observations, a relationship between soft tissue changes or segmental (i. e., somatic) dysfunctions and diseases of internal organs has been suggested (Beal, 1984; Beal and Dvořák, 1984; Larson, 1976). Perl (1975) views this mechanism as a partial explanation of so-called referred pain. Wyke (1979b) suspects multisynaptic intra-

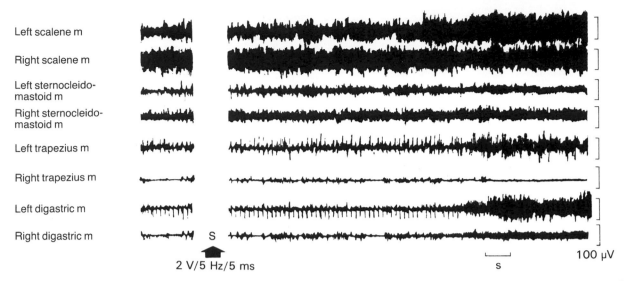

Left scalene m

Right scalene m

Left sternocleido-
mastoid m

Right sternocleido-
mastoid m

Left trapezius m

Right trapezius m

Left digastric m

Right digastric m

S

2 V/5 Hz/5 ms

100 µV

s

Fig. 2.3 The reflexogenic mechanoreceptor effects of a cervical apophyseal joint on the musculature of the neck. At the location indicated by the arrow (S) a single articular nerve of the left C3–C4 apophyseal joint was stimulated for 3 seconds with an electrical impulse (2 v, 5 Hz, 5 ms) that selectively excited the mechanoreceptive afferent fibers in the exposed nerve. The simultaneous electromyographic tracings show a long-lasting effect on the homologous pairs of the neck musculature (after Wyke, 1979)

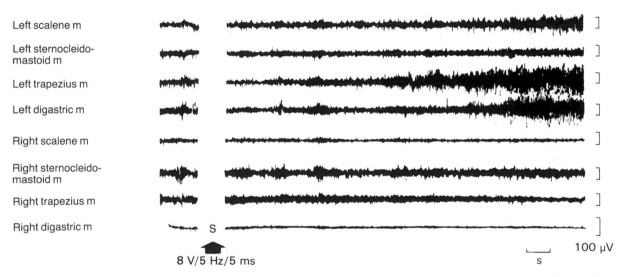

Left scalene m

Left sternocleido-
mastoid m

Left trapezius m

Left digastric m

Right scalene m

Right sternocleido-
mastoid m

Right trapezius m

Right digastric m

S

8 V/5 Hz/5 ms

100 µV

s

Fig. 2.4 The same experimental arrangement as in Fig. 2.3, except with a stimulus of 8 v, 5 Hz, 5 ms, which selectively stimulates not only the mechanoreceptive, but also the nociceptive afferent fibers (after Wyke, 1979)

Fig. 2.5 Reflex effects of the mechanoreceptors of the cervical ▶ apophyseal joints on limb muscles. At the signal (S), a single, exposed ramus of the articular nerve was repetitively stimulated for 3 seconds selectively exciting the mechanoreceptor afferent fibers in the corresponding nerve. The simultaneous electromyographic tracings of the upper and lower limbs muscles display the reflexogenic effects of varying duration and indicate that such inputs affect not only the limb muscles but also the neck muscles (see Fig. 2.3). Stimulation with a nociceptive impulse produces a different muscle potential response (after Wyke, 1979)

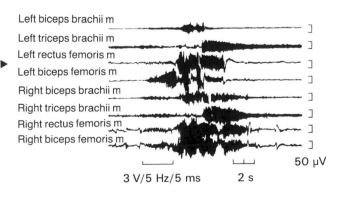

Left biceps brachii m
Left triceps brachii m
Left rectus femoris m
Left biceps femoris m
Right biceps brachii m
Right triceps brachii m
Right rectus femoris m
Right biceps femoris m

3 V/5 Hz/5 ms   2 s   50 µV

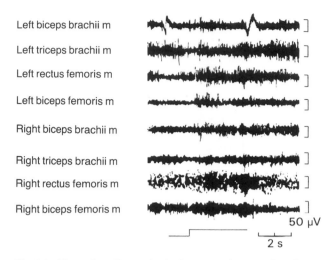

Left biceps brachii m

Left triceps brachii m

Left rectus femoris m

Left biceps femoris m

Right biceps brachii m

Right triceps brachii m

Right rectus femoris m

Right biceps femoris m

50 μV

2 s

Fig. 2.6 The reflex effects of articular manipulation at C3−C4. At the signal, a rapid vertical traction procedure was applied across the isolated joint. The simultaneous electromyographic tracings of the homologous pairs of the upper and lower limb muscles display the reflex effects of such cervical manipulation on the peripheral musculature (after Wyke, 1979)

spinal tracts, both ascending to the brainstem and descending to the basal nuclei of the lower levels of the spinal cord.

2.3 Functional Pathology of Muscle

2.3.1 Morphology and Function of the Slow Twitch Fibers (Type I) and Fast Twitch Fibers (Type II)

Human skeletal muscle is comprised of thousands of muscle fibers. The individual muscle fiber is about as thin as a strand of hair and can be as long as 10−15 cm, depending on the size of the muscle. Two major types of fibers are differentiated, namely, the slow twitch (type-I) fibers and the fast twitch (type-II) fibers. In addition to these two distinctive sets of fiber types there exist intermediary representatives, the so-called type-IIa and type-IIb fibers, which will not be described in detail in this chapter. The two major types can be distinguished from each other by histochemical means, not only qualitatively but also quantitatively. Thus, the proportion of type-I and type-II fibers in a muscle can be determined using ATPase staining techniques.

The postural muscles, also known as the tonic muscles, are charakterized by having a significantly greater proportion of slow twitch (type-I) fibers than fast twitch fibers. In contrast, the phasic muscles are primarily made up of fast twitch (type-II) fibers. As the name implies, the contraction or twitch speed of the slow twitch fibers is slow especially when compared to their counterparts, the fast twitch fibers. The slow twitch fibers are high in oxidative enzymes and low in myosin ATPase activity. They rely predominately on the aerobic mechanism, with glycogen and fat being the major energy supplies. There is low production of lactic acid. The slow twitch fibers are resistant to fatigue and do so only after several hundred contractions. In contrast, the fast twitch fibers, which are high in glycolytic enzymes as well as myosin ATPase activity, rely more on the anaerobic metabolism and tend to accumulate lactic acid much faster than the slow twitch fibers. The fast twitch fibers fatigue much more rapidly, and may do so after only a few contractions.

Vascular and nerve supply is also different for the two fiber types. The number of capillaries in the slow twitch fibers is significantly higher than that in the fast twitch fibers, with 4.8 capillaries per fiber in the slow twitch group in contrast to 2.8 capillaries per fiber in the fast twitch group. The slow twitch fibers receive their innervation primarily through th $\alpha2$-motor neuron and show a high concentration of muscle spindles. In contrast, the fast twitch fibers are supplied by $\alpha1$-motor neurons with relatively few muscle spindles present (Richmand and Abrahams, 1979).

The uneven distribution of muscle spindles most likely plays a role in the functional pathology of the different muscles. Table 2.2 summarizes the major charakteristics of the slow and fast twitch fibers.

Studies in high performance athletes seem to indicate that the type of activity and therefore specific use of certain muscle groups may alter the proportional

Table 2.2 Characteristics of slow twitch and fast twitch muscle fibers

Flexion	Slow Twitch (I)	Fast Twitch (II)
Function	tonic (postural)	phasic
Twitch speed	slow	fast
Metabolism/enzymes	oxidative	glycolytic
Myosin ATPase	low activity	high activity
Fatigability rate	slow	rapid
"Color"	red	white
Capillary density	high	low
Spindle number	high	moderate
Innervation	α_2-motor neuron	α_1-motor neuron
Reaction to functional disturbance	shortening	weakening

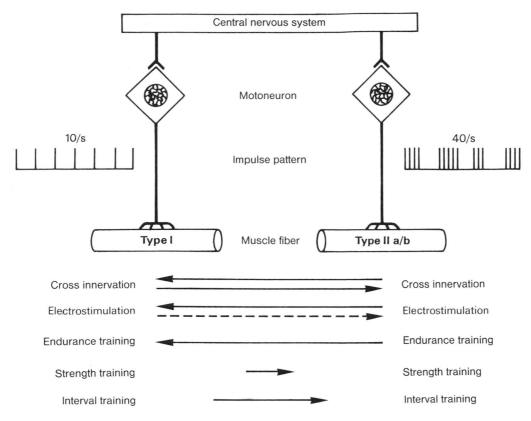

Fig. 2.**7** Transformation of the slow twitch fibers (type I) and the slow twitch fibers (type II) as a result of various different activities (loading) and electrostimulation (after Howald)

relationship between the slow and fast twitch fibers in the muscle (Howald, 1982) (Fig. 2.**7**). It was observed that 93% of the fibers in the quadriceps muscle of a marathon runner were of the slow twitch type. In contrast, only 48% of the fibers were of the slow twitch type in the quadriceps muscles of an untrained person.

Histochemical studies of the multifidus muscle (Jowet and Fidler, 1975) show that both hypomobility in the lumbar spine and nerve root compression change the proportion of slow and fast twitch fibers in favor of the slow twitch fibers. The same study shows further that there is a predominance of slow twitch fibers on the side of convexity in patients with idiopathic scoliosis as compared to the concave side. It would be plausible then to assume that a clinically shortened muscle (i. e., a muscle with primarily postural function) would show a significantly higher proportion of slow twitch fibers than normal. However, no such morphological transformation of the individual muscle fibers from one type to another in a patient with a so-called functional muscle imbalance has been histochemically demonstrated thus far.

Table 2.**3** presents the major muscle groups according to their primary function of either postural support (also known as the tonic muscles) or phasic function (Schneider and Tritschler 1981). Clinically, the various groups are examined for either shortening (primarily the postural muscles) or weakening (the phasic muscles).

2.3.2 Muscle Receptors

Five types of receptors are recognized in the striated musculature, namely:

- muscle spindles
- Golgi tendon organs
- Pacinian corpuscles
- free nerve endings (nociceptors, type IV)
- mechanoreceptors (type III)

The three-dimensional free nerve endings and the type-III mechanoreceptors that are primarily located at the tendon-bone junction have already been described. The two most important muscle receptors — the muscle spindles and the Golgi tendon organs — will be described in greater detail below.

Table 2.3 Overview of the important muscles with primarily phasic or tonic function (from Schneider and Tritschler, 1981)

Primarily Postural (tonic) muscles	Primarily phasic muscles
Pelvic Region	
Biceps femoris m	Vastus medialis m
Semitendinosus m	Vastus lateralis m
Semimembranosus m	
Iliopsoas m	Gluteus medius m
Rectus femoris m	Gluteus maximus m
	Gluteus minimus m
Tensor fasciae latae m	
Adductor longus m	
Adductor brevis m	
Adductor magnus m	
Gracilis m	
Piriformis m	
Calf and Foot	
Gastrocnemius m	Tibialis anterior m
Soleus m	Peroneal mm
Shoulder Girdle	
Pectoralis major m	Rhomboid mm
Levator scapulae m	Trapezius m (ascending)
Trapezius m (descending portion)	Trapezius m (horizontal)
	Pectoralis m (abdominal)
Biceps brachii m (short head)	Triceps brachii m
Biceps brachii m (long head)	
Trunk	
Erector spinae muscles in Lumbar and cervical region	Erector spinae Muscles in mid-thoracic region
Quadratus lumborum m	
Scalene muscles	

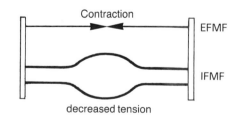

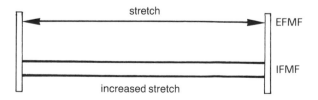

Fig. 2.8 Function of the muscle spindle
EFMF Extrafusal muscle fibers
IFMF Intrafusal muscle fibers

2.3.2.1 Muscle Spindles

Morphologic studies by Richmond and Abrahams (1979) clearly demonstrate that there is great variation in the distribution of the muscle spindles in the striated musculature. Muscles responsible for fine and precise movement have a significantly higher concentration of spindles than those muscles that must accomplish more gross movement. The small suboccipital muscles, for instance, have approximately 150−200 muscle spindles per gram of muscle tissue, whereas the rectus femoris muscle has only 50 muscle spindles per gram of muscle tissue.

An exceptionally high concentration of muscle spindles is found in the paraspinal musculature, that is, the intertransverse muscle in the cervical spine, where it is not uncommon to find 200 − 500 spindles per gram of muscle tissue. Furthermore, the muscle spindles are not evenly distributed throughout the muscles; rather, they appear to be organized predominantly around the slow twitch muscle fibers (Richmond and Abrahams, 1979). This may help explain the reaction of the primarily postural muscles in a state of overload. As mentioned above, there is a greater proportion of slow twitch fibers in those muscles whose primary task is that of maintaining posture. Clinical experience has shown that the postural muscles have a tendency to shorten. This is in contrast to the phasic muscles, which are mostly made up of fast twitch fibers and tend to become weak rather than short.

The muscle spindles are comprised of three to eight slender, specialized muscle fibers, which have been assigned the name "intrafusal muscle fibers." The intrafusal muscle fibers are arranged in parallel to and surrounded by the extrafusal muscle fibers, the regular skeletomotor fibers that make up the bulk of the muscle (Freeman and Wyke, 1967). With contraction of the muscle through the action of the extrafusal fibers, tension is reduced in the noncontractile elements of the muscle spindles (Fig. 2.**8**). Tension is increased in both the extrafusal and intrafusal fibers when the muscle is being stretched (Brodal 1981; Simons, 1976).

2.3.2.2 Golgi Tendon Organs

The Golgi tendon organs consist of a group of broad, myelinated nerve fibers (12−18 µm) (Copper and Daniel, 1963; Schoulitz and Swett, 1972). They end freely between the collagenous fibers of the tendons and are usually found at the muscle-tendon junction. In contrast to the spindles, they are arranged in series with the extrafusal muscle fibers; this is an important point in regard to their function. The tendon organs react to tension changes, both during muscle contraction and relaxation. This is important as both of these situations cause tension in the Golgi tendon organs.

In other words the Golgi tendon organs function as a tension receptor, whereas the muscle spindles primarily register changes in muscle length (Granit 1955, 1975).

2.3.3 Alpha-Gamma Coactivation
(Granit 1955, 1975)

Despite its complexity, this mechanism is presented here for its importance in the understanding of the function of the α- and γ-motor neurons and their role in manual medicine. A graphic representation has been reproduced in Figure 2.**9** (after Hassler, 1981). Here, the right half of the diagram represents the circuit responsible for reflexive muscle length changes, while the left half represents events associ-

ated with the circuit of muscle tension control and external stretching force application.

Components of the reflex arc of the phasic proprioceptive reflex include the nuclear bag and the intrafusal muscle fibers, which undergo contraction when stimulated through the γ-1 neurons. This causes the noncontractile central portion of the muscle spindle, the nuclear bag, to also become stretched. Subsequently, the surrounding spiral endings of the Ia-fibers (the primary or annulospiral endings) also become distracted. This mechanism is responsible for the proprioceptive reflex, which, via the Ia-fibers and the direct reflexive collateral branches, connects with the α1-motor neurons, resulting in contraction of the extensor muscles. Innervation of γ1-assures that the very sensitive nuclear bag can be reset for a shortened length, which is then automatically maintained through the proprioceptive reflex. The strength of the phasic proprioceptive reflex is directly dependent on the external stretching force, as well as on the activity of the γ1-system.

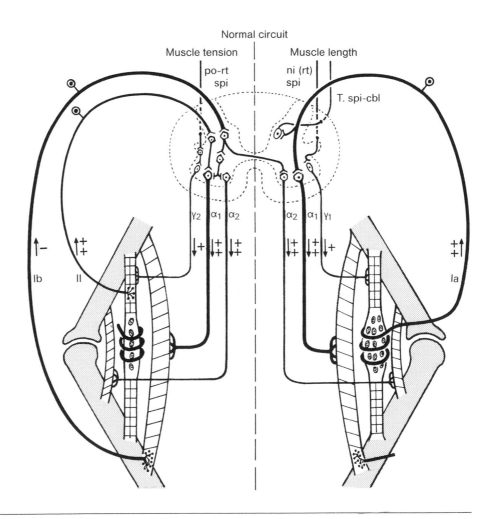

Fig. 2.**9** Control of muscle length (circuit on the right) and muscle tension (left) with the appropriate reflex arc (after Hassler). (Details in text)

Circuit for muscle tension control. It is the intrafusal muscle fibers of the thin nuclear chain fiber that will contract when the tonic γ2-fibers are stimulated. The spindle afferents of the smaller size (type-II) fibers terminate primarily on the polar segments of the nuclear chain fibers via the secondary or flower spray endings (II in Fig. 2.**9**). External stretch induces these endings to fire; this is relayed to the α2-motor neurons in the anterior horn cells via the afferent type-II fibers and multiple synapses at the spinal cord level. It is these α2-motor neurons that cause the slow postural muscles to contract. The length of the postural muscles is maintained as long as the nuclear chain fibers are held at a particular length through the influence of the γ2-neurons. Another important regulatory component of muscle tension, in addition to and in feedback with the action of the tonic stretch reflex, are the Golgi tendon organs. Originating from the tendon organs are fast Ib-fibers that convey information to the spinal cord and, by way of several interneurons, have an inhibitory effect on both the α1- and α2-motor neurons. This leads to the inhibition of the contraction of the postural muscles via the α2-efferent neurons, thus countering the effect of the tonic stretch reflex (a "relief reflex", in a sense). The α1-efferent motor neurons terminate on those contractile muscle fibers that are involved in the phasic extensor action. The conclusion, then, is that muscle tension, even under the influence of external stretching forces, is regulated by a feedback mechanism between the regular stretch reflex (originating from the secondary endings) and the so-called relief reflex (Hassler, 1981). Rethelyi and Szentagothai (1973) observed that the afferent fibers originating from the muscle spindles send off collaterals at the dorsal root level to more than one spinal segment. This is especially useful information when correlating it with principles involving alpha-gamma coactivation (Brodal, 1981). Furthermore, it may be clinically relevant and of use in the understanding of segmental (somatic) dysfunction and the spondylogenic reflex syndrome. Therefore, it may be possible that the afferent fibers from a muscle spindle influence motor neurons of several spinal segments (Brodal, 1981).

2.3.4 Postcontraction Sensory Discharge

Several authors have investigated the role of the post-contraction sensory discharge in clinically shortened postural (tonic) muscles (Brown et al., 1976; Eldred et al., 1976; Hnik et al., 1973). Buerger (1983) suggests that this phenomenon may explain some of the therapeutic effects of various manual medicine techniques.

In single fiber studies from a single annulospiral ending, as well as studies from the entire root portion, the following observation was made: tetanic stimulation of a single muscle spindle or its gamma-efferent fiber caused an increased discharge pattern at the respective annulospiral ending. A shortening in the muscle spindle led to a decrease in discharge. *Rapid overstretch of the involved muscle spindle, however, causes the effect of a tetanic gamma stimulation to be absent.*

The importance and role of these experimental observations, especially as they relate to the mechanism of shortening of the postural muscles, cannot be conclusively interpreted at this time.

However, it can be assumed that at least to some extent, the postcontraction sensory discharge phenomenon is involved when postural muscles shorten or when there is transformation of the fast twitch fibers to slow twitch fibers.

2.3.5 The Influence of Nociceptive Muscle Afferents on Muscle Tone

It has been stated above that the Ia-fibers supply the primary muscle spindles, whereas the Ib-fibers innervate the Golgi tendon organs.

Furthermore, the type-II muscle afferents also innervate muscle spindles and have been referred to as the secondary spindle afferents. Little is actually known about the three-dimensional free nerve endings of these nociceptors and their afferent fibers originating from the muscles. It can be assumed that these nerve endings serve the purpose of registering actual tissue damage or noxic stimuli (stimuli that potentially could damage the tissues). Studies by Mense (1977) indicate that the nociceptors of the muscle are not a uniform population of receptors. They can be activated either mechanically or chemically (bradykinin, potassium, serotonin). They have also been found to fire with prolonged muscle contraction or in the presence of ischemic changes.

Schmidt et al. (1981), studying the α-motor neuron system in response to painful muscle stimulation in animals, found that the small-caliber muscle afferent fibers (nociceptive afferents), once stimulated by the painful stimuli, have direct entry to the α- and γ-motor neurons at the spinal cord level. Furthermore, the same study showed that this transmission occurs with significant intensity and is by no means only a marginal occurrence. Concluding from this study by

Schmidt et al. (1981), it may be theorized that the small-caliber muscle afferents have a profound influence on the extent as well as the distribution of muscle tone in the standing or moving animal. The findings of these animal studies seem to indicate that both stimulation of the nociceptive muscle receptors by pain induction and chronic irritation of the small-caliber muscle afferents (type-III and -IV afferents) via the gamma loop produce permanent elevation of muscle tone. At this time it is hypothesized that this mechanism may play a specific role in the human being as well, especially in relationship to the so-called localized muscle spasm (myotendinosis or the hard, palpable band of muscle) secondary to a segmental dysfunction. In addition, this mechanism may explain reports of regressive muscle damage caused by a chronic myotendinosis (localized muscle spasm, palpable band) (Fassbender, 1980). Figure 2.10 demonstrates the vicious cycle between the stimulation of the nociceptive receptors of skeletal muscle and the activation of the gamma loop.

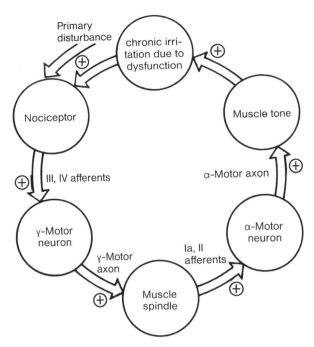

Fig. 2.10 Increase in muscle tone with chronic irritation of the small nociceptor afferents from skeletal muscles (after Schmidt)

3 Differential Diagnosis and Definition of the Radicular and Spondylogenic (Nonradicular) Pain Syndromes

In 1955 Gutzeit identified two important historical starting points documenting the importance of the vertebral factors in the clinical presentation:

- The operation of the herniated intervertebral disk by Mixter and Barr in 1934 by which the "rheumatic" ischialgia could be healed
- The perception by osteopathic physicians and chiropractors that pain caused by the vertebrae can be influenced through manual treatment of the spine

Both points are still of great significance. Diagnosis of the objective radicular failure, clarification through radiology (myelography and computer tomography [CT] scan, including three-dimensional reconstructive recordings [Glen et al., 1979]), as well as precise palpatory examination of the spine and the paraspinal soft tissue are all prerequisites to allow a clear decision as to what procedure is to be applied: either the surgical removal of a radicular compression syndrome, be it the result of a herniated intervertebral disk or bony new growth, or the manual treatment of the spine when a spondylogenic (nonradicular) pain syndrome is present.

As a result of their extensive palpatory experience, manual therapists (Maigne, 1970; Lewit, 1977), osteopathic physicians (Jones, 1981; Mitchell et al., 1979), and chiropractors (Walther, 1981) have made considerable contributions in the field of functional diagnosis of the musculoskeletal system, especially the vertebral column and the paraspinal tissue.

The diagnostic challenge of an acute nerve root compression in patients with overt signs and symptoms should not be a great one. In contrast, it is much more difficult to develop a diagnosis in patients who suffer from chronic back pain. Without an adequate diagnosis, it is no easy task to formulate an appropriate therapeutic plan. This is made even more difficult by the many cases that present with a mixed clinical picture.

The indications for surgery still remain a matter of discussion. Little attention has been paid thus far to large statistical analyses which seem to indicate that conservative measures show satisfactory results in 80% of patients (Jorg, 1982). In West Germany, for instance, 20000 patients underwent lumbar disk surgery in one year (Schirmer, 1981). The question of whether the surgical procedure was indicated in all of these patients remains unanswered. The authors' experience shows that approximately one third of patients who had undergone back surgery were later dissatisfied with the results, and between 10% and 20% of the patients were on partial or complete disability (Dvořák et al., 1988). If complaints continue to be reported by the patient despite therapy (i. e., surgery), the question of psychological overlay may be raised. In some cases then, it may actually be beneficial to arrange for preoperative psychological evaluation (i. e., the Minnesota Multiphasic Personality Inventory [MMPI]), as the results may influence the decision of whether or not to operate (Cashion and Lynch, 1979; Southwick, 1983; Herron, 1985; Dvořák et al., 1988).

These statistical analyses, as well as previous clinical experience should be thought-provoking, since only a few decades ago the criteria for indication of surgery were much stricter. It is interesting to note that residual symptoms are rare in those elderly patients who were seen by a physician at a time when practitioners were more reluctant to use surgical intervention as a means of treating low back pain (Jorg, 1982). In this context, the functional and palpatory examination of patients with back pain assumes a paramount role.

When examining a patient for the possibility of a herniated disk, concentration should be on eliciting objective findings such as motor deficits and changes in the muscle stretch reflexes.

Sensory examination should focus on radicular (segmental) deficits, especially perception to pain (algesia). Hypesthesias (decreased sensation of light touch) and paresthesias (abnormal perception ranging from tingling to overt numbness) are only of limited value, as similar symptoms are also typical for the pseudoradicular syndromes (Brügger, 1977; Feinstein et al., 1954; Kellgren, 1939).

For the classic neurological examination procedure of the root syndromes, the pertinent textbooks should be consulted.

3.1 Radicular Syndromes

3.1.1 Anatomy of the Spinal Nerves

All but three of the 31 pairs of nerve roots exit the spinal column through the intervertebral foramina. The first cervical root exits between the atlas and the occiput, and the last sacral and the only coccygeal nerve exit via the sacral hiatus (Fig. 3.1).

The faster growth rate of the vertebral column results in a height difference between the spinal cord level and the vertebral level. Due to this displacement, the nerve roots in the lumbar and sacral region run laterally and almost vertically to their point of exit in the intervertebral foramen. This is in contrast to the cervical roots, which are mostly horizontal. The length of the roots increases from a few millimeters to about 25 cm (Mumenthaler and Schliack, 1982).

The spinal cord inferior to L2 contains nerve roots only, commonly called the cauda equina.

The spinal nerve roots are positioned for the most part intradurally. The pia mater covers the beginning portions, and the arachnoid runs along the roots, terminating at the root pockets formed by the dura. Both the anterior and the posterior roots exit through separate openings in the dura before they unite to form the spinal nerves. After leaving the intervertebral foramen, the spinal nerve divides into four typical rami (Fig. 3.2).

The meningeal nerve, which is both sensory and autonomic, returns to the spinal cord. The white communicating branch (sympathetic fibers) is directed to the corresponding ganglion of the sympathetic trunk in the paravertebral region. A section of the postganglionic, less-myelinated sympathetic fibers returns to the nerve roots as the gray communicating branch. The remaining fibers continue to the visceral organs. The rami communicantes contain sensory fibers in addition to autonomic fibers that pass through the ganglion and terminate at the visceral organs. Furthermore, the nerve root divides into a dorsal ramus and a ventral ramus. With the exception of the first and second dorsal rami (suboccipital nerve and greater occipital nerve, respectively), the ventral rami are substantially thicker than the dorsal rami.

Important for practical purposes is the topographical relationship of the nerve root to the intervertebral canal or the intervertebral foramen. The vertebral bodies, the vertebral arches, and the articular processes determine the bony limitations, and the joint capsule and the intervertebral disk are the soft tissue borders. Fat tissue (noted in a CT-scan) and the

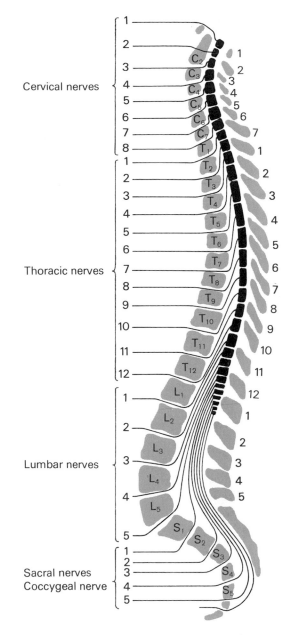

Fig. 3.1 Diagram of the position of the spinal cord segments of the nerve roots with reference to the bodies and spinous processes of the vertebrae (after Borovansky, 1967)

venous plexi cushion the spinal nerve against the wall. It is of clinical significance that the diameter of the intervertebral foramina decreases from L1 to L5, whereas the circumference of the nerve roots increases severalfold.

In addition to radicular pain caused by compression, any of the surrounding structures (soft tissue, bones) can be a source of pain (Wyke, 1967). The joint capsule of the small apophyseal joints seems to play a

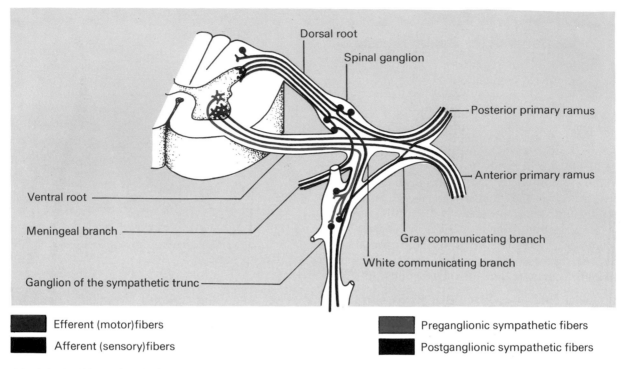

Dorsal root

Spinal ganglion

Posterior primary ramus

Anterior primary ramus

Ventral root

Meningeal branch

Gray communicating branch

White communicating branch

Ganglion of the sympathetic trunc

▉ Efferent (motor)fibers	▉ Preganglionic sympathetic fibers
▉ Afferent (sensory)fibers	▉ Postganglionic sympathetic fibers

Fig. 3.2   Individual fibers of a spinal nerve (after Borovansky, 1967)

special role in the nonradicular pain character or the so-called referred pain (Brügger, 1977; Feinstein et al., 1954; Hockaday and Whitty, 1967; Kellgren, 1938; Korr, 1975; Reynolds, 1981; Sutter, 1975; Wyke 1967, 1979b).

3.1.2 Important Radicular Syndromes

The topographic relationship between the nerve roots and the intervertebral canal and disk, as well as the differing loads on the individual spinal segments (also known as vertebral units), is primarily responsible for disk protrusion (or prolapse) that occurs most frequently at the lower lumbar and first sacral root levels. The relationship between the diameter of the nerve root and the intervertebral canal is significantly unfavorable in the lumbosacral junction in comparison to other segments of the spinal cord.

Apart from the limited spatial arrangement, it is the vertical course of the nerve roots in the lumbosacral junction that can cause the next root to come into contract with the intervertebral disk as well.

The posterolaterally herniated intervertebral disk of L4−L5 primarily compresses the fifth lumbar nerve, whereas the disk of L5−S1 compresses the first sacral nerve. The nerve root leaving the intervertebral fora-

men in this vertebral unit can exit without compression. When the hernia of the disk is substantial, a combined L4−L5 and L5−S1 or a radicular syndrome can arise (Fig. 3.3).

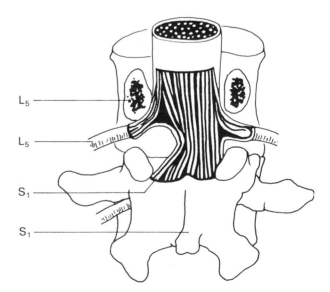

L_5

L_5

S_1

S_1

Fig. 3.3   A large, postero laterally herniated disk in the lumbosacral junction compresses both the first sacral and the fifth lumbar roots (Dubs, 1950)

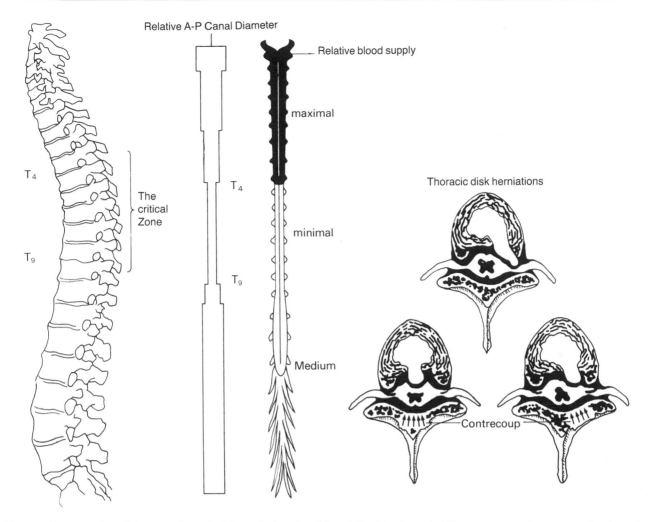

Fig. 3.4 Cross-section of the central canal of the spinal cord and its relative blood supply. The contrecoup phenomenon for thoracic herniated disks. The relatively small cross-section and the minimal blood supply in the thoracic spine between T4 and T9 are responsible for the catastrophic nature of thoracic disk disease (after White and Panjabi, 1978b)

The occurrence of the radicular syndrome from cervical nerve roots is about 0.01 that in the lumbar region. The root of C6 is involved most frequently due to the great mobility of the segment C5−C6. The thoracic root syndromes are extremely rare. The clinical presentation of a herniated disk in the center of the thoracic spine, however, can be very dramatic, since the diameter of the canal of the spinal column between T4 and T9 is quite small, and the vascular supply is markedly decreased in comparison to the remaining segments of the spinal cord (White and Panjabi, 1978).

These two factors can result in the increased likelihood of injury as the consequence of a "contrecoup" mechanism involving the spinal cord and the nerve roots (Fig. 3.4).

3.1.3 Symptomatology of the Root Syndromes

Compression of the individual nerve roots is normally accompanied by the following symptoms (Table 3.1).

- Pain in the region supplied by the nerve roots
- Radicular loss of sensitivity according to the dermatomes
- Motor loss of the muscles innervated by the corresponding roots
- Deep tendon reflex changes

3 Differential Diagnosis of Radicular Pain Syndromes

Table 3.1   Review of root syndromes (after Mumenthaler and Schliack, 1982)

Segment	Sensation	Muscles Involved	Tendon Reflex	Remarks
C3/4	Pain (hypalgesia) in shoulder region (see Fig. 1)	Partial or total paralysis of diaphragm	No detectable changes	Partial diaphragmatic paralysis, C3 more ventral and C4 more dorsal
C5	Pain (hypalgesia) over lateral aspect of shoulder, covering deltoid area	Disturbance of innervation of deltoid and biceps brachii muscles	Diminished or absent biceps reflex	
C6	Dermatome on outer aspect of arm and forearm as far as the thumb	Paralysis of biceps brachii and brachioradialis muscles	Diminished or absent biceps reflex	
C7	Dermatome lateral and dorsal to C6 dermatome, including index finger to ring finger	Paralysis of triceps brachii, pronator teres and occasionally the finger flexors; often visible atrophy of the thenar eminence	Diminished or absent triceps reflex	Differential diagnosis of carpal tunnel syndrome: note the triceps reflex
C8	Dermatome to C7, extending to include little finger	Small muscles of hand, visible atrophy especially of hypothenar eminence	Diminished triceps reflex	Differential diagnosis of ulnar nerve palsy: note the triceps reflex
L3	Dermatome extending from greater trochanter over the extensor surface to the medial side of the thigh and knee	Paralysis of quadriceps femoris muscle	Absent quadriceps reflex (knee jerk)	Differential diagnosis of femoral nerve palsy: area of saphenous nerve innervation remains intact
L4	Dermatome extending from lateral surface of thigh across the knee to the anterior and medial quadrant of the leg, including the medial part of the sole	Paralysis of quadriceps femoris and tibialis anterior muscles	Diminished quadriceps reflex (knee jerk)	Differential diagnosis of femoral nerve palsy: involvement of tibialis anterior or muscle
L5	Dermatome extending from above lateral condyle of femur, over the anterior and outer quadrant of the leg as far as the great toe	Paralysis and atrophy of extensor hallucis longus, often also extensor digitorum brevis muscles	Absent tibialis posterior reflex, only useful if the opposite reflex can be clearly elicited	
S1	Dermatome extending from flexor surface of thigh to outer and posterior quadrant of leg, and over the lateral malleolus to the little toe	Paralysis of peroneal muscles, frequently also disturbances of innervation of the triceps surae muscle	Absent triceps surae reflex (ankle jerk)	
Combined L4/5	L4 and L5 dermatomes	All extensor muscles of ankle; also disturbances of innervation of quadriceps femoris	Diminished quadriceps reflex. Absent tibialis posterior reflex	Differential diagnosis of peroneal nerve palsy: peroneal muscles escape. Note knee jerk and tibialis posterior
Combined L5/S1	L5 and S1 dermatomes	Extensors of toes, peroneal muscles, occasionally also disturbances of innervation of triceps surae muscles	Absent tibialis posterior and triceps surae reflex	Differential diagnosis of peroneal nerve palsy: tibialis anterior muscle escapes. Note the reflex findings

3.2 Neurologic Diseases Accompanied by Back Pain

(An excellent review of the literature has been presented by Mattle, 1988)

3.2.1 Extramedullary, Intraspinal Tumors

In the presence of prolonged and prominent radicular symptoms, differentiation must be made between a cervical herniated disk and an extramedullary, intraspinal tumor. Schwannomas (neurilemmomas) are the most frequently encountered tumors (Burger and Vogel, 1982; Herd, 1973). The recognition of this benign tumor in a patient with radicular symptoms is beneficial in that surgical intervention has produced good results. However, the prognosis is worse in a patient in whom a transection-type of injury to the spinal cord has occurred. Causes of such an injury may include prolonged compression of the spinal cord by a tumor or, as in an acute situation, occlusion of the anterior spinal artery.

Schwannomas may grow along the nerve root and extend beyond the intervertebral foramen which, as a result, becomes enlarged. This can be visualized on oblique radiographs, but better yet on axial CT scans.

3.2.2 Intramedullary Space-Occupying Lesions

Intramedullary space-occupying lesions can be present for weeks or even months, causing neck pain or back pain, or both, before neurological deficits are clinically detected. There is usually segmental, radiating pain corresponding to the level of tumor involvement, as well as distal paresthesias and peripheral paralysis or paresis. Segmental muscle weakness and atrophy or fasciculations are sometimes found on physical examination. Below the level of involvement, a central palsy and dissociated sensory changes can occur (loss of pain and temperature sensation with preserved proprioceptive and touch modalities). Frequent causes of a space-occupying lesion include astrocytomas and ependymomas. If the symptoms extend over years, a syringomyelia should be suspected, the causes of which may include malformations such as basilar impression, Klippel-Feil or Arnold-Chiari syndromes. The diagnosis is made either by CT or magnetic resonance imaging (MRI).

3.2.3 Radiculopathies and Neuropathies

Amyotrophic lateral sclerosis, when principally involving the spinal cord and lower motor neurons, is characterized more by shoulder pain than neck pain. Frequently, it is not until the original sharp pain has subsided that the patient realizes the presence of weakness, atrophy, or even paralysis in the upper arm. Sensory changes are rarely present. An electromyogram (EMG) of the involved muscles reveals a neurogenic pattern in almost all cases (i. e., profuse fibrillations, fasciculations, increased amplitude motor unit action potential firing). Nerve conduction velocities (NCV) are usually normal.

The polyradiculopathy in Guillain-Barré syndrome usually progresses, except for initial paresthesias at the onset, without significant pain (Loffel, 1977; Guillain-Barré, 1981). It has been occasionally observed that a patient complains of nonspecific lumbagolike pain for days to weeks preceding the muscle weakness.

A polyradiculitis caused by spirochetes is usually characterized by monosegmental or plurisegmental pain and may reveal severe, pronounced peripheral muscle weakness (Bacher, 1985; Schmitt, 1985; Steer, 1983). By specific questions during the history interview, it may be elicited that the patient had been stung by an insect, followed by skin changes consistent with erythema chronicum migrans. Laboratory examination of the spinal fluid of the patient infected with spirochetes usually reveals an increased cell count. Confirmation of a diagnosis of spirochete infection, however, requires serological testing.

It is difficult to differentiate dermatomal pain from other causes in a patient who suffers from a herpes zoster infection but who has not progressed beyond the prodromal period, until the vesicles actually appear (Mumenthaler, 1985).

3.2.4 Bone Metastases

Diffuse pain developing over a short period of time and localizable to a specific region in the spine with possible dermatomal radiation may be caused by metastatic carcinoma of the bone (Harner, 1982). The metastases usually reach the spinal cord anteriorly, therefore causing more destruction on the anterior components of the cord than the posterior ones. Clinically, there may be paraparesis with loss of pain and temperature sensation, whereas touch and positional sensation are usually preserved. Conventional X-rays, in particular the anteroposterior projection, may reveal bony changes, particular attention should be paid to the arches of the roots.

3.2.5 Circulatory Changes Affecting the Spinal Cord

The vessel most frequently involved is the anterior spinal artery. Occlusion of this artery may lead to a central monoparesis with contralateral dissociated sensory disturbances, that is, Brown-Sequard-syndrome. These neurological symptoms are often accompanied by acute back pain which radiate segmentally. There is flaccid paresis in the segmentally related muscles in the presence of circulation abnormalities.

3.2.6 Spontaneous Spinal Epidural Hematoma

The occurrence of a spontaneous spinal epidural hematoma is rare (Feet and Food, 1981). Immediate diagnosis of this disorder and prompt laminectomy will prevent the patient from becoming permanently disabled (Mattle, 1985). The first clinical symptoms the patient complains about are usually severe neck pain or back pain, or both, soon followed by pain radiating along the distribution of a root. Within minutes to hours, or even days, the patient may develop a transection-type of cord injury with paraplegia. The possibility of a spontaneous spinal epidural hematoma should always be considered when there is acute pain, especially when the patient is on anticoagulation medication. The diagnosis is usually confirmed by myelography or CT.

3.2.7 Spinal Epidural Abscess

Extremely severe and well-localizable pain in patients with signs of a systemic infection and fever may be due to an epidural abscess. In most cases staphylococcus is the offending organism (Kaufmann, 1980; Bakker, 1975). The dura to bulge, applying mechanical pressure on the spinal cord which in turn may decrease the spinal circulation. A rapidly progressive paraplegia may ensue. The diagnosis can usually be made by myelography. Therapeutic intervention includes surgical decompression by laminectomy and appropriate antibiotic coverage.

3.2.8 Lumbar Spinal Stenosis

In elderly patients complaining of chronic back pain, radicular symptoms, and intermittent neurogenic claudication, a lumbar spinal stenosis should be sus-

pected (Blau, 1978; Benini, 1981; Hohmann, 1984). The patient's history usually reveals the need for frequent rest periods after walking a short distance. Furthermore, a change in posture, such as leaning forward (i. e. supporting one self over the cart when shopping), or assuming a sitting position is necessary to bring about some relief. To demonstrate possible deep tendon reflex changes or alteration in sensation, as well as muscle weakness, it is often necessary to have the patient move until the state of claudication is reproduced. CT and MRI are very valuable tools in the diagnostic workup. A recent monography by Postacchim (1989) deals in detail with this disease, which is increasingly affecting aging patients.

3.3 Spondylogenic (Pseudoradicular) Syndromes

The observations of the nonradicular pain syndromes, to date empirical only, have been gaining more importance through the experimental neurophysiological work by Korr (1975), Simons (1976), and Wyke (1967 and 1979b). Different authors attempted to organize and categorize the painful soft-tissue changes (often described as inflammatory soft-tissue rheumatism) and furthermore to correlate them with the functional disturbances of the spinal cord or the peripheral joints (Brügger 1962, 1977; Feinstein et al., 1954; Hohermuth, 1981; Jones, 1981; Mitchell et al., 1979; Sutter, 1975; Sutter and Fröhlich, 1981; Waller, 1975; Dejung, 1985; Dvořák et al., 1987a; Dvořák et al., 1987b; Southwick and White, 1983; Herron and Turner, 1985; Mattle, 1986). The ultimate goal is to assure clear diagnostic differentiation from the actual radicular syndromes and consequently to specify the appropriate therapy, be it manipulation on the joints or stretching and rehabilitation of the muscles.

Even though similar somatic phenomena are described, the language and terminology used by the different authors reflect the individual's opinion and school of thought. The diversity of terminology and neurophysiological theories – understandable from a historical viewpoint (Dvořák, 1982; Gibson, 1980; Wardwell, 1980) – led to the result that these valuable clinical observations have found only limited diagnostic utilization in the mainstream of medicine. At an international seminar in 1983, an attempt was made to unify the terminology used internationally in the field of manual medicine (Dvořák, 1984).

In the following chapter, five concepts of the spondylogenic syndrome are presented. Despite the difference in terminology, the attentive reader will not miss the similarities. In order to appreciate the phenomena of the soft-tissue changes in daily practice, a good working knowledge of the topographic anatomy and palpation on the living human being is required.

3.3.1 Referred Pain

Kellgren (1938), Sinclair et al. (1948) and Hockaday and Whitty (1967) demonstrated in clinical experiments that local and referred pain occurs upon mechanical or chemical stimulation of different spinal and paraspinal structures.

When injecting hypertonic sodium chloride solution into the paravertebral musculature, ligaments, and apophyseal joints, or when scratching the periosteum with a needle, local and referred pain was elicited in every instance according to the segmental innervation (Kellgren 1938, 1939; Lewis and Kellgren, 1939) (Fig. 3.5).

When deep structures were stimulated, a diffuse pain distant from the origin of stimulation could be

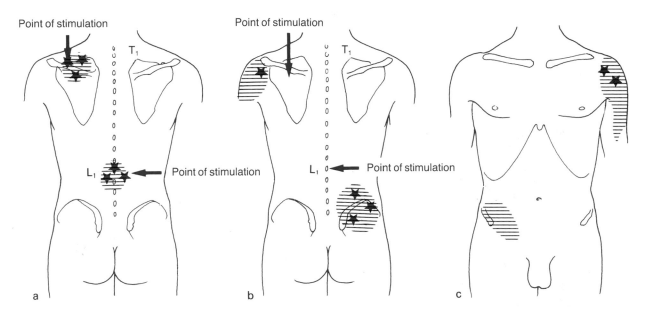

Fig. 3.5 Pain pattern upon injection of hypertonic sodium chloride solution into superficial (a) and deep structures (vertebral arches, fossa infraspinata scapulae) (after Kellgren, 1939)

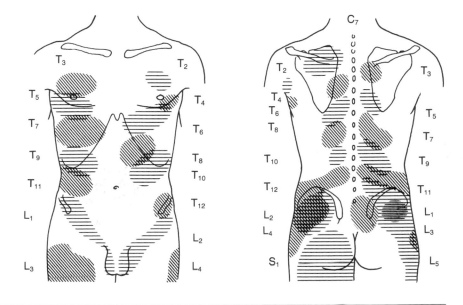

Fig. 3.6 Diagram of the patchwork distribution of referred pain after stimulation of deep structures of the thoracic spine (vertebral arches, joints) (after Kellgren, 1939)

3 Differential Diagnosis of Radicular Pain Syndromes

observed. Stimulating structures of the thoracic spine produces pain similar to skin hypersensitivity on both the anterior and posterior side of the trunk in a patchwork manner (Fig. 3.6) (Hockaday and Whitty, 1967). This is in contrast to a bandlike pain encircling the body in a girdle fashion when nerve lesions are present (for instance with herpes zoster).

Upon stimulation of structures of the lumbosacral junction, patients perceive a deep pain in the gluteal region and in the thigh, but seldom reaching below the knee.

Palpation can detect the differences between the structures affected by referred pain (muscles, liga-

ments, fascia) and the surrounding tissue. Local anesthesia in these secondarily altered structures reduces the referred pain. The spontaneous local pain of the originally stimulated tissue (i. e. supraspinous or interspinous ligaments) is thereby influenced very little. As local anesthesia is applied around the irritated ligament, both local and referred pain disappear (Kellgren, 1939).

The outcome of the experimental observations is summarized by Kellgren as follows:

"The superficial fascia of the back, the spinous processes, and the supraspinous ligaments induce local pain upon stimulation, while stimulation of the su-

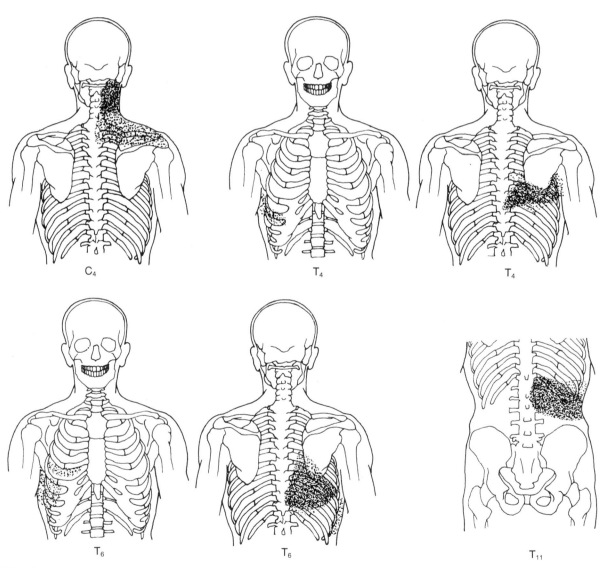

Fig. 3.7   Schematic representation of referred pain after injection of hypertonic sodium chloride solution into the infraspinous soft tissue (after Feinstein et al., 1954)

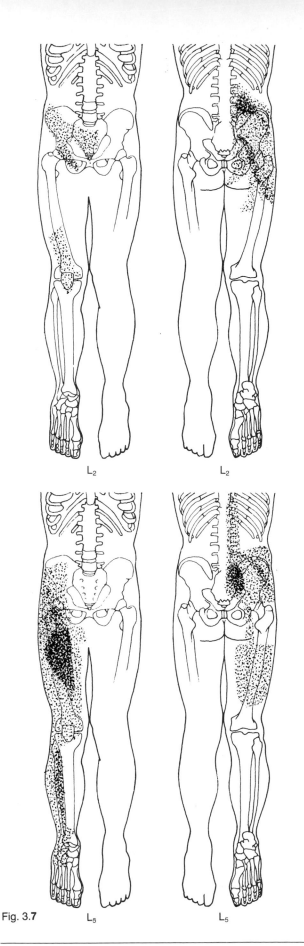

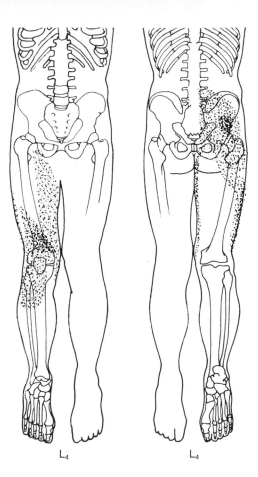

L₂ L₂

L₄ L₄

Fig. 3.7 L₅ L₅

perficial portions of the interspinous ligaments and the superficial muscles result in a diffuse type of pain. The deep muscles, ligaments, and periosteum of the apophyseal joints, as well as the joints themselves, can cause referred pain according to the segmental innervation when sufficiently stimulated."

Feinstein et al. (1954) also injected a hypertonic sodium solution into the paravertebral structures of the vertebral units C1−S3 (deep muscles, ligaments). The manifestation of referred pain and the localization of zones with decreased sensitivity to pain did not always correlate with the radicular supply (Head zones).

Upon injection of the sodium solution, pain was felt mostly in the reflexogenic hypertonic muscles and was accompanied by autonomic symptoms, such as paleness, excessive sweating, decreased blood pressure, fainting, and nausea.

Figure 3.7 depicts the observed patterns of referred pain corresponding to the level of segmental stimulation (i. e., C4, T4, T6, T11, L2, L4, L5).

Pain distribution evoked by injecting the zygapophyseal joints of the cervical spine has been described recently by Bogduk et al. (1988).

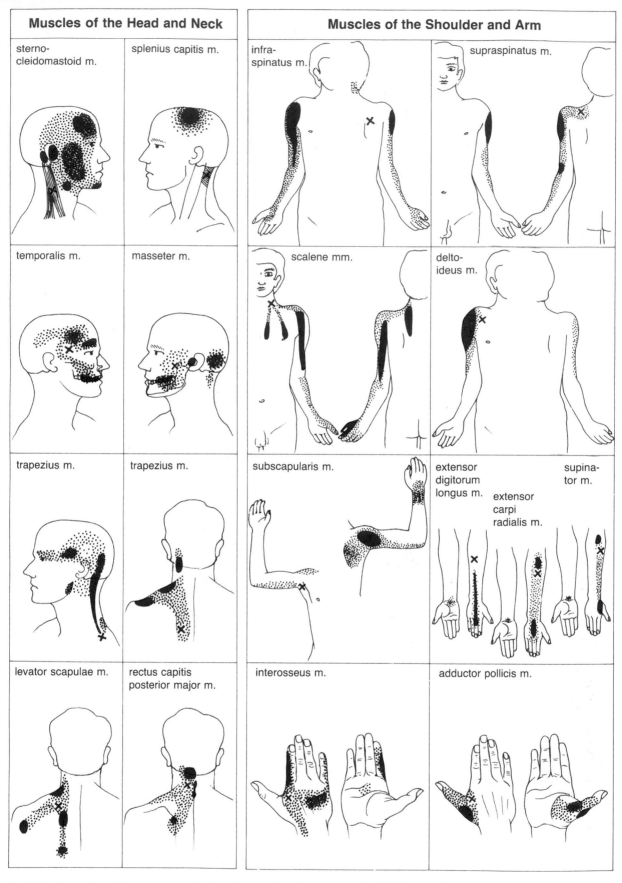

Muscles of the Head and Neck

sterno-cleidomastoid m.

splenius capitis m.

temporalis m.

masseter m.

trapezius m.

trapezius m.

levator scapulae m.

rectus capitis posterior major m.

Muscles of the Shoulder and Arm

infra-spinatus m.

supraspinatus m.

scalene mm.

delto-ideus m.

subscapularis m.

extensor digitorum longus m.

supina-tor m.

extensor carpi radialis m.

interosseus m.

adductor pollicis m.

Fig. 3.8 Examples of trigger points and referred pain in the reference sites (Pain Reference Pattern; after Travell and Rinzler, 1952)

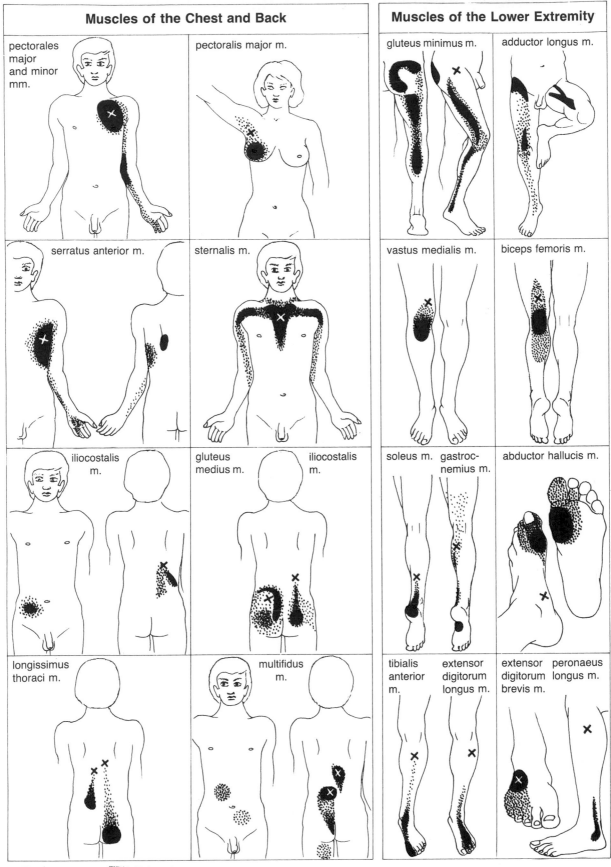

Muscles of the Chest and Back

pectorales major and minor mm.

pectoralis major m.

serratus anterior m.

sternalis m.

iliocostalis m.

gluteus medius m.

iliocostalis m.

longissimus thoraci m.

multifidus m.

Muscles of the Lower Extremity

gluteus minimus m.

adductor longus m.

vastus medialis m.

biceps femoris m.

soleus m.

gastrocnemius m.

abductor hallucis m.

tibialis anterior m.

extensor digitorum longus m.

extensor digitorum brevis m.

peronaeus longus m.

✖ Trigger point   ▰▰▰∴ Pain pattern

57

3.3.2 Myofascial Trigger Point (TP) Syndromes

As a result of research over many decades, the myofascial trigger point (TP) has been reported by several investigators (Melzack, 1978; Reynolds, 1981; Rubin, 1981; Simons 1975/1976; Travell and Rinzler, 1952; Travell 1976, 1983).

The points are painful either spontaneously or upon pressure and can cause referred pain in the muscles. The painful response is consistently observed in that musculature that is correlated with the TP (Fig. 3.**8**).

The anatomical substrate (analogous to the zones of irritation) of the trigger points and the neurophysiological interaction with the referred pain in the muscles are unknown.

3.3.2.1 Trigger Points

The TP is a small (0.5 to 1 cm) area of muscle that is hypersensitive to pressure and is noticeably different from the surrounding region when palpated.

The *active* TP has a low threshold for mechanical stimulation. With normal physiological motion, local pain appears, but it is the referred pain in the reference musculature that is perceived by the patient as being more irritating.

The clinically asymptomatic *latent* TP refers pain only when considerable palpatory pressure is applied or when an acupuncture needle is inserted into the TP (Melzack, 1981). Characteristics of a muscle with a TP are weakness of contraction but no atrophy. Contraction leads to decreased motility of the corresponding joint (Travell, 1981).

In normal muscle, a TP cannot be demonstrated and pain cannot be initiated with normal palpatory pressure.

Even though little is known about the etiology of the TP, the list of main causes includes direct muscle or joint injury, chronic muscle overload, or lengthy periods of hypothermia (Travell, 1981). Latent TPs can be activated by small impulses, such as the overstretching of muscle, momentary overload, or immobilization. The formation of TPs in the segmental musculature is also known to occur with compression of the nerve root (Travell, 1976). As a rule, they are not reversible, even after successful operative management (caution: postlaminectomy syndrome) (Travell, 1976).

Reports exist that hypomobility of the joints, due to segmental dysfunction or inflammatory processes, can contribute to the formation of a TP in a muscle (Reynolds, 1981).

3.3.2.2 Referred Pain in the Reference Zone

Referred pain, either with an active or latent TP, can usually be well-localized by the patient. Using palpation, the painful muscle or part of the muscle (myotenone) can be demarcated. It is described as a "palpable band" (Simons 1975/1976), which should be palpated perpendicular to the direction of the fibers (similar to the myotendinoses). Palpation often causes a local, painful twitch response in the muscle involved (Simons, 1976; Travell, 1952).

One TP can cause pain in one or in several reference sites (Fig. 3.**9**).

The induction of several so-called satellite TPs by a primary TP is described by Travell (1981). For instance, a TP in the sternal region of the sternocleidomastoid muscle can cause a satellite TP in the sternalis muscle, pectoral muscle, and the serratus anterior major muscle.

In addition to causing referred pain, the active TP can influence autonomic functions in the reference site (cooling by local vasoconstriction, increased sweat secretion, increased pilomotor activity).

Occasionally, hyperalgesic skin regions can be observed (Travell, 1981).

3.3.2.3 Treatment

The activity of the TP can be reduced through maximal stretching of the involved muscles. The "spray-and-stretch" method has proven to be valuable (Travell, 1981). With the help of a cooling spray (fluorimethane), afferent nociceptive impulses of the skin are initiated. Due to the nociceptive reflexogenic influence, the shortened muscle can be stretched more easily. This stretch stimulus in turn is able to block the activity of the TP via the reflexogenic pathway through the spinal cord or possibly the higher central nervous system (CNS) center. Additionally, the TP activity can be reduced or even brought to a complete halt by injection of local anesthetics, such as procaine. The muscle involved is stretched passively during the injection.

3.3.3 Pseudoradicular Syndrome

Brügger (1962, 1977) makes a clear distinction between the radicular syndrome and the pseudoradicular syndrome. The pseudoradicular syndrome is based on the reflexogenic arthromuscular aspect of the disease. It is the result of the nociceptive somatomotoric blocking effect (Brügger, 1977) attributable to the painfully stimulated tissues, especially the joint capsule, origins of tendons, and other soft tissues. Not only the muscles with their corresponding tendon junctions (tendomyoses), but the skin as well, can be reflexogenically painful (Brügger, 1958). Tendomyosis is described as the reflexogenic functional change in the muscle in the presence of concurrent functionally dependent muscle pain. These reflexogenic reactions are initiated by nociceptor stimulation.

3.3.3.1 Sternal Syndrome

The changes associated with the sternal syndrome are the result of the body's reactions (i. e., greater sensitivity) to abnormal posture and concomitant loading abnormalities in the thoracic area. This is primarily true for the slouched posture, versus the erect straight posture, where the sternocostal and sternoclavicular areas along with the surrounding soft tissues are especially involved (Fig. 3.**9**).

The clinical tendomyotic presentation of the sternal syndrome develops in those muscles that support the sternocostal and sternoclavicular joints (intercostal muscles, pectoralis major muscle, sternocleidomastoid muscle, scalene muscles, posterior neck muscles). The reflexogenically contracted and thus painful muscles are palpatorily examined both in the upright and in the abnormal thorax position.

Involvement of the pectoralis major muscle may very well imitate the parasternal pain caused by organic heart disease (Fig. 3.**10**).

Brügger considers the effort syndrome as a part of the sternal syndrome.

The reflexogenically hypertonic neck musculature may cause a secondary spondylogenic cervical syn-

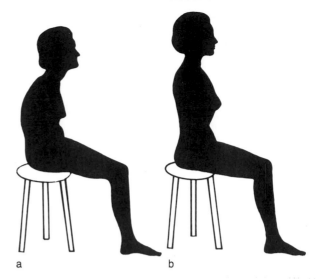

Fig. 3.**9 a** Slouched position **b** Erect (straight) thorax position (after Brügger, 1977)

drome. Sternocostal and sternoclavicular stimulation can also lead to the reflexogenic contraction of all arm muscles (myotendinosis). The clinical presentation of the reflexogenic tendomyoses is significantly different for the upright and normal thorax positions. This observation can be explained by the mechanoreceptor and nociceptor reflex mechanisms (Wyke, 1979b).

Disturbances in the acromioclavicular joints can induce reflexogenic tendomyoses in the anterior serratus muscle, the trapezius muscle, the biceps brachii muscle, the coracobrachialis muscle, and the hand and finger extensors (Brügger, 1977).

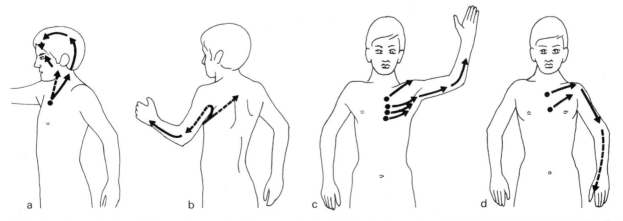

Fig. 3.**10** Overview of pain radiation patterns when the sternoclavicular joints (**a, b, c, d**) and different sternocostal joints (**c, d**) are irritated through puncture (Brügger)

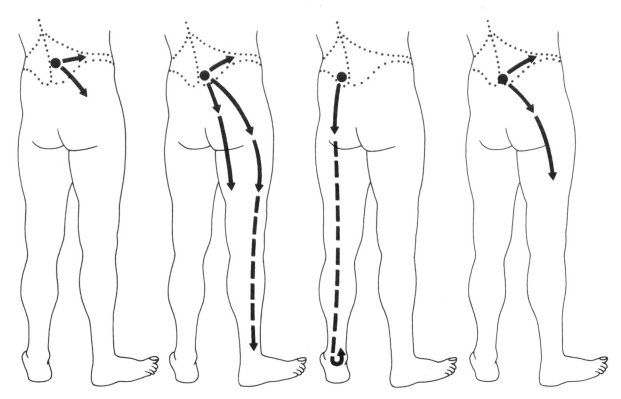

Fig. 3.11   Pain radiation patterns when puncturing different apophyseal joints (after Brügger, 1962)

The sternal syndrome may lead not only to tendomyoses of the musculature of the shoulder, neck, chest wall, or arm acroparesthesias, but also to trophic disturbances of the skin. According to an important observation by Brügger (1977), it is possible that primarily brachial syndromes (including carpal tunnel syndrome and overload injuries) induce a secondary reflexogenic sternal syndrome (Brügger, 1977; Gerstenbrand et al., 1979).

3.3.3.2 Syndrome of the Trunk

Functional disturbances of the locomotive apparatus in the region of the trunk and diseases of inner organs can lead to arthrotendomyotic syndromes via nociceptive and somatomotoric reflexes (Brügger, 1965).

A thorough knowledge of soft tissue anatomy, palpatory determination of painful tendomyoses, analysis of body posture and movement patterns, and local infiltration with anesthetics in the originally disturbed joints (apophyseal joints, costovertebral joints) all help distinguish the primarily functional disturbances of the locomotive apparatus from primarily organic diseases (Wyke, 1979a).

It is known that a primary segmental dysfunction of the locomotive apparatus can cause referred pain in the inner organs (Schwarz, 1974b). The reverse is also observed, that is, diseases of inner organs can reflexogenically induce tendomyotic changes (somatovisceral, viscerosomatic reflexes) (Korr, 1975; Beal, 1984).

3.3.3.3 Syndromes of the Lower Body

According to Brügger, the functional unit of the lower body consists of the thoracolumbar spine and posterior and anterior back, as well as the abdominal muscles, the pelvis, and the legs.

Abnormal mechanical strains on the locomotive apparatus in the lumbosacral junction evoke tendomyotic reactions in the abdominal, pelvic, and leg muscles. Brügger believes that this can result in edematous swelling and reactive inflammatory changes in the regions of the tendinous insertions, tendinous sheaths, and interstitial tissue of the musculature (Fassbender and Wegner, 1973; Fassbender, 1980). The efficiency of the locomotive apparatus is further decreased by the nociceptive somatomotoric inhibiting effect. According to Brügger, this mechanism explains the numerous lumbar algesias and leg pains, and partially explains the syndromes of the small pelvis (iliopsoas muscle).

Subcutaneous inflammatory processes, hemorrhages, and scars can also cause arthrotendomyotic presentations (Reynolds, 1981).

The differentiation between cause and effect is difficult until the reflexogenic arthrotendomyotic manifestations are recognized as such and can be differentiated from the real nidus of disease.

Stimulation of the apophyseal joints in the thoracolumbar and the lumbosacral junctions can cause pain in the abdominal wall muscles and the paravertebral and leg muscles according to their tendomyotic pattern (Fig. 3.**11**).

Radiation of pain into the abdominal organs is also described (Schwarz, 1974b).

3.3.3.4 Symphyseal Syndrome

It is observed that the infiltration of the symphysis with local anesthetics can lead to the immediate disappearance of pain in the small pelvis or legs. This would indicate that both the symphysis and the pelvis can play a role in disease. With irritation of the symphysis or with functional disturbances of the pelvis, tendomyotic reactions are observed in the paravertebral muscles (symphyseal lumbar algesias), the muscles of the pelvis and the abdomen (symphyseal abdominal wall pain), and leg muscles (quadriceps femoris muscle, sartorius muscle, tensor fasciae latae muscle) (Brügger, 1962, 1977) (Fig. 3.**12**).

It is often impossible to distinguish the primary symphyseal disturbance from secondary, reflexogenically affected, painful changes of the ligaments and tendoperiosteal tissue of the symphysis, that is, caused by disturbances in the thoracic spine.

In the slouched posture, as described by Brügger (Fig. 3.**13**) the balance of the synergism between the sacrospinalis muscle and the abdominal wall muscles is displaced in favor of the abdominal muscles, which in turn can lead to irritation of the symphysis.

In order to recognize a true radicular syndrome, it is necessary to understand the reflexogenic tendomyotic reactions resulting from irritation of the symphysis or a slouched position (Fig. 3.**14**).

The *longissimus thoracis muscle* between the sacrum and the central thoracic spine is hypotonically tendomyotic (pain between the shoulder blades and in the lumbar region). To prevent backward tilt, the iliopsoas muscle contracts. The tensor fasciae latae, sartorius, and rectus femoris muscles act synergistically. The hamstring, calf muscles and peroneal muscles become painfully hypotonic.

When a tendomyotic pain syndrome develops in this fashion, it can very well simulate a radicular lumbar sciatica. The palpatory examination of the affected muscle groups is to be performed in the slouched, erect, or supine positions. The tendomyotic reactions often disappear with upright posture.

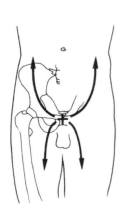

Fig. 3.**12** Pain radiation with irritation of the symphysis (after Brügger)

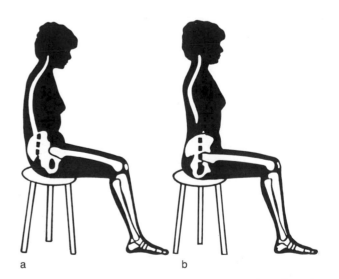

Fig. 3.**13** A torque acting in the posterior direction when the patient is in the slouched position (**a**). The disappearance of the torque in the pelvic region when patient is sitting erect (**b**) (after Brügger)

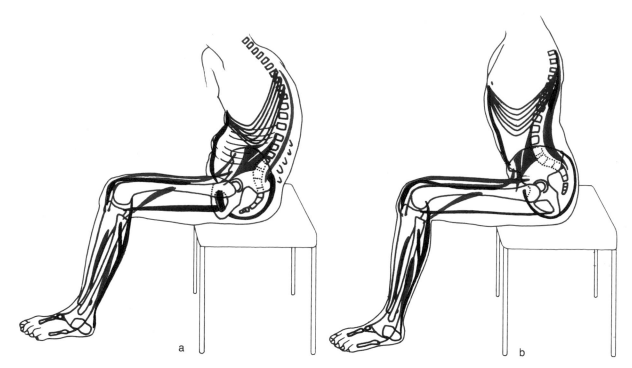

Fig. 3.**14**   Muscles involved in extension of the trunk (red), muscles involved in the slouched position (blue).

a   Slouched position
b   erect position (after Brügger)

Figure 3.**15** provides an overview of the pseudo-radicular pain radiation patterns encountered with irritation of different joint capsules.

3.3.4   Tender Points

In the osteopathic literature and practice, the entity called "somatic dysfunction" is the basis for segmental diagnosis and treatment (Korr, 1975; Mitchell et al., 1979; Jones, 1981).

This term is defined as the impaired or altered physiological function of related components within the somatic (body framework) system: the skeletal, arthrodial, and myofascial structures, and the related vascular, lymphatic, and neural elements.

As a result of this definition, the "osteopathic lesion" was registered with the International Classification of Diseases under the number 739.

The *tender points* (Jones, 1964; Kellgren, 1938) provide important information for the diagnosis of joint function, both of the apophyseal and peripheral joints, and consequently the reflexogenic changes in the soft tissues.

The tender points, which are painful upon pressure (stabbing pain), are usually found in the proximity of the affected joint as swollen, flat regions in specific parts of the body. They are located in the deeper muscle layers, and their size does not normally exceed 1 cm in diameter.

With spondylogenic dysfunction, they often appear multiply, primarily in the paravertebral region (articular processes), but also on the anterior side of the trunk (Fig. 3.**16**).

Tender points have been described for all joint dysfunctions. Even with subclinical disturbances, they can be demonstrated by careful palpation (compare latent phase of the intervertebral insufficiency according to Schmorl and Junghanns [1968]). The results of the *positional examination* indicate the direction of the manual therapeutic approach. When the joint is positioned so that pain is absent, the painfulness of the related tender point decreases significantly, and sometimes diminished tissue tension can be noted with palpation. After proper therapy, they are no longer evident (compare the definition of the zone of irritation).

The understanding of the segmental diagnosis and the experience with soft-tissue palpation led to the "muscle energy" (Mitchell et al., 1979), and later the "strain and counterstrain" techniques (Jones, 1964,

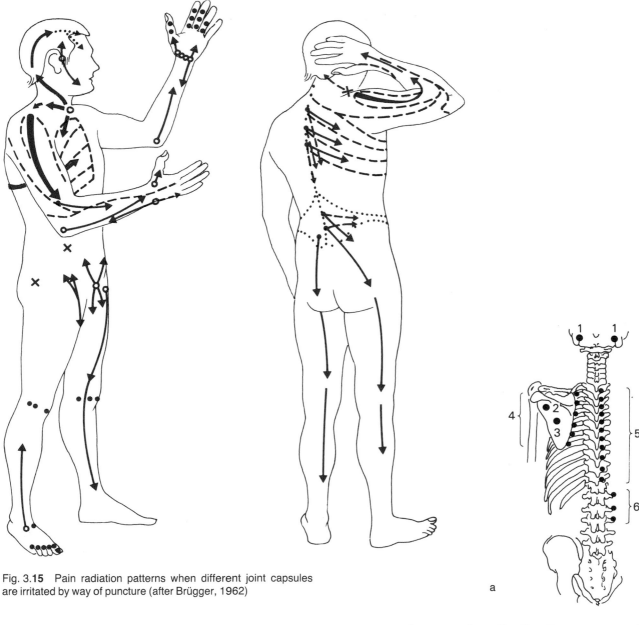

Fig. 3.**15** Pain radiation patterns when different joint capsules are irritated by way of puncture (after Brügger, 1962)

Fig. 3.**16a** Localization of tender points, posteriorly (examples) ▶
(after Jones, 1981)
1   C1
2   T2
3   T3
4   Ribs
5   T1−T12
6   L1−L3

b Localization of the tender points, anteriorly (examples) (after Jones 1981)
1   Acromioclavicular joint
2   C7
3   Sternoclavicular joint
4   T1−T6

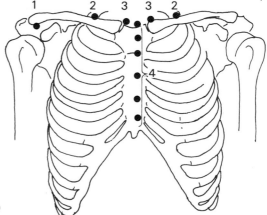

1981). Similar to these techniques is the so-called muscle facilitation and inhibition techniques introduced by Lewit (1981).

3.3.5 Spondylogenic Reflex Syndrome

Empirical clinical observations showed that relationships exist between the axial skeleton and the peripheral soft tissues that are not easily explained on the basis of radicular, vascular, or humoral reasoning.

Sutter (1975) defines these clinical, empirically determined interrelationships as the spondylogenic reflex syndromes (SRS).

Being mediated through the reflexogenic pathway of the CNS, the SRS is defined as the reproducible, causative relationship between the reciprocal functionally abnormal position (segmental dysfunction) of skeletal parts of the axial skeleton and the local, anatomically determined noninflammatory rheumatic soft-tissue changes. The term "functionally abnormal position" (segmental dysfunction) is understood as a disturbance of the so-called internal function of the vertebral unit. The well-balanced interaction between the bony structures (skull, vertebrae, pelvis) and the corresponding muscle-tendon apparatus is impaired. Maigne (1970) describes these disturbances as "dérangements intervertebrales mineurs".

The functionally abnormal position (segmental dysfunction), however, is not always identical to those changes of the skeletal parts that can be detected spatially on radiographs (such as scoliosis and deformities). The dysfunction leads to reversible, objectively demonstrable impairments of mobility in the appropriate skeletal segment.

The afferent source of the SRS is primarily the intervertebral joints. Reflexogenically induced disturbances (via CNS) in the appropriate peripheral soft tissue can develop (Waller, 1975) as a result of permanently suprathreshold stimulations of the numerous mechano- and nociceptive receptors in the joint capsules and ligamentous structures (Wyke, 1976 b).

The first demonstrable clinical manifestation is the so-called zone of irritation (Caviezel, 1976), also known as segmental point (Sell, 1969), paravertebral point (Maigne, 1970), or TP (Jones, 1981).

These are painful swellings, tender upon pressure, and detectable with palpation, located in the musculofascial tissue in topographically well-defined sites (refer to chapter). The average size varies from 0.5 to 1 cm, and the main characteristic is the absolutely

timed and qualitative linkage to the extent of the functionally abnormal position (segmental dysfunction). As long as a disturbance exists, the zones of irritation can be identified, yet disappear immediately after the removal of the disturbance. This is extremely important for therapeutic control. It is emphasized that a clinical-palpatory term is being dealt with. To date, no anatomic-histologic substantiation for the zones of irritation has been found.

Among the most important causes of the functionally abnormal position (segmental dysfunction) are uncoordinated movement, trauma, muscular imbalance, acute and chronic mechanical overload of the vertebrae, and osteoligamentous insufficiency. Additionally, inflammatory, arthrotic-degenerative irritations, as well as neoplastic infiltrations must be considered to be pathological afferences from the intervertebral joints (Northup, 1966).

The functionally abnormal position (segmental dysfunction) in a vertebral unit results in the reflexogenic pathological change of the soft tissue, the most important being the "myotendinoses," which can be identified by palpation.

3.3.5.1 Myotendinoses

The healthy muscle displays normal plasticity and homogeneity such that the individual muscle bundles cannot be differentiated from each other by palpation.

Myotendinotic changes are charakterized by permanently increased tone, elevated consistency, resistance, and decreased plasticity. A whole muscle or only a few muscle bundles in the longitudinal direction can be affected. When palpating perpendicularly to the muscle fibers with average pressure, myoses or myotendinoses are painful and can easily be differentiated from the surrounding area of the same muscle not immediately affected. Myotendinotic changes can be palpated from the origin to the insertion of the muscle. "Nervous misinformation" of certain muscle bundles (Fassbender, 1980) arriving in the reflexogenic pathway is responsible for the origin of the involuntary isometric increase of tonus in the muscle bundle (Fig. 3.**17**).

It is possible, then, that these myotendinotic changes affecting the muscle or its insertions are simply the result of, or caused by, segmental dysfunctions. This has become known as noninflammatory soft-tissue rheumatism (Fig. 3.**18**).

Myosis is the state of increased painful changes in texture that can be caused by pressure or appear spontaneously. Myoses exist mostly in the center of

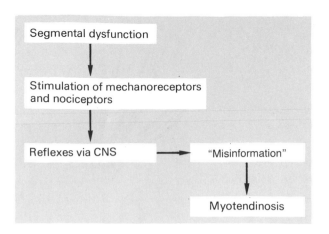

Fig. 3.**17** Development of myotendinosis (after Fassbender, 1980)

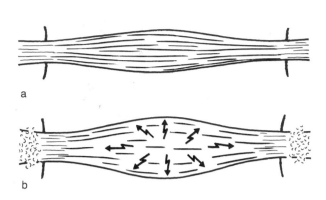

Fig. 3.**18a** Normal muscle **b** Tendomyotically altered muscle

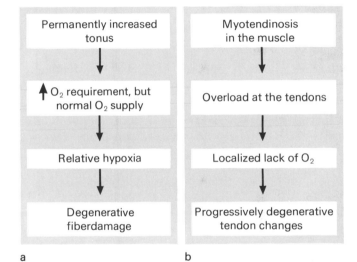

Fig. 3.**19** Pathology of noninflammatory soft-tissue rheumatism (after Fassbender)
a Muscle myosis
b Tendinosis (ligaments and tendon)

the muscle mass. They are often found at sites where the course of the whole muscle is changed or at the free muscle borders (e.g. trapezius muscle, pectoralis major muscle). With continued, nonphysiological stimulatory impulses and the presence of permanently increased tonus, degenerative changes appear (Fassbender 1973, 1980), resulting in the damage of the muscle fibers (Fig. 3.**19**).

Attachment tendinoses are local swellings of tendons that are well-defined at the origin and insertion and are extremely painful upon palpatory pressure in the direction of the inserting tendinous fibers. The typical hallmark is their mirror-image appearance. In addition to these typical sites at the points of origin and insertion, tendinoses can also appear at the muscle and tendon junction.

Abnormal growth of the mesenchymal connective tissue cells (Fassbender, 1980; Fassbender and Wegner, 1973) caused by relative hypoxia can be detected morphologically (Fig. 3.**20**).

Due to their reflexogenic nature, the appearance of tendinoses and myoses is delayed. They disappear following a latent period (thus called "latent zones" by Sutter) once the causative disturbance has been eliminated. This is an important differential diagnostic quality distinguishing them from the zones of irritation. Clinically, they must be differentiated from those myotendinoses caused by other mechanisms (such as trauma).

A certain muscle contains the same amount of defined longitudinal sections that can independently undergo tendomyotic changes in a set sequence. Such

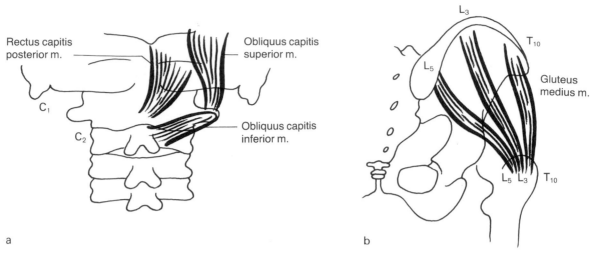

a Rectus capitis posterior m.

Obliquus capitis superior m.

Obliquus capitis inferior m.

C_1

C_2

L_3

T_{10}

Gluteus medius m.

L_5

L_5 L_3 T_{10}

a

b

Fig. 3.**20 a** Individual myotenones

b Myotenones in a fan-shaped muscle

a clinical muscle-unit with the corresponding tendons is named a *myotenone*.

Slender muscles represent a single myotenone. Broad, flat, and fan-shaped muscles comprise several myotenones (Fig. 3.**20**).

Clinical experience shows that certain axial skeletal parts are correlated with certain myotenones, which can be reproduced symmetrically, qualitatively, and objectively. A functional disturbance in one vertebral unit initiates myotendinosis simultaneously in the empirically correlated myotenones. Since the spondylogenic-reflexogenic myotendinoses can be routinely located, they are collectively termed *systematic myotendinosis* (Sutter and Fröhlich, 1981;

Travell and Rinzler, 1952). The primary functionally abnormal position of a vertebral unit, followed by myotendinotic changes, represents the primary SRS.

Under certain circumstances additional secondary, tertiary, and other SRSs can develop in a chain reaction. Thus, factors such as the basic composition of the spine, type of carriage, motion, muscle, muscular imbalance, muscle strength, and joint function play an important role. In clinical practice, an inherently complex picture is most often found.

Often, it is not possible to determine the causative primary SRS, especially in patients with chronic conditions; it may have already healed. In those cases, the induced secondary and other SRSs are consi-

Table 3.2   Important characteristics for the zone of irritation and spondylogenic myotendinosis in the context of the spondylogenic reflex syndrome

	Zone of Irritation	Spondylogenic Myotendinosis
Changes	Skin, subcutaneous tissues, tendons, muscles, joint capsule	muscles, ligaments
Localization	In area of the disturbed spinal segment, topographically defined in region around spinous or articular processes	muscles, ligaments (referred pain?)
Time course (latency)	Immediate reaction to a segmental dysfunction	Apparent after a certain latent period
Qualitative palpatory findings	Decreased ease of skin displacement, increased tissue tension, localized pain	Increased resistence, less resiliency, tender upon pressure with radiation (trigger?)
Quantitative palpatory findings	Related to the degree of abnormal segmental function	Dependent on the duration of segmental dysfunction
Changes observed with successful treatment	Immediate decrease in quality and quantity	May disappear after a certain latency period (possibly reflexively)

dered primary (Travell, 1981). The important characteristic features of a zone of irritation are listed and compared to those of a spondylogenic myotendinosis in Table 3.**2**.

In order to establish the correct diagnosis and to initiate the appropriate therapy, careful examination techniques and precise anatomical knowledge are necessary.

3.3.5.2 Clinical Correlation of Reflexes Associated with Nociceptors and Mechanoreceptors — Spondylogenic Reflex Syndrome

The clinical symptoms of pain, be it spontaneous pain or pain due to palpatory pressure, are defined by Sutter (1974, 1975) as the SRS.

Likewise the authors were able to observe the so-called systematic myotendinoses with a functionally abnormal position or segmental dysfunction involving the individual apophyseal, occipital-atlanto-axial, and sacroiliac joints.

During the course of therapeutic intervention, improvement of these systematic myotendinoses could be seen in the individual patient. It was therefore assumed that, in addition to other helpful physical and therapeutic procedures, the mechanical correction of the vertebral unit plays the primary role (Schmorl and Junghanns, 1968).

The results of articular neurology, according to Wyke, present new views contributing greatly to the diagnostic and therapeutic understanding of manual medicine.

In a clinical study of adolescents, the authors found that the absence of pain is not identical with the absence of soft-tissue findings. It is well known that localized (palpable bands) or systematic myotendinoses can often be detected with palpation in those individuals subjectively free of complaints. According to the authors understanding, this situation is to be considered pathologic and correlates with the latent state of intervertebral insufficiency (Schmorl and Junghanns, 1968). Using the experimental work by Wyke for comparison, this would be equated with the tonic reflexogenic influence of the type-I mechanoreceptors upon the motoneurons of the axial musculature and musculature of the extremities. It has been shown that pain-inducing nociceptors demonstrate a significantly higher threshold than pain-inhibiting mechanoreceptors; this explains the time delay for the subjective perception of the emotional disturbance presenting the patient with pain.

In this situation as well, however, the nociceptive stimulatory conduction can be inhibited presynaptically by adequate stimuli of the mechanoreceptors (mainly type II). This may occur by release of encephalins from cells in the gelatinous substance of the dorsal horns.

It is very likely that this neurophysiological mechanism plays as important a role in the manual therapeutic treatment as the mechanical correction of the segmental dysfunction. Figures 3.**21** and 3.**22** attempt to present this model schematically.

3.4 Differential Diagnosis of Vertigo

Various authors (Lewit, 1977; Hülse, 1981) suggest that manipulative therapy is indicated in those cases where the cervical vertigo or perception of unbalance is caused by functional disturbances (i. e., somatic dysfunction) in the upper cervical spine, including the C0−C1, C1−C2 facet joints. However, this form of vertigo must always be clearly differentiated from other causes of vertigo, especially those not amenable or even contraindicated to manual therapy.

3.4.1 Sensation of Unbalance (Disequilibrium): Dizziness — a Cardinal Symptom

In 1913, Oppenheim described vertigo as an unpleasant sensation resulting from a disturbance in perception of the body in relation to its surroundings and position in space.

To maintain equilibrium, or in other words, to assure an intact awareness of the body in space, three sources of afferent impulses from different systems are required: the optic, vestibular, and proprioceptive systems. In addition, according to studies by Hülse (1981, 1982, 1983) and Wyke (personal communications), the receptors of the facet (apophyseal) joints in the cervical spine assume an important role in the maintainence of equilibrium.

A disturbance or irritation of receptors in the cervical spine may lead to vertigo and cervical nystagmus.

Hülse (1981, 1983) describes the cervical nystagmus as a *sine qua non* condition in patients with complaints of dizziness and findings of functional disturbances in the cervical spine (i. e., somatic dysfunction).

In their experimental studies, Hirosaka and Maeda (1973) suggest that a connection exists between the facet joints and the abducens nuclei. It has been shown that impulses originating from joint receptors

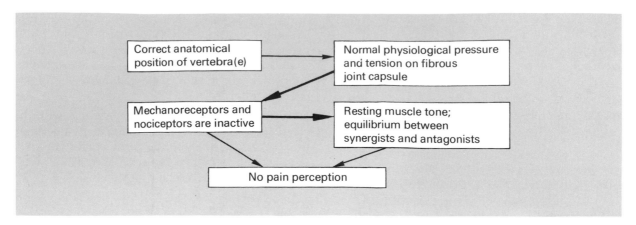

Fig. 3.**21** Model for the receptor activity when vertebrae are in the correct position

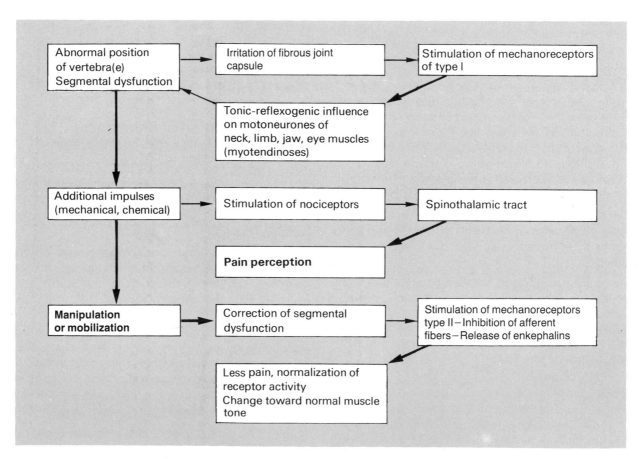

Fig. 3.**22** Model for receptor activity when vertebrae are in abnormal position (segmental dysfunction)

in the cervical spine can be projected to the area of the vestibular nuclei (Fredrikson et al., 1965; Maeda, 1979) along with a connection to the abducens nuclei; this may explain the occurrence of cervical vertigo. This type of presentation, however, makes it more difficult to differentiate these disturbances from those associated with abnormalities in or damage to the vestibular apparatus secondary to, for instance, vascular aberrations.

3.4.2 Evaluation of the Patient with Vertigo

A careful case history is of utmost importance. One of the main tasks for the examiner is to pay particular attention to those patient symptoms that help in the differentiation between the so-called systematic and nonsystematic types of vertigo. The systematic form of vertigo is most often being dealt with when the patient complains about such sensations as head and body rotation or whirling, (known in the European literature as "rotary vertigo"), nonrotatory swaying or to-and-fro movements ("sway vertigo"), or up-and-down movement ("lift vertigo"). This form of vertigo is usually due to a disturbance in the vestibular system. In contrast, nonsystematic vertigo is associated with such patient complaints as unsteadiness, lightheadedness, and general unpleasant feeling of discomfort.

During the neurological examination, particular attention should be paid to the sensory branch of the trigeminal nerve and the other more caudal cranial nerves.

The patient should also be evaluated for the presence of nystagmus, including the spontaneous nystagmus (Pfaltz, 1983), vestibular nystagmus by use of provocative testing, as well as postural nystagmus, and that nystagmus elicited with head positioning or induced movement (using fitted Frenzel spectacles; Hess, 1983). However, it must be emphasized, that, in association with head rotation, it is easy to mistakenly diagnose a postural nystagmus that in reality is a cervical nystagmus (Hülse, 1983). Kornhuber (1974) rejects the idea that a postural nystagmus can be caused by a disturbance in the somatosensory proprioceptors located in the C0–C1 or upper cervical spinal joints.

A detailed functional examination of the cervical spine, including a careful search for zones of irritation as well as localized muscle changes (i. e., palpable bands), is especially indicated in patients in whom receptor irritation may have led to cervical vertigo.

Radiographic evaluation includes the conventional anteroposterior and lateral views of the cervical spine. In the presence of segmental or regional joint dysfunctions, additional views should be utilized, such as the functional lateral and transbuccal anteroposterior views. Reich and Dvořák (1984) suggest that atlantoaxial instability may be demonstrated on functional transbuccal views.

Otoneurologic studies, including electronystagmography, aid in the differentiation between peripheral and central abnormalities of the vestibular apparatus. Based on studies by Hülse (1983), electronystagmography is also very helpful in distinguishing between vascular and cervical nystagmus or vertigo.

CT-scans of the head and cervical spine have become very useful in the diagnostic workup, especially when a tumor (intracranial or extracranial) is suspected.

3.4.3 Important Disorders Associated with Vertigo

- Ménière's disease: labyrinthine disease characterized by whirling or rotational vertigo, tinnitus, unilateral deafness, autonomic changes (i. e., nausea, vomiting); nystagmus is present during the acute attack
- Vestibular neuronitis (neuropathy): disturbance in vestibular function (mostly unilateral vestibular paresis) characterized by suboccipital headaches, rotatory vertigo (hours, days, weeks), autonomic symptoms (i. e., nausea, vomiting), the feeling of unsteady gait (i. e., "off balance"); tinnitus and deafness are usually absent
- Oculomotor disorders: diplopia, possible brief sensation of vertigo accompanied by mild nausea; may be seen in persons with error of refraction (astigmatism, myopia, hyperopia)
- Tumors in posterior cranial fossa: including meningeoma, ependymoma
- Acoustic neuroma: loss of hearing, tinnitis, vertigo (usually of the nonsystematic type and rarely observed as initial symptom), ipsilateral ataxia of limbs, nystagmus, involvement of the trigeminal nerve (corneal reflex), increased intracranial pressure
- Ischemia (labyrinthine apoplexy): basilar insufficiency, orthostatic vertigo, usually a single precipitous attack with nausea and vomiting but without tinnitus or hearing loss
- Multiple sclerosis: when localized to the bulbopontine region, vertigo is usually of the nonsystematic type
- Epilepsy due to abnormalities in the temporal cortex

- Trauma: brain injury, cervical spine trauma, including hyperextension/hyperflexion at the cervical spine due to deceleration accidents
- Craniocervical malformations: basilar impressions, assimilation of the atlas
- Neurotic or psychogenic
- Cervical vertigo

Differentiation between the proprioceptive and vascular types of cervical nystagmus is very important, since manipulative therapy is contraindicated with the vascular type due to possible complications associated with the procedure. According to Hulse (1983), proprioceptive nystagmus occurs immediately upon turning the head (i. e., there is no latent period). In contrast, the vascular type of nystagmus is usually not evident until the patient's neck is turned to the extreme position in which case it takes from seconds up to three minutes to become apparent. Thus, a certain latent period is more characteristic of the vascular type of nystagmus.

An additional differentiating quality is the clearly decrescendo character of the nystagmus seen with the proprioceptive type, in contrast to the crescendo character of the nystagmus observed with the vascular type.

4   General Principles of Palpation

A thorough, well-founded knowledge of anatomy is necessary in order to understand the nature and principles of the spondylogenic reflex syndrome and to be able to utilize it at the patient (see chapter 3).

The practice of manual medicine requires a good, three-dimensional perception of anatomy so that it can be applied clinically to the process of palpation. Palpation usually proceeds layer by layer, starting with the skin and followed by an individual assessment of the subcutaneous tissues, fasciae, intermuscular septa, and superficial and deep musculature. During palpation, the skin is evaluated for its thickness, moisture, and ease of displacement in all directions. The ease of displacement, also known as the skin rolling test or Kibler-fold test, assumes great significance when examining the skin over the back. Abnormal autonomic skin reactions, such as erythematous changes, increased sweat production, and pain that can be induced with minimal palpatory pressure, may indicate a segmental dysfunction (somatic dysfunction). Individual muscles may be identified and distinguished from each other by palpating along the septal divisions.

Muscle palpation always proceeds from origin to insertion, but the direction of palpation follows different paths at the site of attachment to bone and at the muscle belly. At the attachment site, the individual bundles are palpated along the course of the tendon, whereas at the muscle belly the fibers are palpated from a direction perpendicular to their course. With these principles in mind, a practitioner should be able to palpatorily differentiate healthy muscle tissue from painful, pathological muscle changes, as found, for instance, with a hard, palpable band.

Palpation is started at that area indicated by the patient as painful. The palpating finger usually remains at the same tissue level when searching for a painful or pathologic change. This pain may be either already present or elicited with certain movement. The patient is usually able to localize the pain to one specific point or some broader area. He or she may point to a contracted muscle band as well, which may be tender either at rest or upon introduction of movement. It is the task of the practitioner of manual medicine to localize, evaluate, and correlate the painful manifestation with an anatomic structure and differentiate it from the surrounding healthy tissues. Again, a good, three-dimensional anatomic understanding of the various soft-tissue structures and their relationships is absolutely vital.

In the examination of a muscle, both its origin and insertion are palpated. The painful structure is then identified by a process of exclusion, whereby all the muscles, ligaments, tendons, and other soft-tissue structures confined to the specific area in question are palpated.

Palpatory assessment of the landmarks on the living human being is often very different from that learned in anatomy laboratory sessions. Again, patience and continued practice will be required in order to acquire the clinical skills necessary for adequate functional assessment of the locomotor apparatus.

Principles of Palpation
- Objective palpation: findings observed (palpated) by the examiner
- Subjective palpation: sensation perceived by the patient when palpated

Objective palpation is guided by a sound anatomic knowledge with case-specific palpatory pressure dictated by the area, force, and direction of restrictive changes.

Requirements for Adequate Palpation:
- The painful sites reported by the patient must be correctly localized
- Palpatory force must be along a path perpendicular to the bone where the tendon inserts. This technical detail is a crucial prerequisite for palpation to be successful
- Comparison of symmetrical skeletal parts should not be done, since disturbances are usually present symmetrically (in a quantitative measure). Qualitatively, they always present in a symmetrical fashion. Thus, comparision should be limited to the same side of functional abnormality, or, if appropriate, to locations with the same or very similar anatomic arrangement and to unaffected sites
- In order to prevent confusion, parallel changes of adjacent, similar structures must be differentiated from each other. This can be done by palpating

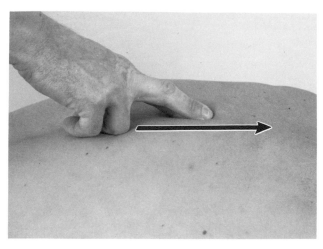

Fig. 4.**1**

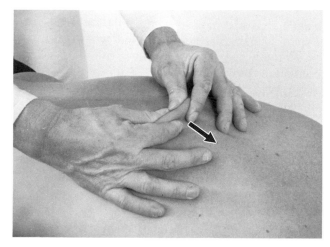

Fig. 4.**2**

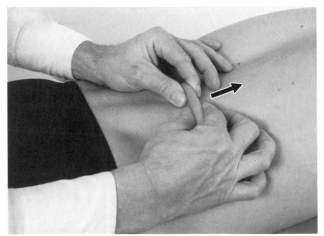

Fig. 4.**3**

their course, shape, and opposite poles of muscle attachments (i. e., muscle origins and insertions)
- Myotendinotic changes or hard, palpable bands are best detected by palpation using a pressing-stroking type of motion, not unlike that of "ploughing." Palpatory direction is perpendicular to that of the muscle fibers. This process is repeated over and over again in order to eventually cover the entire muscle from origin to insertion, where anatomically possible

Before the novice in this field becomes all too confused with the many details of the spondylogenic reflex symptoms, it is emphasized once more that palpation must be practiced repeatedly and performed as precisely as possible. Unfortunately, the authors have seen many negative palpatory findings resulting from improper palpatory technique and deficient anatomic knowledge.

4.1 Palpation of the Skin over the Spine

Examination of the skin overlying the spine has been found very helpful, as certain skin changes in a particular location may point in the direction of a dysfunctional spinal area. The examination of the skin is part of the so-called scan, which is an intermediate, detailed examination of specific body regions that have been identified by findings emerging from the initial screen (initial general somatic examination). The scan focuses on segmental areas for further definition or diagnosis (Ward and Sprafka, 1981).

There are basically two variations of the skin examination: the one-handed skin stroke test; and the skin rolling test, which utilizes both hands for palpation simultaneously. In both of these examinations, the patient lies prone on the examination table. In the skin stroke test, the examiner produces a skin bulge in front of the palpating fingers by gently pressing the middle finger (superior) and index finger (inferior) against the skin. Applying a constant downward and cephalad force, the two fingers are pushed, along with the bulge in front, from inferior to superior on either side of the spine along a line parallel and slightly lateral to it (Fig. 4.**1**). With this test, the ease of skin displacement or resiliency, amount of moisture present in the various spinal regions, and pain provocation are evaluated. A distinct difference in skin thickness may sometimes be palpated. Findings consistent with a segmental or regional (somatic) dysfunction include increased resistance to displacement or decreased laxity, increased moisture production, and skin tenderness or pain. Repeating this test two to three times in a patient with a segmental dysfunction may actually produce erythematous reactions of the skin in the area of segmental dysfunction due to autonomic alterations. This test is then followed by the skin rolling test. A skin fold extending just lateral to either side of the midline of the spine is formed between the thumb and index finger of each hand (Figs. 4.2 and 4.3). Starting from below and following the course of the spine, this fold is rolled upward towards the head. The ease of fold displacement, skin thickness, and pain provocation are also of interest here. This test is often more than an intermediate or preliminary examination, as it may actually aid in the localization of a specific segmental or regional dysfunction.

4.2 Palpation of Bony Landmarks

4.2.1 Occiput
(Fig. 4.4)

- External occipital protuberance: this is the most prominent bony structure at the occiput in the midline
- Superior nuchal line: palpable by following the external occipital protuberance laterally
- Inferior nuchal line: located approximately 1 ½ finger widths below the superior nuchal line. Of significance is the area between the two nuchal lines, where the insertion of the semispinalis capitis muscle can be palpated
- Mastoid process: palpation begins behind the ear; From there the palpating finger descends towards the tip of the mastoid process. Starting from the medial portion of the tip, the palpating finger is moved superiorly where it reaches the upper pole of the mastoid sulcus, an important area in the evaluation of the irritation zones for C0 and C1

4.2.2 Upper Cervical Spine
(Fig. 4.4)

- Transverse process of the atlas: starting from inferior, this bony landmark is palpated by placing the finger in the area between the mastoid process and the descending ramus of the mandible. Due to anatomic variations, it is not always easy to palpate the transverse process of the atlas. In some cases, palpation of this area may be very painful (insertion tendinoses) and should therefore always be performed gently. It may sometimes be beneficial to palpate both transverse processes simultaneously.

- Posterior arch of the atlas: due to the strong muscles in this area and the deep location of the atlas, palpation of the lateral portion is possible only in a limited number of patients and is therefore dependent on the individual's anatomy
- Spinous process of C2: this is the first prominent bony landmark that is accessible to palpation below the occiput. The palpating finger localizes the external occipital protuberance first and then moves inferiorly along the midline until it encounters the protruding spinous process of C2

4.2.3 Lower Cervical Spine
(Fig. 4.4)

- C6 and C7: localization of these two vertebrae is important for exact level determination and is usually best accomplished by introducing passive flexion and extension to the cervical spine. The most prominent vertebra is not always C7; on occasion, it is C6 that is most prominent. The superior joint surfaces of C7 are still relatively flat (more horizontal), whereas its inferior joint surfaces show an arrangement resembling that of a thoracic vertebra. This explains why during maximal neck extension the cervical vertebrae, except the C7 vertebra, move deep or away from the palpatory hand. This clinical observation is an important criterion for exact level localization at the cervical spine

4.2.4 Thoracic Spine
(Fig. 4.5)

- Scapular triangle: this bony landmark is palpated by following the spine of the shoulder blade medially until the scapular triangle is encountered at the medial border of the scapula

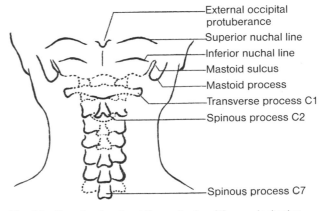

Fig. 4.4 Bony landmarks at the occiput and the cervical spine

External occipital protuberance
Superior nuchal line
Inferior nuchal line
Mastoid sulcus
Mastoid process
Transverse process C1
Spinous process C2
Spinous process C7

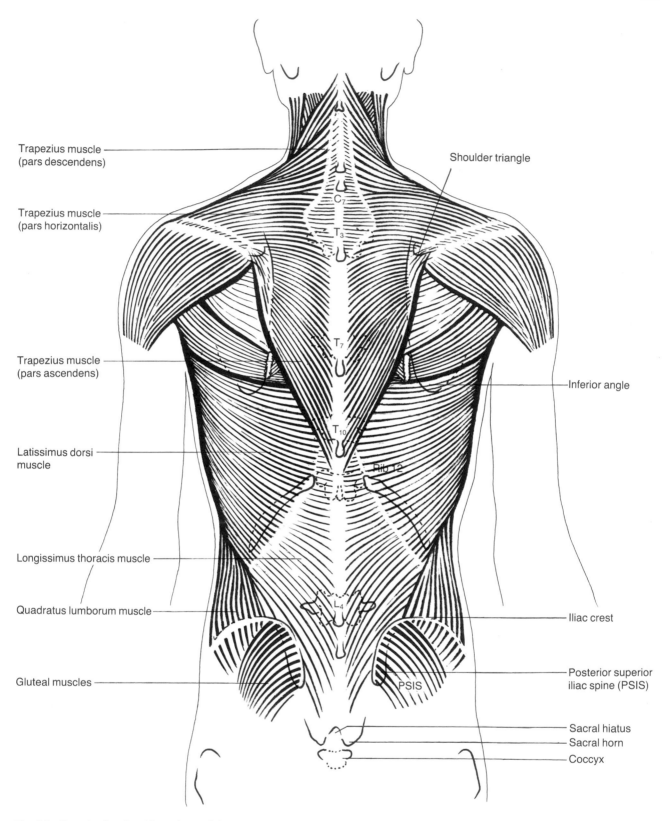

Trapezius muscle
(pars descendens)

Trapezius muscle
(pars horizontalis)

Trapezius muscle
(pars ascendens)

Latissimus dorsi
muscle

Longissimus thoracis muscle

Quadratus lumborum muscle

Gluteal muscles

Shoulder triangle

C₇

T₃

T₇

T₁₀

Rib 12

L₄

PSIS

Inferior angle

Iliac crest

Posterior superior
iliac spine (PSIS)

Sacral hiatus
Sacral horn
Coccyx

Fig. 4.5   Bony landmarks at the spine and the pelvic region

- T3: this vertebra lies on a line connecting the two scapular triangles (patient supine)
- T7: the seventh thoracic vertebra can be localized by drawing a line connecting the inferior angles of the scapula. T7 lies in the center of this line
- T10: this vertebra is localized by hypothetically following the course of the lowest set of ribs medially. Along with its spinous process, T10 is then located just above the point of intersection of these lines. Palpation in the thoracic spine must be guided by the understanding of the changes of relationship between the levels of the transverse processes and the articular processes at the various levels. The spinous processes of T1 and T2 are one fingerwidth below the corresponding articular processes, while at T3 and T4 the difference measures two fingerwidths, at T5 to T7 three fingerwidths, T8 and T9 two fingerwidths, and T10 and T12 one fingerwidth

4.2.5 Lumbar Spine
(Fig. 4.5)

- Spinous processes of L1 to L5: these bony landmarks are very easily accessible to palpation
- Spinous process of L4: lies on a line connecting the pelvic crests
- Transverse process of L4: best palpated with the patient supine. Starting laterally, the L4 transverse process is palpated between the iliocostalis lumborum muscle and the abdominal musculature below
- Transverse processes of L3, L2 and L1: these are two fingerwidths apart from one another (starting inferiorly). They may also be localized by finding the lower pole of the spinous process of the vertebra above, that is, the transverse process of L3 is at the same level as the lower pole of the spinous process of L2

4.2.6 Pelvic Girdle
(Fig. 4.5)

- Iliac crest: this landmark is best palpated on either side, starting laterally and moving medially
- Posterior superior iliac spine (PSIS): following the posterior curve of the iliac crest downward to its tip, the so-called posterior superior iliac crest is reached. This must not be mistaken for the posterior inferior iliac spine, which is more laterally and, as the name implies, more inferior. It may also be sometimes mistaken for the free margin of the sacrum. It is extremely important that the practitioner is familiar with the correct palpation of the PSIS not only because of its role in the functional examination of the sacroiliac joint, but also for localization of the zones of irritation at the sacrum
- Sacral hiatus: located at the lower pole of the sacrum, the lateral borders are formed by both sacral horns
- Coccyx: palpation of this landmark is usually performed without difficulty
- Lateral sacral angle (border): this angle is palpated approximately one fingerwidth lateral to a line connecting the PSIS and the sacral horn on either side

5 Functional Examination of the Spine

Examination	Symbol
Fixation	
Palpation	
Active Flexion Extension Rotation	
Passive Flexion Extension Rotation	

Examination: Inclination/reclination, active and passive motion testing

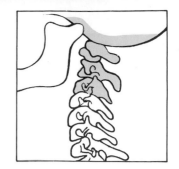

Examination Procedure

While in the seated position, the patient is requested to perform flexion and extension movements in this portion of the spine that have specifically been termed inclination and reclination movement, respectively (Figs. 5.**1**, 5.**2**). These particular movements require the examiner to give precise instructions to the patient, since only the joints of the upper cervical spine should be engaged. These movements are different from the more generalized flexion/ extension movements in the remainder of the cervical spine. The inclination movement (specific flexion motion in the upper cervical spine) involves nodding the head. With this movement, the occipital condyles move posteriorly on the atlas while the atlas is displaced anteriorly on the axis. During the reclination movement (specific extension movement in the upper cervical spine, that is, "nodding" the head backwards), the occipital condyles glide anteriorly on the atlas, which itself is being displaced posteriorly.

In the passive examination, the examiner cradles the patient's head with one hand. Using the index finger and the thumb of the other hand, the examiner then fixates (stabilizes) the axis and therefore the vertebrae below. It is important to remember that the fixating forces are directed towards the articular processes only, so that the soft tissues, in particular the muscles, are not compressed during this procedure. Poor localization of forces often causes pain, limiting the conclusions that can be drawn from the findings elicited with this examination.

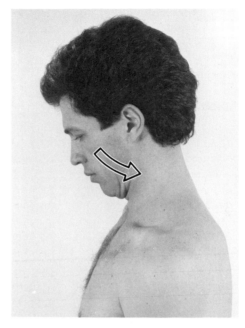

5.**1**

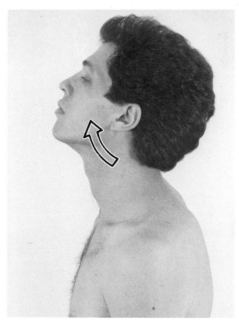

5.**2**

Examination: Inclination/reclination, active and passive motion testing

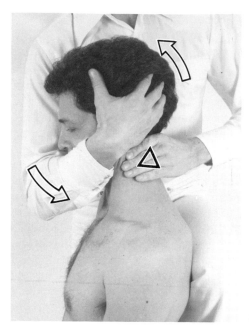

Inclination (Fig. 5.**3**) and reclination (Fig. 5.**4**) movements are tested passively in sequence. Range of motion, which measures 15° to 20° in the normal adult, is of particular interest here. Pain at the end of motion should also be noted.

Possible Pathological Findings

1. Decreased range of motion either during inclination or reclination with hard or soft *endfeel.* A hard *endfeel* is most likely associated with articular (structural) degenerative changes, whereas a soft *endfeel,* together with decreased range of motion, is probably due to shortened suboccipital muscles.
2. Suboccipital pain either with movement or at the end of movement. This may indicate a somatic dysfunction, but the possibility of C0—C3 instability must be included in the differential diagnosis; inflammatory changes in this area of the spine must be excluded as well.
3. Autonomic symptoms are reported. It is important that these be further investigated, especially when accompanied by complaints of vertigo.

5.3

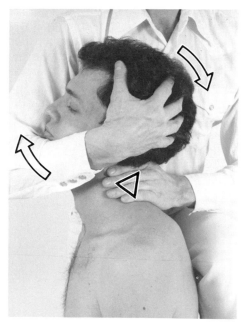

5.4

Examination: **Axial rotation at C1–C2 (rotation around the y-axis), active and passive motion testing**

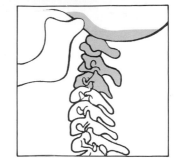

Examination Procedure

The seated patient flexes the cervical spine maximally, including maximal inclination at the C0–C3 portion. The lower cervical spinal segments are "locked" in maximal flexion, that is, they are brought into their extreme or end position, thus allowing rotation to occur only in the upper cervical spine (C0–C2). The patient is subsequently requested to turn the head from one side (left, Figs. 5.**5, 5.6**) to the other (right, Figs. 5.**7, 5.8**). The patient rests his or her thorax against the thigh of the examiner, who stands behind the patient, during passive motion testing. This exaggerates the normal thoracic kyphosis and flexion at the cervicothoracic junction. The examiner places one hand over the parietal region of the patient's head and gently introduces flexion to maximum. The other hand, cradling the mandibles introduces rotation with slight lateral bending to the opposite side to lock the distal segments. The induced motion should follow along the lines of the clavicles. Normal range of motion is between 40° and 45° to either side (Figs. 5.**9, 5.10**).

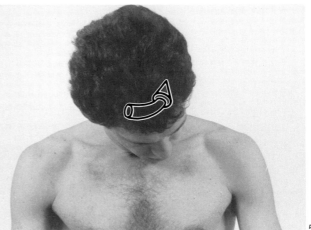

5.5

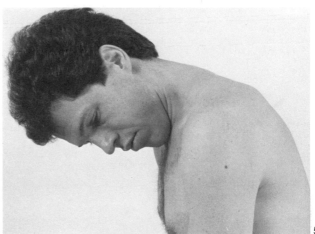

5.6

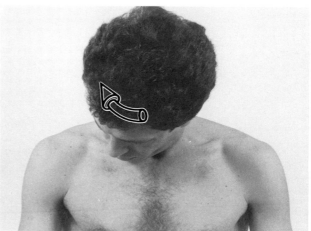

5.7

Examination: **Axial rotation at C1—C2 (rotation around the y-axis), active and passive motion testing**

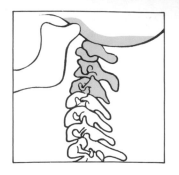

Possible Pathological Findings

1. Decreased rotation with hard or soft *endfeel*, in combination with neck pain. A hard *endfeel* may indicate articular (structural) degenerative changes, whereas a soft *endfeel* is most likely associated with shortened suboccipital muscles.

2. Vertigo at the extreme or end position of rotational movement. This requires further work-up for causes of vertigo, including the possibility of vertebral artery compromise.

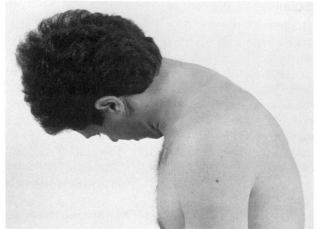

5.8

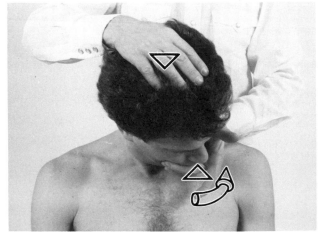

5.9

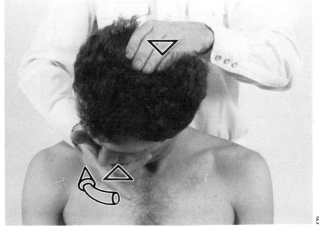

5.10

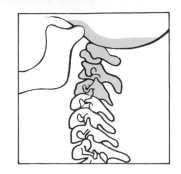

Examination: **Passive motion testing of axial rotation at C1–C2, joint play**

Examination Procedure

The head of the seated patient is cradled by one of the examiner's arms in such a manner that the forearm supports the facial bones and the hypothenar eminence, while the small finger rests on the transverse process of the atlas. The index finger and thumb of the other hand gently fixate (stabilize) the axis (Fig. 5.**11**). The examiner introduces rotational movement to the head (passive rotation), which is accompanied by anterior and posterior gliding movements at these spinal segments (Fig. 5.**12**).

Possible pathological findings

1. Decreased angular range of motion or diminished joint play, either with hard or soft *endfeel*. A hard *endfeel* is most likely due to articular (structural) degenerative changes, while a soft *endfeel* is usually associated with shortened suboccipital muscles.
2. Vertigo during the procedure. This should raise the suspicion of cervical spine instability, changes in the vertebral artery blood flow, or inflammatory processes affecting the upper cervical spine.
3. Pain in conjunction with introduced motion indicates a segmental somatic dysfunction.

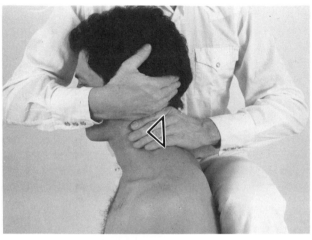

5.**11**

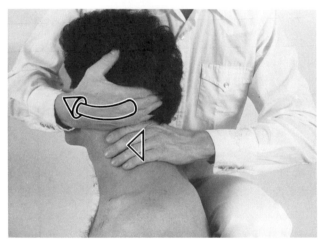

5.**12**

Examination: Active and passive motion testing: flexion, extension, rotation, and lateral bending

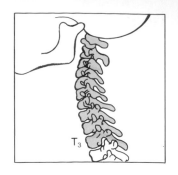

T₃

Examination Procedure

The patient is requested to actively perform movements of flexion (Fig. 5.**13**), extension (Fig. 5.**14**), rotation (Figs. 5.**15**, 5.**16**), and lateral bending (side bending) (Figs. 5.**17**, 5.**18**). The examiner evaluates symmetry, range of motion, and substituted movements. For passive motion testing, the examiner fixates the patient's shoulder with one hand while introducing the above named motion components to the cervical spine with the other hand (Figs. 5.**19**—5.**24**).

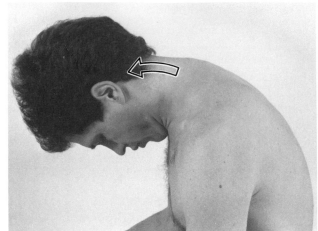

5.**13**

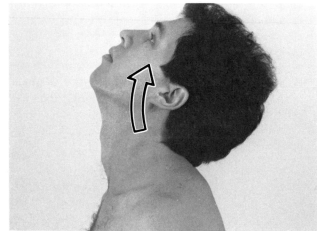

5.**14**

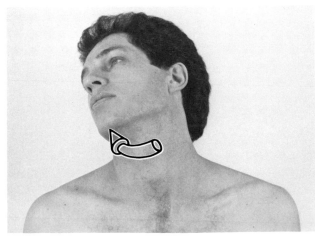

5.**15**

Examination:　**Active and passive angular motion testing: flexion, extension, rotation, and lateral bending**

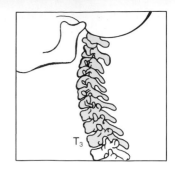

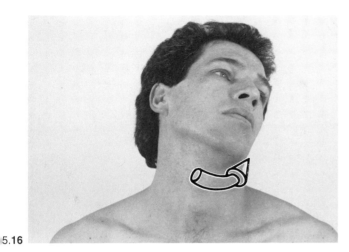

5.16

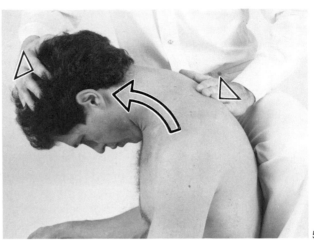

5.19

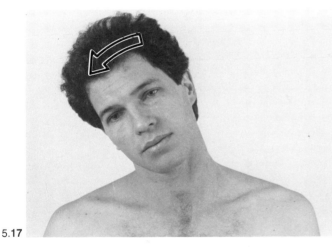

5.17

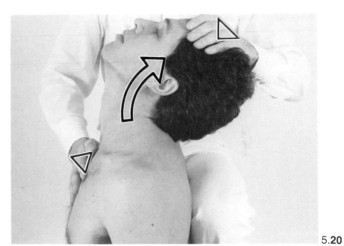

5.20

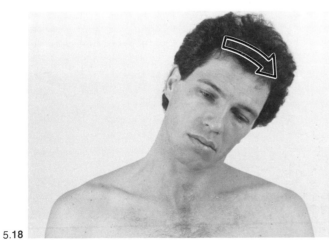

5.18

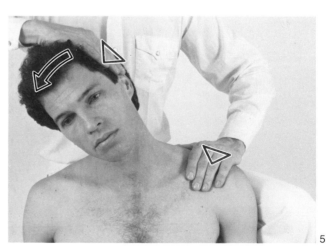

5.21

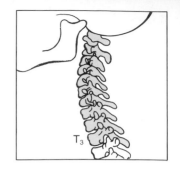

Examination: Active and passive angular motion testing: flexion, extension, rotation, and lateral bending

Possible Pathological Findings

1. Generalized loss of motion without pain at the extreme of the movement (the motion barrier) is more indicative of degenerative problems. At the time of the examination, this finding is of less crucial importance. In contrast, pain that is elicited with movement, either during or at the end of the introduced motion, must be further investigated.
2. Vertigo that appears immediately with movement and disappears rapidly is more likely to be due to cervical-spondylogenic causes. Vertigo of the crescendo type is more indicative of peripheral or central-vestibular disturbances.
3. An isolated finding of restricted lateral bending is often due to a spondylosis in the uncal region.

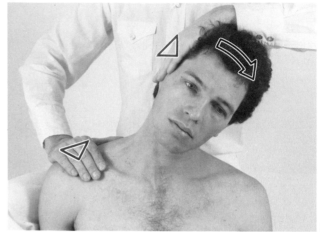

5.22

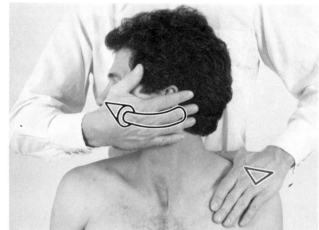

5.23

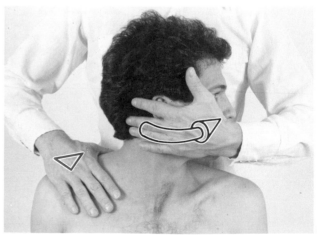

5.24

Examination: **Forced rotation of the axis with lateral bending, axis rotation**

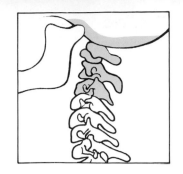

Examination Procedure

While the patient is sitting, the examiner places an index finger over the spinous process of the axis and a middle finger over the spinous process of C3. The other hand is placed at the patient's parietal region so that lateral bending to either side (Fig. 5.**25**) and rotation (Fig. 5.**26**) can be introduced. At the moment lateral bending is initiated, the axis starts to rotate, typically in the same direction as lateral bending (the spinous process rotates in the opposite direction). In contrast, the axis does not start to rotate immediately with the induced rotation of the head, but only after about 20° to 30° does it do so (coupling patterns).

Possible Pathological Findings

1. Forced rotation of the axis during sidebending may be absent due to lesions of the ligaments, in particular the alar ligaments; differential-diagnostically, the possibility of segmental instability is important.
2. If the axis begins to rotate immediately upon cervical spine rotation, it may be due to a segmental dysfunction at the C1—C2 spinal segment, and is most likely a functional motion restriction.

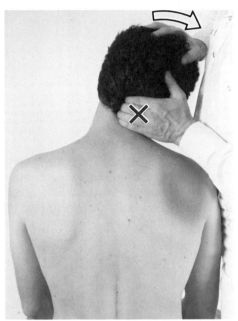

5.**25**

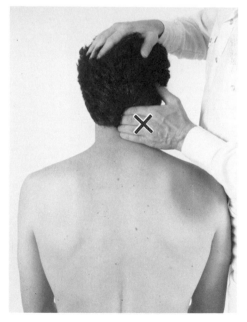

5.**26**

Examination: End rotation and springing test of the atlas

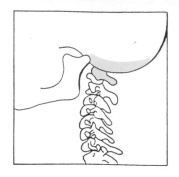

Examination Procedure

With the patient in the seated position, the examiner places the index finger of the monitoring hand over the transverse process of the atlas and the index finger over the mastoid process. With the other hand, which is placed broadly over the side of the patient's face, the examiner introduces maximal rotation (passive rotation). At the extreme of rotation, a spring-like motion can be perceived. In the absence of pathology, this is a sign of normal and unaltered rotation between the occiput and the atlas. Occasionally, a diminished distance between the mastoid and the transverse process of the atlas can be observed (Fig. 5.**27**).

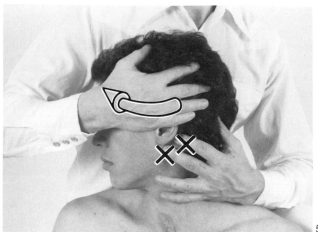

5.27

Possible Pathological Findings

1. The spring-like motion of the atlas in absent. Lewit (1970, Caviezel (1976), and Dvořak (1986) report that this absence is due to a functional disturbance (somatic dysfunction) in the upper cervical spinal joints.
2. Pain and vertigo. Pain may indicate the presence of a segmental somatic dysfunction. Vertigo elicited with movement may be related to a disturbance in the vertebral artery.

Examination: **Lateral bending at the C0—C1 and C1—C2 segments**

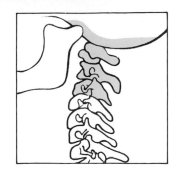

Examination Procedure

The patient is either seated or in the supine position. The index finger of either of the examiner's hands localizes the transverse processes of the atlas on either side. The other fingers fixate the patient's head at the face and temporal region. Examining one spinal segment at a time, passive lateral bending is introduced, there by evaluating the ease of side-to-side gliding (Fig. 5.**28**). There is minimal lateral displacement of the occipital condyles on the joint surfaces of the atlas in the direction opposite to where sidebending is introduced. In contrast, the atlas glides in the same direction as that of gross lateral bending (Dvořák 1986; Reich and Dvořák, 1986).

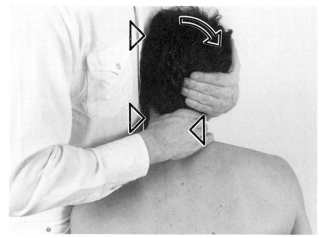

5.**28**

Possible Pathological Findings

The atlas does not glide in the same direction as lateral bending or, paradoxically, even moves in the direction opposite that of sidebending. This may indicate a segmental somatic dysfunction as well as instability. Passive lateral bending was not introduced starting from the neutral position. If the head is excessively extended (reclined), paradoxical gliding movement may take place.

Region: C0—C3

Examination: Translatory gliding at C0—C3

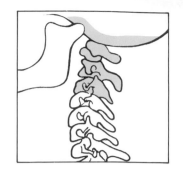

Examination Procedure

The patient is in the supine position. The examiner palpates the patient's transverse process on either side with each middle finger, while the index fingers rest over the mastoid process (Fig. 5.**29**). While simultaneously introducing longitudinal traction, the patient's head is shifted (translatory movement) from side to side (Figs. 5.**30**, 5.**31**).

Possible Pathological Findings

1. Increased resistance (or decreased resiliency) during the translatory side-to-side movement.
2. Total absence of translatory motion with hard or soft *endfeel,* or both.

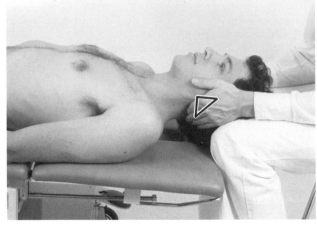

5.**29**

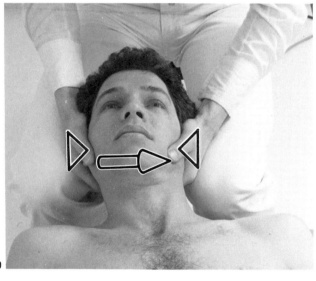

5.**30**

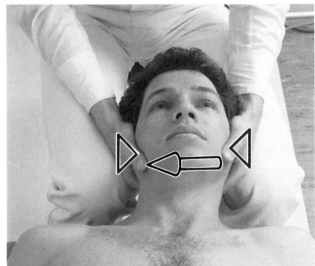

5.**31**

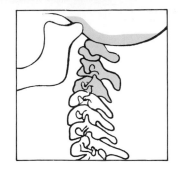

Examination: **Provocative testing by position and motion testing, rotation, and reclination at C0–C3 (vertebral artery)**

Examination Procedure

The patient is in the seated position. While the examiner's hand rests on top of the patient's head, the cervical spine is passively rotated and reclined or extended (Fig. 5.**32**). The patient is then requested to look into the opposite direction while focusing on the examiner's index finger. The examiner should note the presence of nystagmus in order to exclude the possibility of a latent-type of nystagmus. The patient should remain in the above-described position for at least 20 to 30 seconds. However, if the patient begins to complain of vertigo or nausea during the examination, or if a possible nystagmus does not abate, the examination procedure must be terminated immediately.

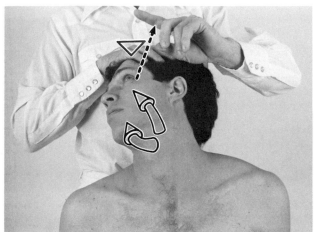

5.**32**

Possible Pathological Findings

1. Vertigo gradually progressive with positioning; occasionally accompanied by nonresolving nystagmus, more of the crescendo type; this may be indicative of either a peripheral, central, or vestibular disturbance, or a combination there of, in the presence of decreased circulation of the vertebral artery.
2. Vertigo that appears at the beginning of the examination, yet improves during the procedure, may occasionally be accompanied by spontaneously resolving nystagmus. This is more indicative of either cervical vertigo or nystagmus, or both. However, clinical interpretation is difficult, and further follow-up by a neuro-ophthalmologist or otoneurologist is indicated.

Examination: Rotation in extension

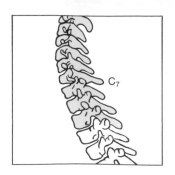

Examination Procedure

The patient is in the seated position with the thoracic spine held as straight as possible. With both hands placed over the patient's parietal region, the examiner introduces reclination and extension (passive movement) to the cervical spine (Fig. 5.**33**). Through this maneuver, the upper cervical spinal joints (C0−C3) are maximally extended, reclined, and fixated by the action of the alar ligaments (which, in this position, are rather taut). Passive rotation of the head, coupled with slight cervical spine sidebending, introduces rotation primarily to the joints below the upper cervical spine, as well as to those at the cervicothoracic junction (Figs. 5.**34,** 5.**35**). From previous clinical experience, "normal" rotation values have been reported at approximately 60° to either side (Caviezel, 1976; Lewit, 1970).

Possible Pathological Findings

1. Decreased range of motion with hard or soft *endfeel.* Degenerative changes that occur with great frequency in the midcervical spine, and include spondylosis, spondyloarthopathy, and arthrosis, may cause motion restriction with a hard *endfeel;* if decreased, range of motion in the presence of a soft *endfeel* is most likely due to shortened long neck extensor muscles.
2. Pain. May be the result of segmental somatic dysfunction.
3. Vertigo and other autonomic signs or symptoms. These suggest a diminished blood supply or an irritation of the vertebral artery (please refer to the provocative testing described for the vertebral artery, p. 89).

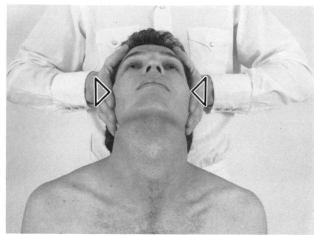

5.**33**

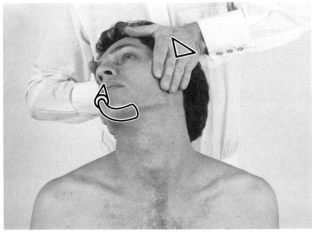

5.**34**

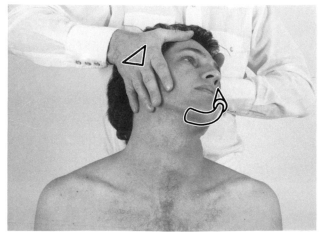

5.**35**

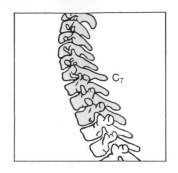

Examination: Passive angular motion of flexion, extension, lateral bending, and rotation; palpation of the spinous processes

Examination Procedure

The examiner, standing behind the seated patient, places four fingers over the spinous processes in the midcervical spine and then, alternatingly, the cervicothoracic junction. By moving the patient's head, the other hand introduces flexion and extension (passive movement) to this area (Figs. 5.**36**, 5.**37**). This is then followed by the introduction of lateral bending (Fig. 5.**38**) and rotation (Fig. 5.**39**). With each motion component introduced, the examiner evaluates the movement of the spinous processes, with particular attention being paid to the coupled movements.

Possible Pathological Findings

Asymmetric movement as a result of segmental somatic dysfunction or abnormal coupling patterns.

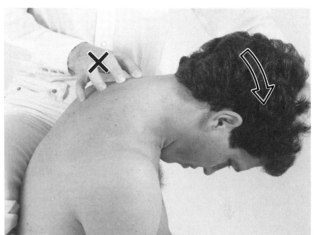

5.36

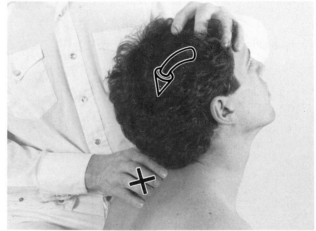

5.37

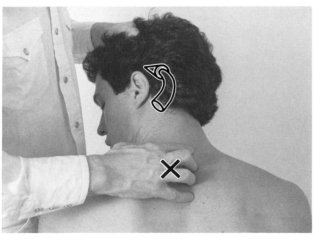

5.39

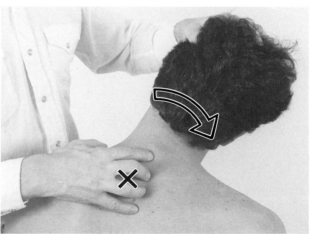

5.38

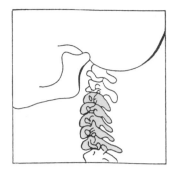

Examination: Passive angular motion rotation, flexion, extension, lateral bending: palpation of the articular pillars

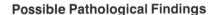

Examination Procedure

The index finger and thumb of the monitoring hand palpate the area over the facet joints, making as much contact with the bony structures as possible (Fig. 5.**40**). Care must be taken, however, not to press on the soft tissues too forcefully, especially those muscles overlying the bone. Entry to the articular processes in this area is between the semispinalis capitis muscle and the longissimus capitis cervicis muscle (see *cervical zone of irritation*). The examiner's guiding hand is placed over the vertex of the patient's head, and then passive flexion/extension, lateral bending, and, finally, rotation are introduced. The examiner determines if movement of the facet joints is symmetrical, in particular if the joints "open" and "close" symmetrically with the respective movement (Fig. 5.**41**).

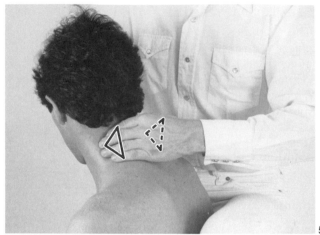

5.40

Possible Pathological Findings

1. Asymmetric joint contours during the individual movements are most likely due to a segmental somatic dysfunction. This examination plays a cardinal role in the segmental diagnosis.
2. Pain exacerbated with movement is probably the result of a segmental zone of irritation.

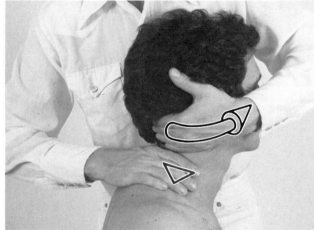

5.41

Region: C3–C7

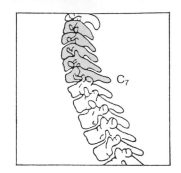

Examination: Translatory gliding

Examination Procedure

With the patient in the supine position, the examiner palpates the area over the facet joint in question (Frisch, 1983). The examiner's hands are placed to either side of the patient's occipital-temporal region. While longitudinal traction is being carefully introduced, the examiner performs a translatory side-to-side movement at the particular joint (Fig. 5.**42**).

Possible Pathological Findings

Movement is asymmetrical, that is, side-to-side movement is "easier" in one direction than the other. A hard *endfeel* is most likely due to structural or degenerative changes in the joint itself.

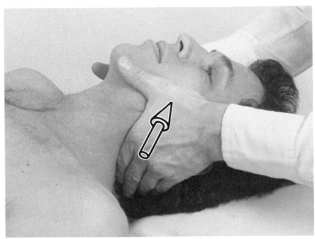

5.**42**

Examination: **Testing of active motion of upper thorax during inhalation and exhalation**

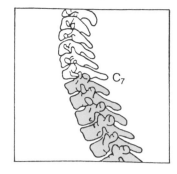

Examination Procedure

The supine patient is requested to deeply inhale and exhale. Motion of ribs I–IV is visually inspected, as well as palpated. The axis of rotation for the first four ribs coincides with the x-axis of the three-dimensional axis system (Figs. 5.**43,** 5.**44**).

Possible Pathological Findings

Decreased thoracic excursion with inhalation and exhalation may be the result of pulmonary disease. Also, motion loss in this part of the thorax may be caused by muscular imbalance in the shoulder and neck region. It is important to include ankylosing spondylitis in the differential diagnosis.

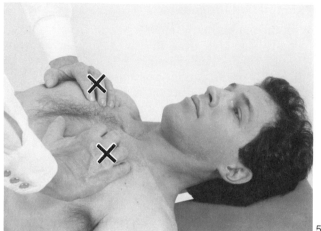

5.43

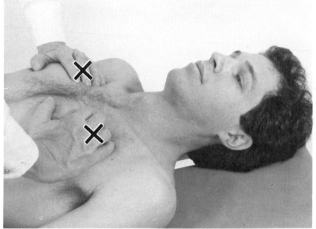

5.44

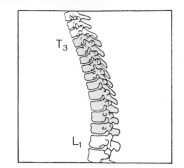

Examination: **Evaluation of thoracic excursion during inspiration and exhalation**

Examination Procedure

The patient is requested to maximally inhale and exhale. Excursion of both the upper and lower half of the thorax are evaluated during the respiratory cycle. The examiner also looks for asymmetrical movement (Figs. 5.**45**, 5.**46**).

Possible Pathological Findings

1. Decreased thoracic excursion. This may be due to various bronchial or pulmonary diseases. The possibility of ankylosing spondylitis must be included in the differential diagnosis. Asymmetric movement may also be seen in the presence of spinal scoliosis.
2. Pronounced abdominal breathing is almost always associated with a decreased thoracic excursion.

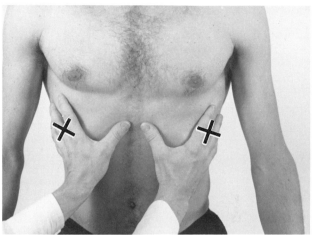

5.**45**

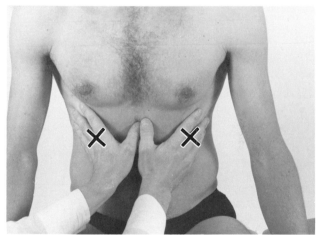

5.**46**

Region: T3–T10

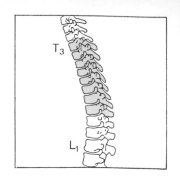

Examination: Passive thorax mobility (testing for resiliency)

Examination Procedure

The examiner places one hand over the sternum and the other hand over the midthoracic spine of the standing patient (Figs. 5.**47**, 5.**48**). During the respiratory movement, the examiner simultaneously compresses the thorax, evaluating both the range of thoracic excursion and the end feel after deep inhalation and exhalation. The inferior portion of the thorax is compressed obliquely at an angle following the thoracic diameter along the costovertebral axes.

Possible Pathological Findings

1. Diminished thoracic excursion in the superior or inferior portion of the thorax. This may be due to bronchial or pulmonary disease. It should be remembered, however, that thoracic elasticity or resiliency decreases with advancing age. In young patients, the finding of decreased thoracic resiliency necessitates measuring (recording) thoracic excursion for later comparison.
2. Pain may be present with initiation, during, or at the extreme of movement.

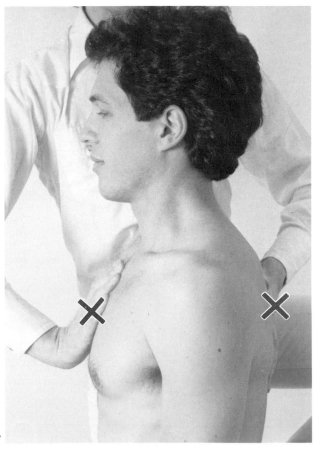

5.47

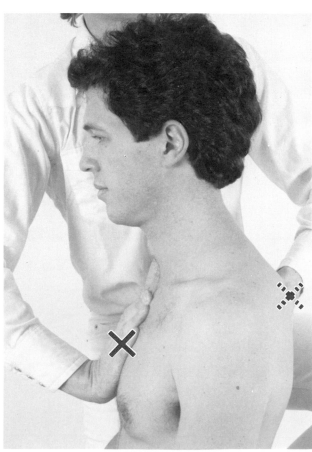

5.48

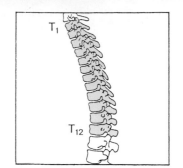

Examination: **Passived motion testing of flexion and extension**

Examination Procedure

The patient is sitting, with hands crossed behind the neck. Through the patient's arms, the examiner introduces further passive flexion and extension at the end of the respective movements that have been performed by the patient. This assures that the area examined is actually in its extreme of flexion or extension.

The fingers of the monitoring hand palpate the movement of the individual spinous processes (Figs. 5.**49**, 5.**50**). Special attention must be paid to the gliding motion of the individual thoracic spinous processes in relation to each other (not unlike that of interrelated roof-top tiles).

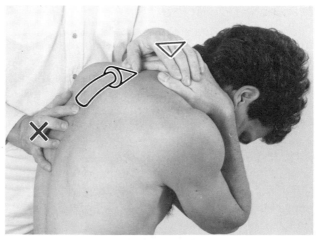

5.**49**

Possible Pathological Findings

1. The spinous processes either do not approximate during extension or do not separate during flexion, or both may occur. Two or three spinal segments are usually affected. Typically, this is due to functional disturbances (somatic dysfunctions) secondary to degenerative changes. In a young patient, it may be related to Scheuermann's disease (juvenile kyphosis).
2. Pain with movement, especially in the cervicothoracic junction and during extension, may be due to a segmental somatic dysfunction.

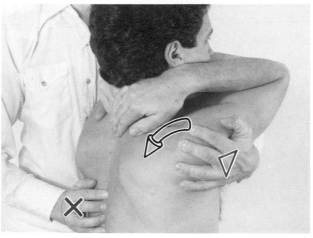

5.**50**

**Examination: Motion testing of lateral bending
(coupling patterns)**

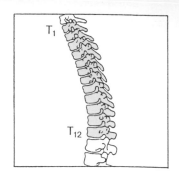

Examination Procedure

The seated patient crosses the hands behind the
neck. The examiner reaches across the patient from
below and places the stabilizing hand over the
patient's shoulder. The fingers of the monitoring
hand palpate the spinous processes (Figs. 5.**51**, 5.**52**).
When sidebent passively to one side (i.e., the right)
the spinous processes in the healthy adult usually
rotate to the same side (i.e., the right), that is,
towards the side of the convexity of the thoracic
spine. During this maneuver it is important that the
patient rests against the operator's chest, through
which the force for sidebending movement is introduced.

Possible Pathological Findings

A segmental dysfunction may be suspected when the
spinous processes do not exhibit coupled rotational
movement with induced lateral bending. Movement
at the various levels in the thoracic spine should
always be compared.

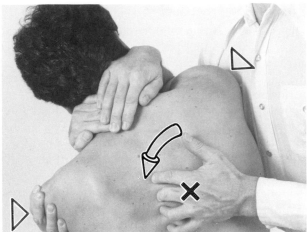

5.51

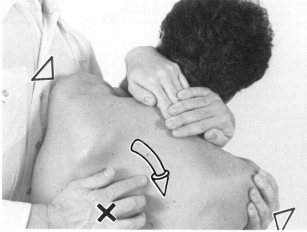

5.52

Examination: Motion testing of rotation

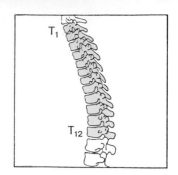

Examination Procedure

The seated patient crosses the hands behind the neck. The examiner, who is standing at the patient's side, reaches across the patient's chest and axilla in order to take hold of the opposite shoulder. The patient, thus stabilized against the operator's chest, is then rotated maximally to either side. The fingers of the monitoring hand palpate the coupled rotatory movement of the spinous processes (Figs. 5.53, 5.54). The examiner evaluates both range of motion and, if present, pain induced with this maneuver.

Possible Pathological Findings

The spinous processes do not rotate with passive rotation (absence of coupled motion); there may be regional extension in the thoracic spine that could be exaggerated and possibly caused by segmental or regional somatic dysfunction.

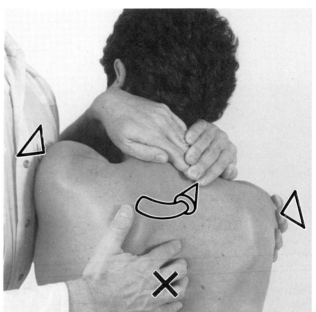

5.**53**

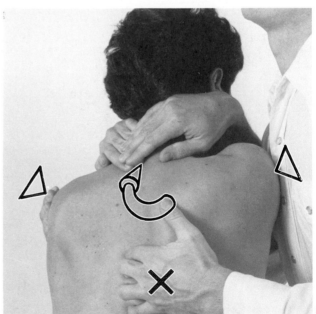

5.**54**

Examination: Springing test

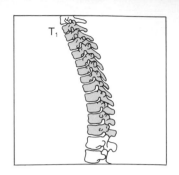

Examination Procedure

The index and middle fingers of the examining hand palpate the area over the articular processes, making as much bony contact as possible. With the hypothenar eminence of the other hand, the examiner introduces a spring-like (up and down) force (Fig. 5.**55**). The palpating fingers are then pushed over to the costotransverse joint, where a similarly directed springing force is introduced (Fig. 5.**56**).

Possible Pathological Findings

Pain, either localized or referred, induced with this maneuver indicates the presence of a segmental instability. At this point, the presence of intervertebral or costovertebral instability, or both, must be determined.

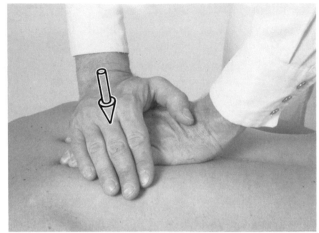

5.**55**

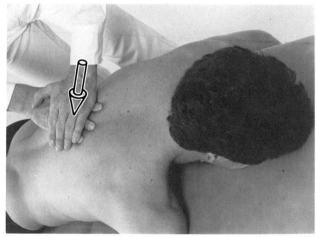

5.**56**

Region: First Rib

Examination: Active and passive motion testing

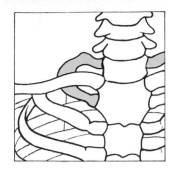

Examination Procedure

The cervical spine of the seated patient is passively flexed, and rotated away from and laterally bent towards the side that is to be examined (Fig. 5.**57**). The index finger of the examiner's monitoring (opposite) hand palpates the first rib on one side. After making contact with that rib, the examiner introduces a springlike force while evaluating the ease of displacement and resiliency (Fig. 5.**57**). With the palpating finger remaining over the first rib, the patient's head is brought back to midline while exhaling as deeply as possible (Fig. 5.**58**).

Possible Pathological Findings

1. Absence of springlike movement in the first rib due to somatic dysfunction with motion restriction involving the first rib.
2. Immediate localized pain or occasional referred pain to the shoulder or arm, or both, may be elicited with this maneuver. This may suggest the presence of the scalenus anticus syndrome.

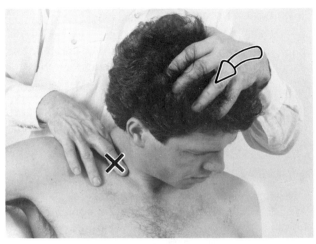

5.57

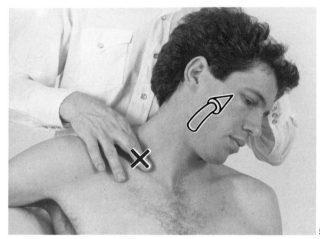

5.58

Examination: Individual rib motion testing during respiration

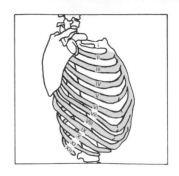

Examination Procedure

The intercostal spaces are evaluated by inspection and palpation, with the patient in either the supine or prone position (Fig. 5.**59**). The examiner looks for the presence of asymmetries during the respiratory cycle. The patient is then examined in the seated position. With arms raised, the patient's rib motion and changes in the intercostal spaces are palpated during inhalation and exhalation (Figs. 5.**60**, 5,**61**).

Possible Pathological Findings

1. Decreased rib motion during respiration, either regionally or segmentally. The possibility of anky-losing spondylitis affecting the thorax must be included in the differential diagnosis.
2. The finding of significant abdominal breathing usually indicates a decrease in thoracic excursion.

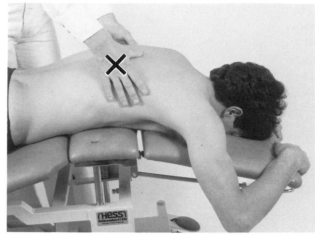

5.**59**

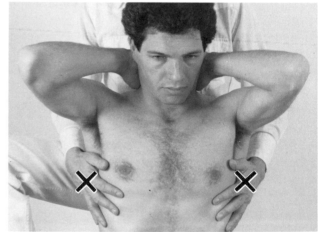

5.**60**

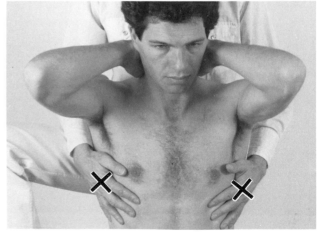

5.**61**

Region: L1—Pelvic Girdle

Examination: Evaluation of posture (static examination) of the lumbar spine and pelvis, patient standing and sitting

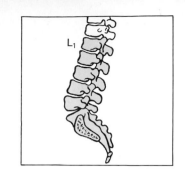

Examination Procedure

The patient's lumbar spine and pelvic girdle are examined for postural abnormalities while the patient is standing or sitting. It may be advantageous to inspect the patient surreptitiously; otherwise, the patient who feels observed may spontaneously assume a different posture.

Possible Pathological Findings

The finding of an increased lordosis (i.e., swayback) in conjunction with a pelvic tilt in the standing patient indicates a muscular imbalance. The lumbar erector spinae muscles, rectus femoris, and psoas major muscles are typically shortened, and the gluteal and abdominal muscles are usually weak. If, in the same patient, the degree of lumbar lordosis decreases when assuming a seated position, inadequate function (i.e., loss of strength) of the entire trunk musculature in the thoracic and lumbar spinal area must be suspected. Also, in the latter case, the abdominal muscles will most likely be weak.

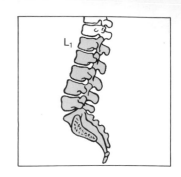

Examination: Motion testing of lumbar flexion, patient standing

Examination Procedure

The patient, standing with legs straight, is requested to bend the trunk forward. The examiner should note if a compensatory scoliosis becomes apparent with this maneuver. The patient is then requested to bend backward, allowing evaluation of the coordination of movement. This is followed by the patient bending the lumbar and thoracic spine laterally. In the healthy adult, this movement causes the spinous processes to arrange themselves in a smooth and symmetric "C-curve".

Possible Pathological Findings

1. Decreased flexion movement must be very carefully investigated since there are various causes. Decreased lumbar spine mobility may be due to degenerative changes. Decreased lumbar spine flexion may be the result of a shortened erector spinae muscle. Decreased lumbar flexion may be caused by lumbar radicular irritation.
2. The presence of a compensatory scoliosis, especially at the extreme of flexion, is highly suspicious of lumbar radicular irritation due to a ruptured lumbar disk.
3. Abnormal coordinated movement while going into extension from the maximally flexed position may possibly be due to a medial ruptured lumbar disk.
4. Regional or segmental loss of sidebending movement may indicate degenerative changes. This should be differentiated from a segmental somatic dysfunction.
5. Nonradiating pain concomitant with flexion or extension movement must be further investigated. Lumbar radicular irritation is probably unlikely.
6. Radiating pain elicited with flexion movement requires further investigation. For a radicular irritation, observe for the presence of a compensatory scoliosis and pain in a dermatomal distribution. It is often difficult to distinguish a purely radicular problem from pseudoradicular radiating pain of spondylogenic origin.

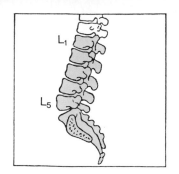

Examination: Passive motion testing of flexion and extension

Examination Procedure

The patient is in the side-lying (lateral recumbent) position. The examiner grasps the patient's legs at the ankle and then introduces 90° of flexion at the knees and hip. The patient's thighs then rest on the thighs of the examiner. The fingers of the monitoring hand palpate the individual spinous processes of the lumbar spine (Fig. 5.**62**). Subsequently, the examiner flexes the hip further, thereby introducing maximal hip flexion, which is accompanied by a reversal (flattening) of the lumbar spine. The changes of the interspinous distance with this movement can be easily detected by palpation, and hence indirectly provides information about the induced rotation about the x-axis (Fig. 5.**63**). Subsequently, the examiner introduces extension (i.e., passive extension) to the lumbar spine by decreasing flexion at the hip (Fig. 5.**63**). Movement of the spinous processes and the interspinous distance between the neighboring vertebrae are again evaluated (Fig. 5.**64**).

Possible Pathological Findings

1. The loss or restriction of either segmental or regional motion, or both, with hard *endfeel* is probably due to degenerative changes.
2. The loss or restriction of either segmental or regional motion, or both, with soft *endfeel* is primarily seen with a shortened longissimus lumborum and thoracis muscle.

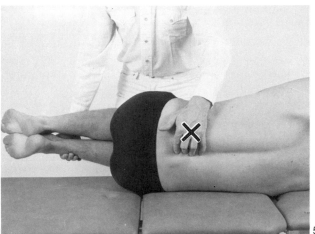

5.**62**

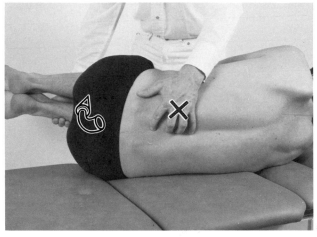

5.**63**

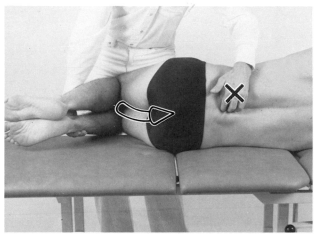

5.**64**

Examination: **Angular motion testing of rotation, lateral bending, flexion, and extension**

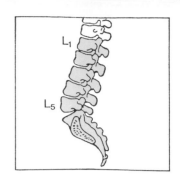

Examination Procedure

The patient is in the side-lying position (lateral recumbent position). The examiner grasps both of the patient's ankles and thus introduces 90° of flexion to both knees and hips. Subsequently, the patient's legs are raised as far off the table as possible, thereby introducing lateral bending (sidebending) to the lumabar spine. The fingers of the monitoring hand palpate the spinous processes, evaluating coupled axial rotation ($\pm$ 0y) as well (Fig. 5.**65**). The same maneuver can be performed with the patient sitting, where passive lumbar sidebending is introduced by the examiner (Fig. 5.**66**). Again, movement of the spinous processes and coupled rotation are evaluated. In a similar fashion, lateral movement can be assessed with the patient assuming a flexed or extended posture (Figs. 5.**67**, 5.**68**).

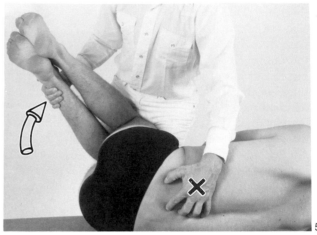

5.**65**

Possible Pathological Findings

Absence of coupled motion indicates a segmental dysfunction. In patients with muscle spasm ("palpable bands") secondary to antalgic postural compensation, coupled motion is usually absent as well.

5.**66**

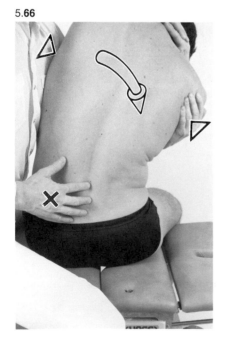

5.**67**

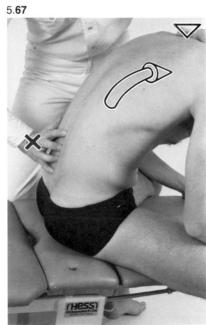

5.**68**

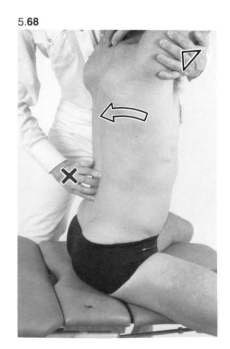

Region: Lumbar Spine

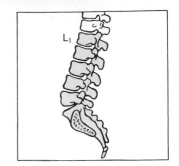

Examination: Springing test

Examination Procedure

The index and middle fingers of the monitoring hand palpate the articular and mamillary processes of the vertebra in question. Through the hypothenar eminence, which rests over the monitoring hand, an anteriorly directed force is introduced (Fig. 5.**69**). The individual vertebrae of the lumbar spine can be examined in this manner.

Possible Pathological Findings

Using this examination procedure, it may be possible to induce either localized or referred pain, or both, segmental instability is present.

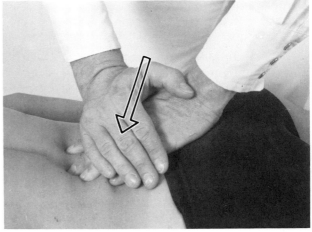

5.**69**

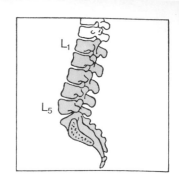

Examination: **Motion testing of rotation at the L5—S1 spinal segment**

Examination Procedure

It is extremely difficult to clinically measure axial rotation, since the movement is no greater than 2° in the upper portion of the lumbar spine. In contrast, rotation movement at the lumbosacral junction is palpable since it measures 5° to 6°. The patient, with hands crossed behind the neck, is seated astride the end of the examination table. The examiner reaches around the patient's trunk at the shoulder level and then introduces passive rotation. The middle finger of the monitoring hand palpates the upper pole of the medial sacral crest while the index finger palpates the motion of the spinous process of L5 (Fig. 5.**70**). The changes of distance between these two landmarks, effected through passive trunk rotation, provide additional information about mobility in the lumbosacral junction and thus about rotation around the y-axis.

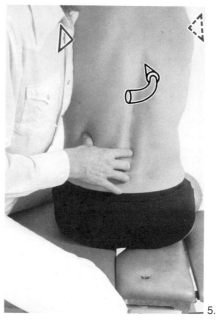

5.**70**

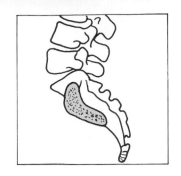

Examination: **Spine test, active motion testing for nutation movement**

Examination Procedure

The patient is standing with his or her back to the examiner. With both feet planted firmly on the ground, the patient is requested to extend both knees. Next, the patient is instructed to push one knee as far forward as possible. While doing so, if there is no SIJ restriction, the ilium on the side where the knee is flexed drops down and simultaneously undergoes a distinct counternutation backwards. While the patient remains in the standing position, the examiner localizes the posterior superior iliac spine (PSIS) on one side with one thumb, and with the other thumb the opposite median iliac crest is palpated at the same level (Fig. 5.**71**). The patient is again requested to push one knee as far forward as possible. If the SIJ is not restricted, the PSIS descends a distance of approximately 0.5 cm to a maximum of 2.0 cm with this induced movement. The angle formed by the body's longitudinal axis and a line connecting the two thumbs increases beyond 90°. When there is an SIJ motion restriction (Figs. 5.**72**, 5.**73**) the ilium does not descend and the above described angle remains at 90° (Dejung, 1985).

Possible Pathological Findings

If motion in one SIJ is lost, the palpated PSIS on that same side moves superiorly due to pelvic tilting.

5.**71**

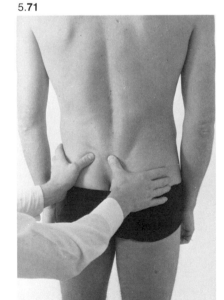

5.**72**

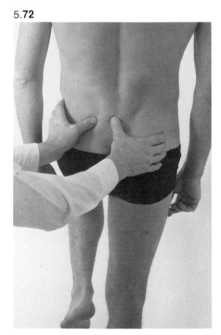

5.**73**

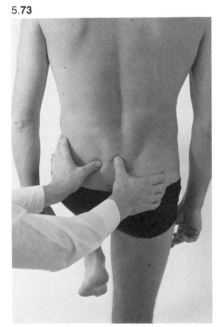

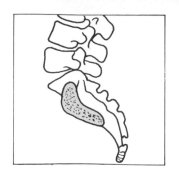

Examination: Standing flexion test, nutation in the SIJ

Examination Procedure

Starting from inferior, the PSIS is palpated on either side with the thumb (Fig. 5.**74**). The respective position is compared when the patient bends forward (Fig. 5.**75**). If nutation movement is impeded in one SIJ, the PSIS on that same side will move more superiorly when compared to the other side. This may, at first, appear paradoxical, yet can be explained, since in the case of SIJ restriction the sacrum and innominate bone move together as a unit due to the loss of normal nutation motion. As a rule, the standing flexion test in called positive on the side where the restriction occurs (greater PSIS excursion in the absence of nutation movement).

Possible Pathological Findings

The clinical finding of greater PSIS excursion with absent nutation movement is, in most cases, indicative of a somatic dysfunction; differential-diagnostically, other causes may include pelvic asymmetry and hip joint asymmetry (epiphysiolysis, dysplasia). A false-positive standing flexion test may be seen in cases of asymmetrical hamstring length or contralateral hamstring shortening.

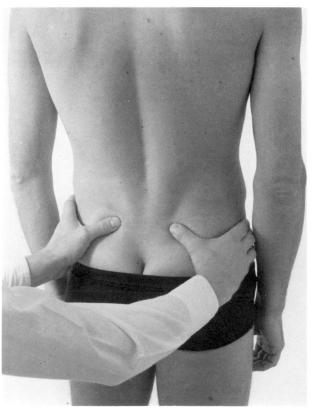

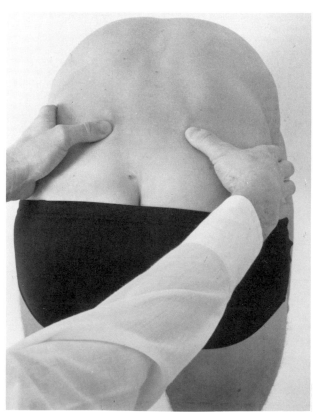

5.74

5.75

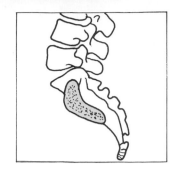

Examination: **Passive motion testing (joint play)**

Examination Procedure

While the patient is in the prone position, the fingers of the examining hand are placed over the SIJ in question and over the short posterior sacral ligaments. Clinically, the SIJ cannot be palpated directly due to its anatomic location. The opposite hand is placed flat over the anterior portion of the iliac bone, subsequently introducing a posteriorly directed force. The palpating fingers register the relative displacement between the iliac bone and sacrum, which should amount to about 2 mm to 3 mm (Fig. 5.**76**).

Possible Pathological Findings

The relative displacement cannot be observed clinically, which is indicative of a functional disturbance in the SIJs.

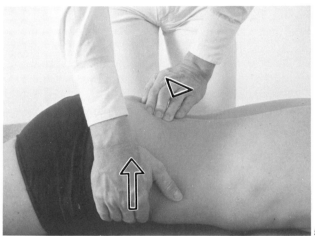

5.**76**

Examination: Leg length difference

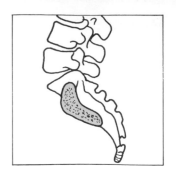

Examination Procedure

With the patient in the supine position, the examiner places one thumb on either medial malleolus (Fig. 5.**77**). The patient, assisted by the examiner, is requested to sit up from the supine position (Fig. 5.**78**). If nutation motion at one SIJ has been found to be absent during the standing flexion test (positive standing flexion test), the leg on the ipsilateral side appears shorter when the patient is supine and becomes relatively longer with sitting up. A difference of less than 2 cm is probably not clinically significant (Fig. 5.**79**).

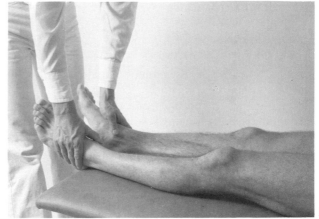

5.77

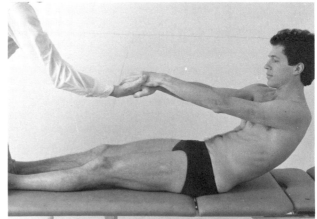

5.78

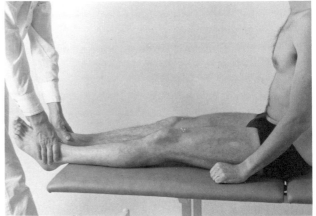

5.79

Region: SIJ, Pelvis

Examination: Patrick or Faber test

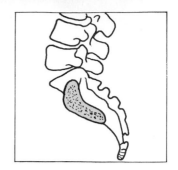

Examination Procedure

The patient is in the supine position. While one side of the pelvis is being carefully fixated by one of the examiner's hands, the leg on the opposite side is flexed, abducted, and externally rotated at the hip as far as possible (please note that the abbreviation of the sequentially introduced movements coin the acronym "**F**lexion-**Ab**duction-**E**xternal **R**otation"). Once in this position, the patient's heal is placed on the opposite knee (Fig. 5.**80**). If the SIJ lacks the normal nutation motion or if there is a functional abnormality, the distance between the patella and the table will be greater than that on the opposite, healthy side (caveat: arthrosis of the hip).

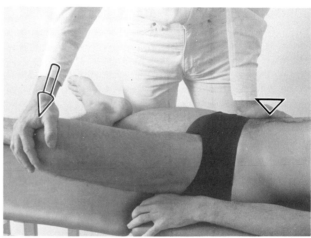

5.80

Possible Pathological Findings

If there is a functional abnormality (i.e., somatic dysfunction) at the SIJ, the distance between the patella and the table will be greater than that on the opposite side. The *end point stop* is soft, which is in contrast to a hard *endfeel* encountered with hip joint problems.

Examination: **Palpation of iliacus muscle**

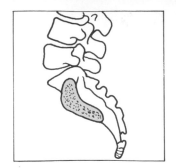

Course and Relations

The muscle originates in the iliac fossa and continues inferiorly, where it joins the lateral margin of the psoas major muscle; together they insert at the lesser trochanter (Fig. 5.**81**).

Innervation

Same as psoas major muscle.

Function

Hip flexion and hip external rotation.

Palpatory Technique

It is difficult to palpate the iliacus muscle in the iliac fossa, and even when it can be done, only partial palpation is possible. The patient should be in a semi-seated position in order to enable relaxation of the abdominal musculature. After locating the anterior superior iliac spine (ASIS) with the palpating thumb, the examiner glides the thumb deeply along the upper portion of the iliac bone. Starting from the ASIS, the iliacus muscle may be followed along the pelvic crest in a superior direction for about three finger widths and in an inferior direction for not more than two finger widths. The ramainder of the fibers at the origin cannot be adequately palpated due to their anatomic position and the overlying abdominal muscles (see p. 297, Fig. 8.**98**).

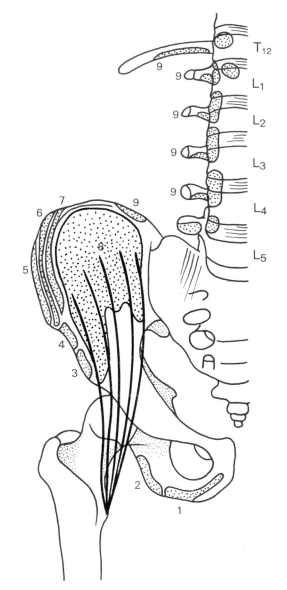

Fig. 5.**81**   Iliac muscle

1   Adductor magnus m
2   Quadratus femoris m
3   Rectus femoris m
4   Sartorius m
5   External abdominal oblique m
6   Internal abdominal oblique m
7   Transversus abdominis m
8   Iliac m
9   Quadratus lumborum m

Region: SIJ, Pelvis

Examination: Position of pubic bones

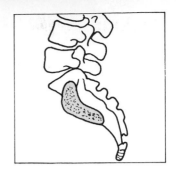

Examination Procedure

The patient is in the supine position. The pubic bone on either side is palpated, and the relative height in regard to the horizontal plane is insepcted (i.e., if the bones are level). Asymmetrical position may be due to a disturbance in the SIJ. There may also be a dysfunction in the symphysis pubis itself. Pelvic dysplasia should always be excluded.

Region: SIJ

Examination: Provocative testing by pressure on the zone of irritation and nutation motion at the SIJ

Examination Procedure

The patient is in the prone position. Pressure of sufficient but not excessive force is applied to the zone of irritation. The patient is requested to remember this pressure pain as "A." In the second phase, the examiner introduces an anteriorly directed pressure force against the sacrum with the other hand. The pressure exerted over the zone of irritation remains unchanged. The patient is instructed to remember this second pain as "B." In the third phase, the anterior force applied to the sacrum is quickly relieved. Pain at that moment is remembered by the patient as "C" (see also p. 228, Figs. 7.**19**−7.**21**).

Possible Pathological Findings

1. Pain C is the worst, with pain B being minimal and with pain A intermediate between pain B and C: this is a strong indication that there is a dysfunction of the SIJ.
2. Pain B is the worst: There may possibly be some psychological overlay.
3. Patient has difficulty providing clear description: interpretation unclear.

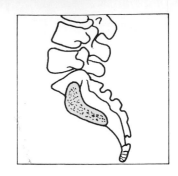

Origin

The inferior and lateral margin of the tips of the costal processes of L4 and L5. These two origins and their corresponding tendons are anatomically independent of each other in their course (iliac tuberosity junction) (Fig. 5.**82**).

Insertion

This ligament inserts in the most medial portions of the iliac crest and the neighboring anterior and posterior surfaces of the ilium (Fig. 5.**83**).

Course and Relations

As mentioned, the tendons arising from L4 and L5 must be considered separately:

L4 segment: Arising from the costal process of L4 this part of the tendon passes steeply inferiorly and laterally reaching the anterior surface of the ilium lateral to the SIJ (Figs. 5.**82**, 5.**83**).

L5 segment: This portion divides in two immediately at the origin of the costal process of L5 (Figs. 5.**82**, 5.**83**).

Fibers arising from the tip pass almost perfectly horizontally to the iliac tuberosity, reaching the anterior side of the ilium where they insert together with the fibers from L4.

Fibers arising from the costal process of L5 pass lateroinferiorly, almost vertically, to the anterior side of the ilium, reaching the linea terminalis, where they insert together with the anterior sacroiliac ligaments.

Function

The iliolumbar ligament transmits the motion of the hip bones to the vertebrae L4 and L5. Thus, it plays an important role in the mechanics of the lumbopelvic junction.

Palpatory Technique

When palpating this anatomically small space, the examiner should be aware that the iliolumbar ligament lies extremely deep. The fibers arising from L4 are still accessible to palpation: from a laterosuperior direction, the origin at the costal process is palpated, whereas the insertion is palpated mediosuperiorly as long as it is accessible at the iliac crest.

When palpating for the fibers arising from L5, only the insertion of the horizontal portion of the fibers is accessible. Palpation, however, presents clear results only after the tendon has become painful.

SRS Correlation

Spondylogenically related to the midthoracic spine. Of great significance is the support function of the iliolumbar ligament at the lumbosacral junction. If spondylogenically affected, it may cause intense back pain, especially when raising the trunk from the flexed position. This ligamentous pain is often persistent and resistant to therapy. The patient often complains about diffuse back pain either during or after performing activities that require flexion of the trunk (e.g., vacuuming, ironing).

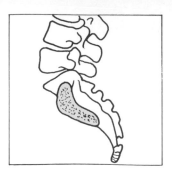

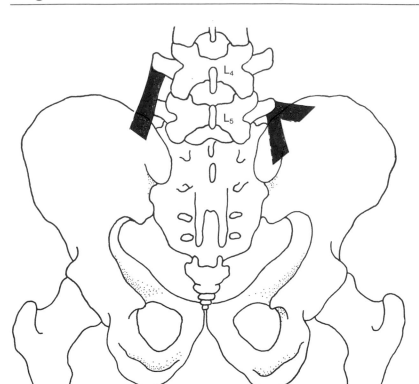

Fig. 5.**82**   Iliolumbar ligament (posterior view)

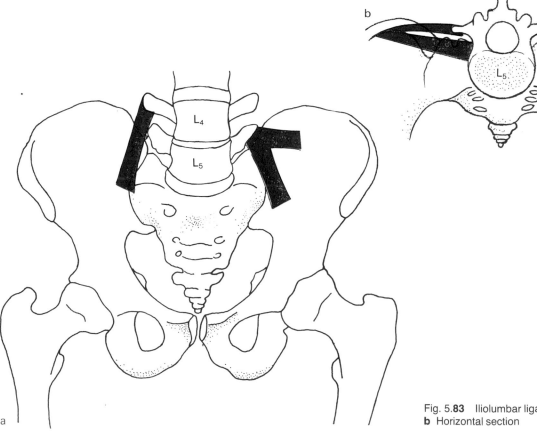

Fig. 5.**83**   Iliolumbar ligament. **a** Anterior view
b Horizontal section

Region: Iliolumbar Ligament

Examination: Functional testing

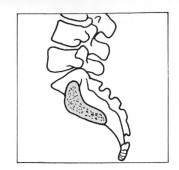

Examination Procedure

With the patient in the supine position, the hip and knee joint are flexed passively and the thigh adducted. During adduction, the examiner introduces an axial loading force onto the femur by leaning onto the patient's knee (Fig. 5.**84**). In the presence of functional shortening involving the ligament, a pathological pain will be elicited that may take 10 to 20 seconds to appear. Differentiation from a functionally shortened piriformis muscle is not possible with this test. It is important to exclude mechanical overload of the ligament due to a pseudospondylolisthesis.

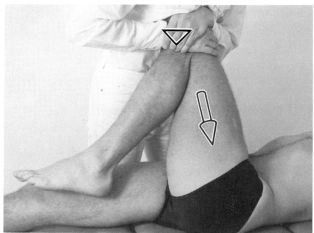

5.84

Examination: **Provocative testing of iliolumbar ligament by pressure and induced movement**

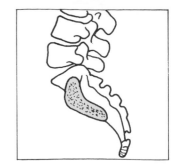

Examination Procedure

The examiner exerts constant pressure over the iliolumbar ligament between the PSIS and the spinous processes of L4 and L5 (Fig. 5.**85**). If pain is elicited with this maneuver, the examiner proceeds to the second phase of the examination. During this phase, progressivley greater pressure is applied by the examiner's thenar eminence in the anterior direction against the spinous processes.

Possible Pathological Findings

1. Localized pain elicited with pressure. This may be due to a functional disturbance of the iliolumbar ligament. Pain in this area may also be caused by a segmental dysfunction with evidence of a zone of irritation, or irritation of the intervertebral joints of L4—L5 and L5—S1 due to degenerative changes.

2. Localized pain is exacerbated by the anteriorly directed pressure against the spinous processes of L4 and L5. This is an apparent indication that there is painful dysfunction associated with the iliolumbar ligament. Differential-diagnostically, it is conceivable that the dysfunction is caused by mechanical stress on these ligaments due to a possible pseudospondylolisthesis.

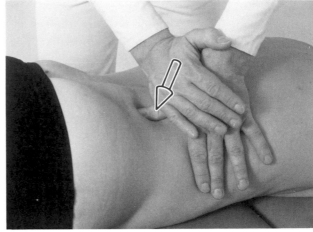

5.**85**

Region: SIJ, Sacrospinous Ligament

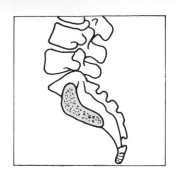

Origin

The lateral margin of the coccyx and the entire free sacral bone up to the level of S3.

Insertion

The spine of the ischium (apex and superior margin). The line of insertion is narrow (about 1 cm).

Course and Relations

The sacrospinous ligament lies anterior to the sacrotuberous ligament. Both ligaments interdigitate at their origin at the free margin of the sacrum. Constructing a vertical line through the posterior superior iliac spine, the spine of the ischium is met inferiorly at the level of the sacrococcygeal junction. From this constructed landmark, the fan-shaped sacrospinous ligament passes to the sacrum and coccyx, that is, in medial to superomedial direction whereby the most inferior fibers are almost horizontal. Laterally, the ligament underlies the muscle mass of the gluteus maximus muscle and medially it is only covered by the thin lining of the abdominal cavity (Fig. 5.**86**).

Palpatory Technique

The origin of the sacrospinous ligament is covered by the origin of the gluteus maximus muscle. Thus, with incorrect palpatory depth this ligament can be confused with the tendinoses of the superficial gluteus maximus layer. The origin can be reached from lateral (bony contact) without any major difficulty. This origin is palpated through the musculature of the gluteus muscle at the correct topographical location (see above) from a posterior direction.

Rectal examination, however, is far superior to external palpation and is the method of choice, especially when definitive clarification becomes necessary.

SRS Correlation

There may be a spondylogenic correlation of the sacrospinous ligament with the cervical spine. The spondylogenic contribution of the sacrospinous ligament is clinically very important.

Often a persistent coccydynia can be caused by the sacrospinous ligament as a result of a functional disturbance in the upper cervical spine region, for instance.

Myotendinosis in the superior fibers can cause an S1 dysfunction, whereas myotendinosis in the inferior fiber tracts can cause dysfunction in S2.

The sacrospinous ligament shows great anatomical variation. Different portions of varying size can develop into contractile muscle fibers, and in very rare cases, the whole tendon can form the coccygeal muscle. In regard to the spondylogenic correlation, it is insignificant whether it is tendon or muscle. Considering the phenomenon of "myotendinosis," no fundamental difference exists between the muscular and ligamentous forms. This fact demonstrates that myotendinosis does not necessarily require myofibril contractility.

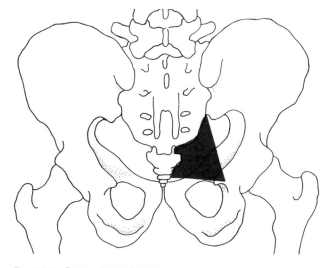

Fig. 5.**86** Sacrospinous ligament

Region: Sacrospinous Ligament

Examination: Functional testing

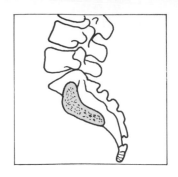

Examination Procedure

With the patient in the supine position, the leg on
one side (testing for the ipsilateral ligament) is maximally flexed at the hip and knee and adducted in the
direction of the opposite shoulder (Fig. 5.**87**). During
this maneuver, the examiner introduces an axial
loading force through the femur by applying pressure
against the knee. This may induce stretch pain, which
might become apparent after a latency period of 10 to
20 seconds, and possibly indicates a functionally
shortened or stressed (overloaded) sacrospinous ligament.

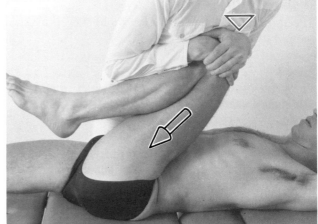

5.**87**

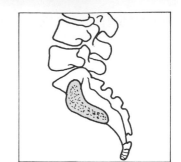

Origin

This ligament arises as a small band from the posterior surface of the sacrum at the level of S3 and S4, between the lateral sacral crest and the sacral foramina. Fibers that arise most laterally intermingle with the fibers of the sacrotuberous ligament, whose origin is at this location as well.

Insertion

The tendon inserts along the entire width (abouth 1 to 2 cm) of the inferior margin of the posterior superior iliac spine (see Palpatory technique).

Course and Relations

The posterior sacroiliac ligament passes almost vertically from its origin at the sacrum to its insertion at the PSIS. The lateral portions of the tendon are in anatomical proximity to the sacrotuberous ligaments, the medial portions to the thoracolumbar fascia (Fig. 5.**88**).

Palpatory Technique

The tendon is located in a groove formed by the insertion of the gluteus maximus muscle and the insertion of the sacrospinous system. Due to this anatomical arrangement, few structures overlie the tendon.

It is possible to misidentify this tendon for the sacral zones of irritation, the origin tendinoses of the longissimus thoracis muscle (sector II), and the most inferior origins of the transverospinous system. The insertion at the PSIS is of practical importance for palpation; this insertion is palpated inferiorly and slightly medially in the direction of the PSIS.

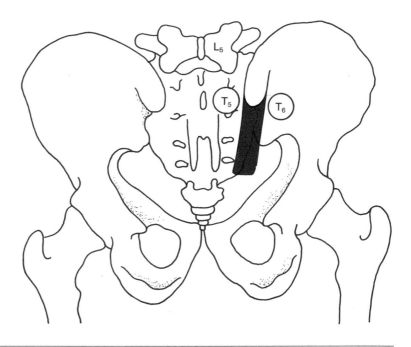

Fig. 5.**88**   Long posterior sacroiliac ligament

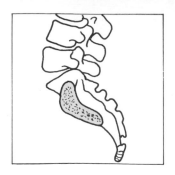

Examination: **Functional testing**

Examination Procedure

The patient is in the supine position. The leg on the side that is to be examined is flexed maximally at the hip and knee joint in order to approximate it with the ipsilateral shoulder. At the same time, the examiner pushes down on the knee in order to introduce an axial loading force on the femur (Fig. 5.**89**). This may induce ligamentous stretch pain, which might become apparent after a latency period of 10–20 seconds, and possibly indicate a functionally shortened or stressed (overloaded) posterior sacroiliac ligament.

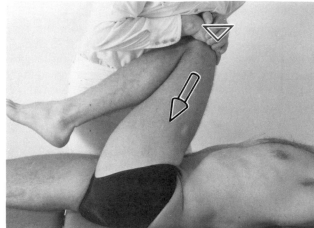

5.89

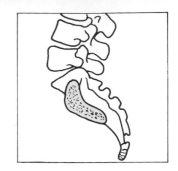

Origin

The sacrotuberous ligament arises above the sacrospinous ligament at the coccyx and the free margin of the side of the sacrum. In contrast to the sacrospinous ligament, the insertion of the sacrotuberous ligament passes further superiorly, reaching the posterior inferior spine; it also joins the fascia lata.

Insertion

From its insertion at the inner surface of the ischial tuberosity a segment of the tendon continues anteriorly along the inner margin of the ramus of the ischium to the posterior margin of the symphysis, forming the so-called falciform ligament. Thus, the insertion is about 5 to 6 cm long.

Course and Relations

The sacrotuberous ligament has a fan-shaped appearance. Its fibers pass in a propellerlike fashion from origin to insertion. Thus, the fiber tracts undergo a changeover with fibers arising most superiorly, cutting across anteromedially (practically vertical) and inserting at the ramus of the ischium most anteriorly. Fibers arising at the most inferior portion, in contrast, ascend posterolaterally to the ischial tuberosity, reaching the line of insertion at the most posterior portion (Fig. 5.**90**).

The sacrotuberous ligament lies posterior to the sacrospinous ligament, which is weaker and shorter.

Portions of the sacrotuberous ligament close to the origin severe as origin for a great part of the gluteus maximus muscle.

Palpatory Technique

When palpating the origin (at the coccyx, sacrum), the examiner must be aware of the anatomical relationship of the sacrotuberous ligament to the sacrospinous ligament and the gluteus maximus muscle. The sacral zones of irritation lie more medial and should not be the cause of confusion. Palpation follows the muscle fiber direction from lateral to the margin of the sacrum. In the prone position, it should not be difficult to palpate the ischial tuberosity. Starting from the ischial tuberosity, insertion tendinoses are then located by palpating along the ramus of the ischium to the posterior margin of the symphysis (the falciform ligament). Rectal examination may again become necessary.

SRS Correlation

The sacrotuberous ligament is spondylogenically related to the upper thoracic spine and similar to the sacrospinous ligament. Myotendinosis or hard, palpable bands of the superior fiber portions favor a disturbance at S1, whereas myotendinosis of the inferior fibers favors a distrubance at S2.

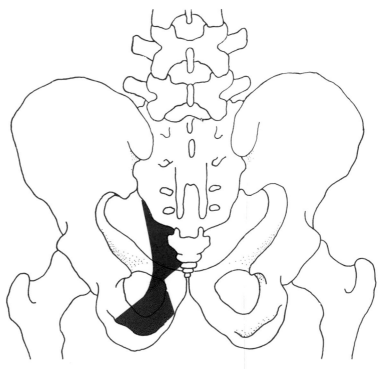

Fig. 5.**90** Sacrotuberous ligament

6 Orthopedic Examination

Joint: Hip

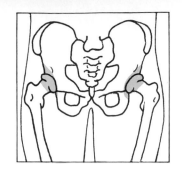

Examination: Trendelenburg test, Duchenne test

Performance

Observe gait (Fig. 6.**1a**). Stands on one leg (Fig. 6.**1b, c**).

Remarks

Limping due to either:

1. Functional weakness (pain)
2. Neurogenic paresis

Trendelenburg: limp due to gluteus medius weakness. Cannot stand on that leg easily; usually tilts to opposite side. *Leans away from* weak side (Fig. 6.**1b**). Tilt of the pelvis.

Duchenne: weakness of tensor fascia lata. Attempts to compensate by using gluteals. *Leans towards* weak side (Fig. 6.**1c**).

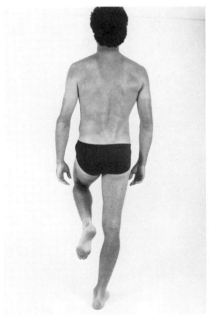

a

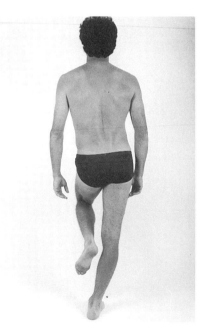

b

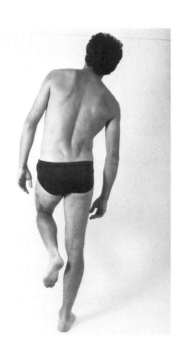

c

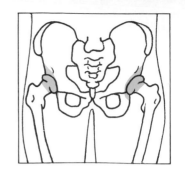

Examination: Screening for leg length discrepancy

Performance

1. *Supine position:* to screen. Flex hips and knees to observe leg length (Fig. 6.**2a**)
2. *Standing:* to observe and compare levels of iliac crest from behind (Fig. 6.**2b**).

Remarks

Standing on two scales at the same time, one foot on each, may indicate imbalance of weight bearing; may indicate functional spinal disorder or leg length difference.

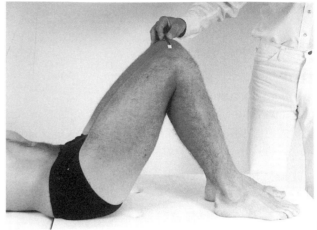

a

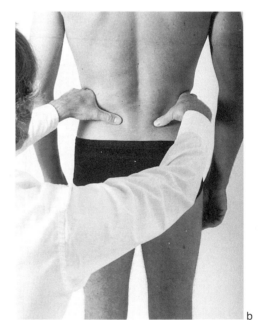

b

Joint: Hip

Examination: Abduction and adduction

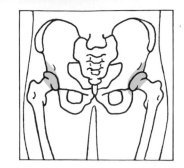

Performance

Supine position. Hold opposite anterior superior iliac spine (ASIS) and monitor at what point it moves. Observe angle of adduction (Fig. 6.**3a**) or abduction (Fig. 6.**3b**).

Remarks

Should be able to achieve 45° to 60° abduction and 30° to 40° adduction.

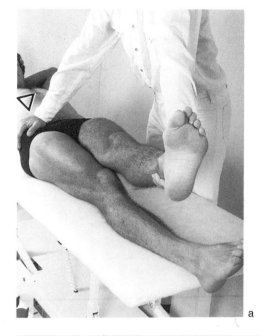

a

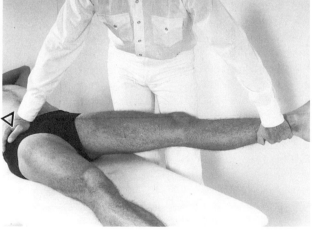

b

Joint: Hip

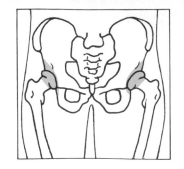

Examination: Flexion

Performance

Flex hip and knee and, with the hand over L4 and L5, monitor when the lumbar spine begins to move. Pelvic rotation finally takes up slack in lumbar spine (Fig. 6.**4**).

Remarks

Approximately 120° to 130° flexion before pelvic rotation occurs.

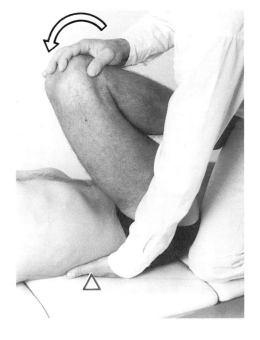

Examination: **Extension**

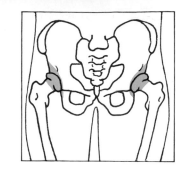

Performance

1. *Supine:* Holding the knee straightens the lumbar lordosis. The other leg should stay on the bed. The monitoring hand over the extended knee ensures this (Fig. 6.**5a**).
2. *Prone:* Keep the pelvis flat with the monitoring hand over gluteus maximus and pelvic crest. Then passively extend the hip joint by lifting just proximal to the flexed knee (Fig. 6.**5b**).

Remarks

Rectus femoris stretched.

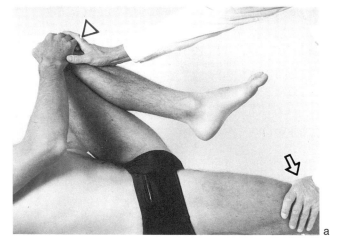

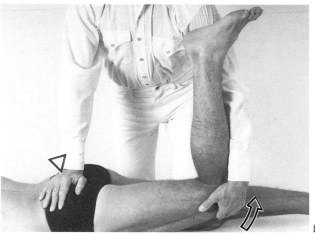

Joint: Hip

Examination: Passive internal and external rotation in extension

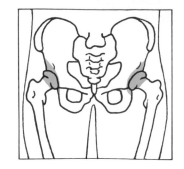

Performance

Prone position. Flex knees. Externally (Fig. 6.**6a**) and internally (Fig. 6.**6b**) rotate by passively crossing flexed legs.

Remarks

While internally rotating, the piriformis is stretched. A shortened piriformis will restrict the range of movement, producing an elastic, often painful end feel. Compare the quality of end feel. Internal rotation approximately 35°−40°. External rotation approximately 40°−50°.

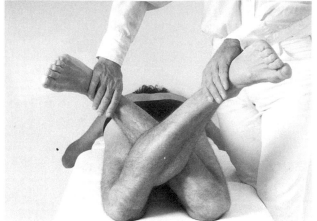

a

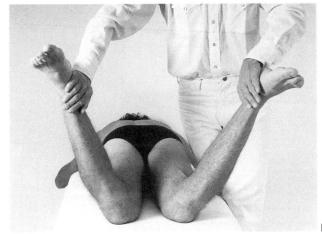

b

Examination: **Passive internal and external rotation in flexion**

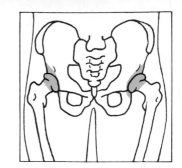

Performance

Supine position. Flexed knees. Passively move leg and observe angle using the monitoring hand on knee and the guarding hand at ankle (Figs. 6.**7a, b**).

Remarks

Internal rotation approximately 30°−45°. External rotation approximately 40°−50°.

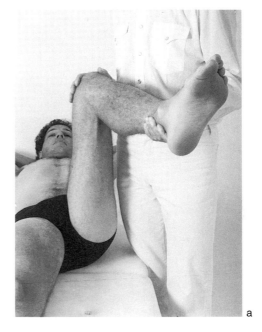

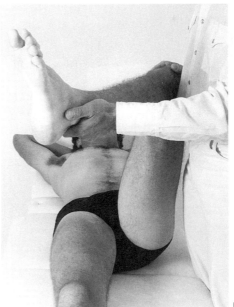

Joint: Hip

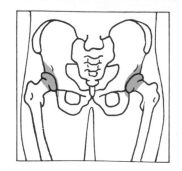

Examination: Active abduction and extension

Performance

1. *Active abduction:* side position. Resistant movement to detect weakness (Fig. 6.**8a**).
2. *Active extension:* prone position. Examine leg actively extended (gravity resists) and held. Muscle outlines, and duration and strength observed (Fig. 6.**8b**).

Remarks

Active abduction tests gluteus medius (anterior part) and tensor fascia lata. *Active extension* tests gluteus maximus and gluteus medius (posterior part).

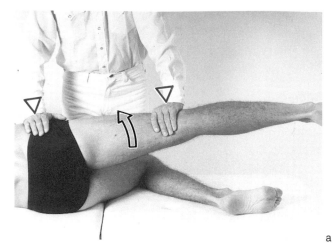

a

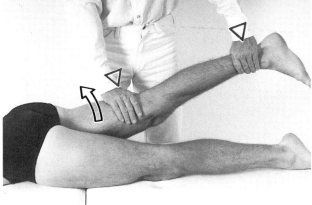

b

Joint: Knee

Examination: Inspection of the axis. Screening. Dynamic active knee movements, especially pivoting

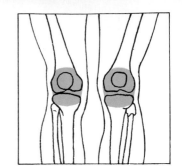

Performance

Standing on one leg. Patient goes through various normal standing positions applying weight to the knee in various degrees of knee angle (Fig. 6.**9a–g**).

Remarks

May evoke position or weight-dependent pain, or both. After standing for static positions, a dynamic test is achieved when the patient jumps sideways from one side to the other. The range and ease with which this is performed is observed. The pain and instability may be obvious. Compare one side to the other.

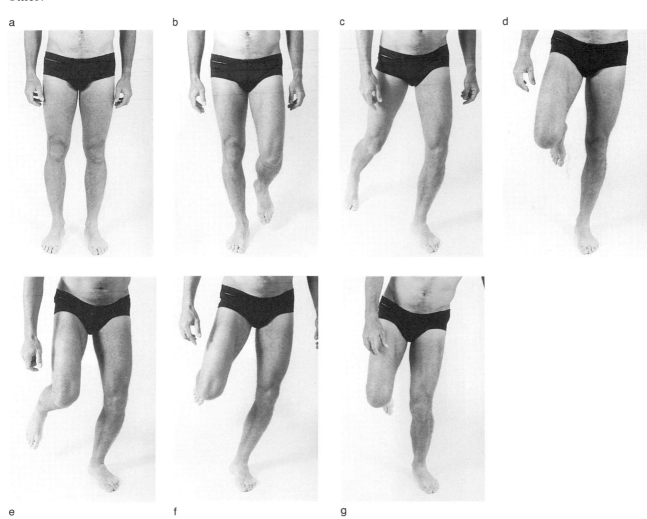

Examination: **Squatting Screening: walking on heels**

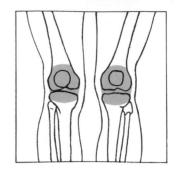

Performance

Roll over from one leg to the other (Fig. 6.**10a, b**).

Remarks

Cannot be performed in:
- knee pathology
- triceps surae shortening

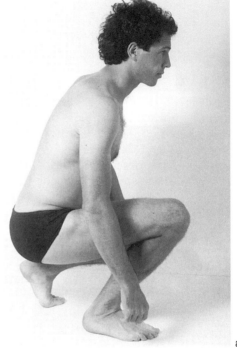

a

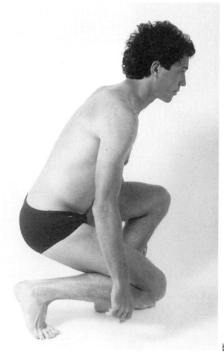

b

Joint: Knee

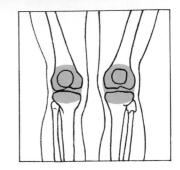

Examination: Translation of patella medially and laterally

Performance

Knee is stabilized in neutral extension. Patella is translated using pincer fingertip grip. Medial and lateral excursions are noted and compared (Fig. 6.**11**).

Palpation of fat pad and peripatellar ligaments.

Remarks

Hypomobility? Hypermobility? Crepitus? Pain with movement?

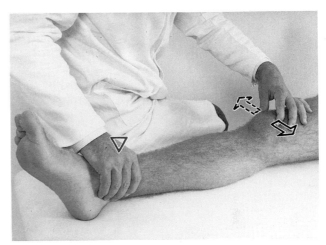

Joint: Knee

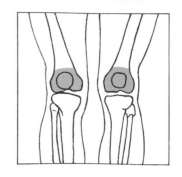

Examination: Coronal and caudal translation of patella

Performance

Straighten relaxed knee. Avoid axial stress perpendicular to condylar surface. Translate patella in caudal (Fig. 6.**12a**), medial (Fig. 6.**12b**), and lateral (Fig. 6.**12c**) directions. With the patella in fully translated position, palpate the articular surface of the patella from below (Fig. 6.**12d**). Palpate peripatellar ligaments and synovium.

Possible Pathological Findings

Myotendinotic tenderness, degenerative changes in articular cartilage?

Remarks

Crepitus? Hypermobility? Motion-induced pain? Swelling? Synovial changes?

Note

Mobilization procedure is almost identical. Mobilization of patella may delay joint replacement, osteotomy, or arthrodesis. However, possibilities of mobilization are relatively limited.

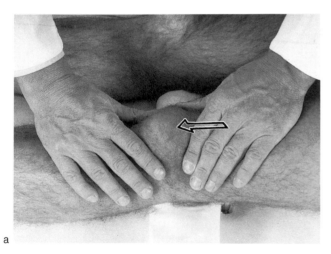

a

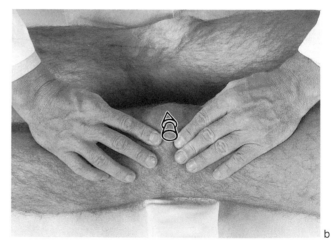

b

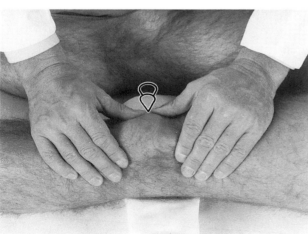

c

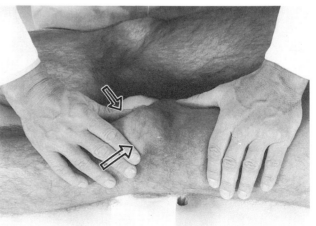

d

Joint: Knee

Examination: Patellar function

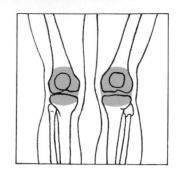

Performance

Observe patellar movement and tracking during various degrees of flexion.

1. Monitor with fingers, using pincer fingertip palpation (Fig. 6.**13a**).
2. Hold hand over patella using palmar surface to monitor patella movements (Fig. 6.**13b**).

Remarks

Observe excursion of patella in all directions—does patella move too far in one direction, or return to normal neutral zone?

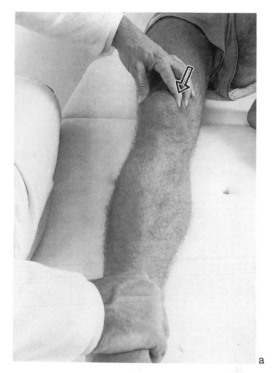

a

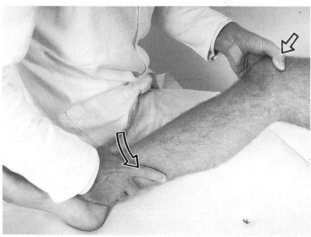

b

Joint: Knee

Examination: Active and passive extension

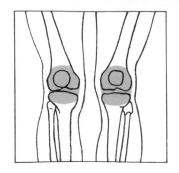

Performance

The knee is fixed by a firm grip above the joint. Active movements are monitored (Fig. 6.**14a, b**).

Remarks

Passive extension beyond the active range is normal and is looked for (approximately 10° extra) (Fig. 6.**14c, d**)

Measure distance (cm) from heel to examination table (Fig. 6.**14e, f**)

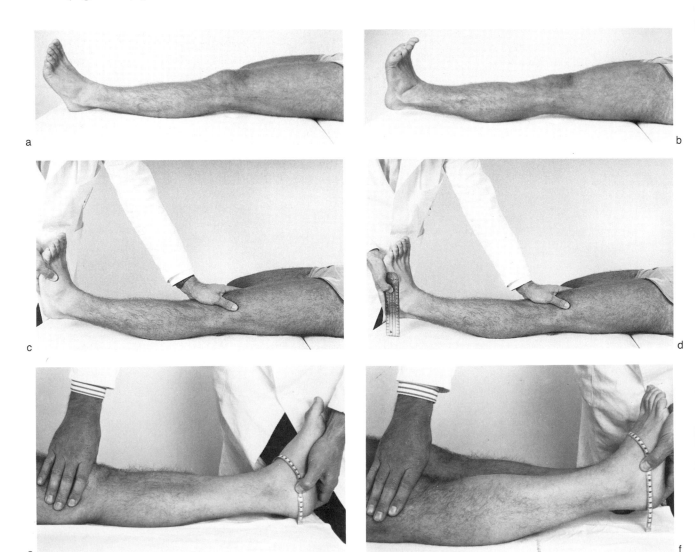

a

b

c

d

e

f

Joint: Knee

Examination: Active and passive flexion

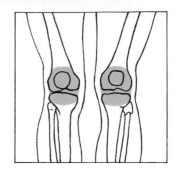

Performance

Patient flexes knee as far as possible; the angle is measured. The examiner holds the goniometer at the level of the joint and increases the flexion. The difference of range of motion is monitored. Passive flexion of 150° is considered normal (Fig. 6.**15**).

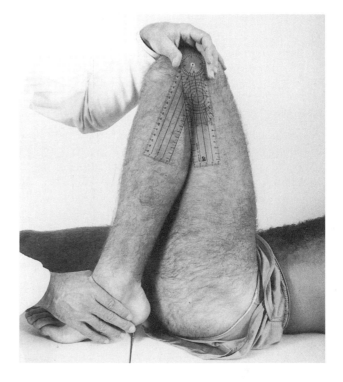

Joint: Knee

Examination: Passive rotations in various degrees of flexion

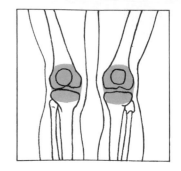

Performance

Monitor joint line with pincer fingertip grip, and perform internal (Fig. 6.**16a**) and external (Fig. 6.**16b**) rotation. Passive rotation maneuvers from slight flexion all the way to full extension.

Remarks

A normal test excludes most articular pathology involving menisci. Pain-provoking pressure is applied to both menisci. *Compare* similar procedure for shoulder.

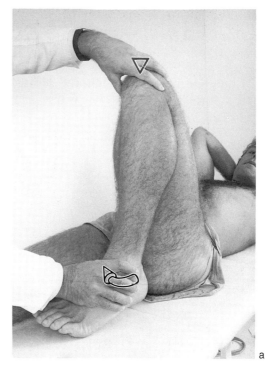

a

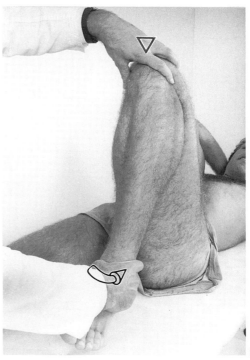

b

Joint: Knee

Examination: Varus and valgus stress-testing of medial and lateral collateral ligaments, and for condition of medial and lateral compartment

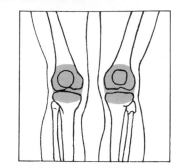

Performance

Medial, lateral, and cruciate ligaments are stretched by valgus (Fig. 6.**17a**) and varus (Fig. 6.**17b**) stresses in slight passive knee flexion. Valgus (Fig. 6.**17c**) and varus (Fig. 6.**17d**) stress in extension.

Remarks

Medial instability usually traumatic.
Lateral instability degenerative or traumatic.
Grinding in varus stress = internal derangement in medial compartment.
Grinding in valgus stress = internal derangement in lateral compartment.

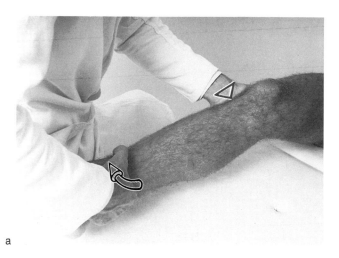

a

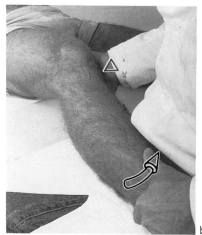

b

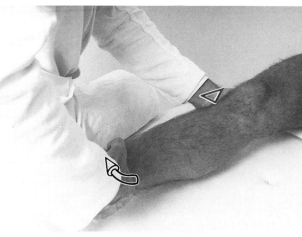

c

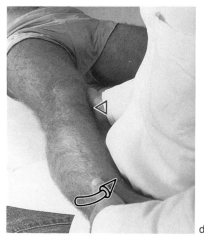

d

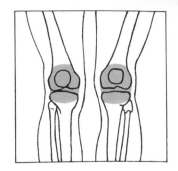

**Examination: Lachman sign for anterior cruciate
ligament (ACL) and
posterior cruciate ligament (PCL)**

Performance

Supine position. Slight knee flexion. Fix femur from
the lateral aspect from below. Fix tibia and glide
tibial head forward over the femoral condyle and
backwards to test ACL and PCL, respectively (Fig.
6.**18**).

Remarks

Translation is normally approximately 5 mm—more
than this is pathological.

Range of movement is observed. PCL or ACL insufficiency can be difficult to determine. Mechanism of
injury, other clinical findings, and lateral stress
X-rays required for diagnosis.

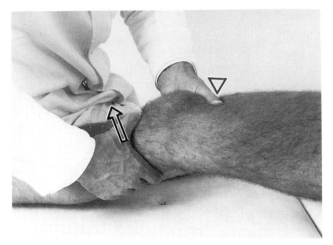

Joint: Knee

Examination: Pivot shift test for anterior cruciate insufficiency (Macintosh)

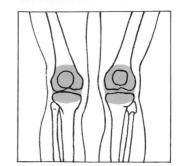

Performance

Two methods are described:

1. Grasp firmly above and below knee with patient on side (Fig. 6.**19a**), with affected side uppermost. Beginning in extension, valgus force and slight internal rotation on the fibula lead is applied during passive knee flexion (Fig. 6.**19b**). A feeling of instability by the patient is experienced and often a click indicating a pivot shift is audible.
   Grasping the thigh can be difficult. The examiner may flex his knee and perform the test over the knee, reducing the requirement of a firm thigh grip.
2. Patient supine (Fig. 6.**19c, d**).

Remarks

More reliable when performed under anesthesia. Too many tests may aggravate the problem of instability. This test usually precedes arthroscopy.

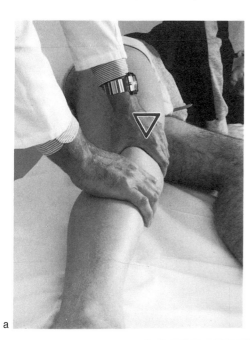

a

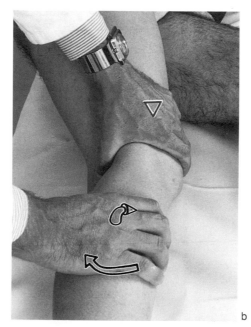

b

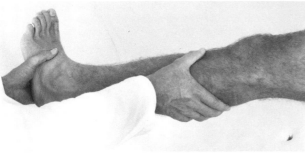

c

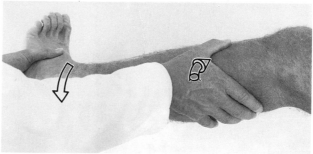

d

Joint: Knee

Examination: Test for anterior cruciate ligament, anterior drawer sign (ADS)

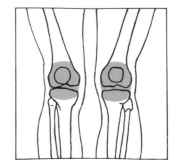

Performance

Supine position. Knee in 70°–90° flexion. Sit on foot. Palpate tibia plateau medial/lateral with thumbs (Fig. 6.**20a**). Test the tightness of hamstrings (should be relaxed!) by palpation with the index finger. Glide tibia anteriorly (Fig. 6.**20b**).

Remarks

Rotatory instability can be found by introducing rotation in both directions at the anterior drawer barrier.

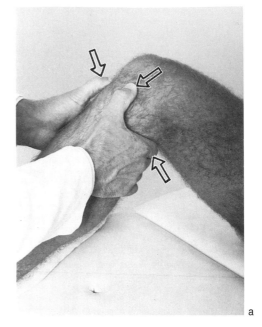

a

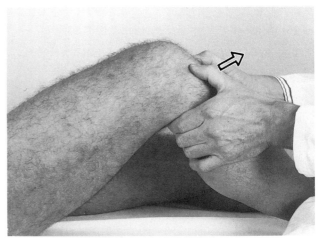

b

Joint: Knee

Examination: Test for posterior cruciate ligament, posterior drawer sign (PDS)

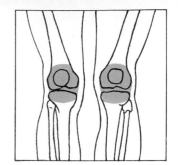

Performance

Posterior drawer sign (PDS). Supine position. Sit on foot. Grasp tibia and fibula close to knee joint (Fig. 6.**21a**) and glide tibia posteriorly (Fig. 6.**21b**).

Remarks

Posterior translation. Good hard stop is normal.

Note

In chronic posterior cruciate ligament (PCL) insufficiency, the tibia is subluxed posteriorly; posterior and anterior drawer can be misinterpreted!

Before testing, bring tibia to neutral position (thumbs on tibia plateau). In doubtful neutral position: lateral stress x-rays!

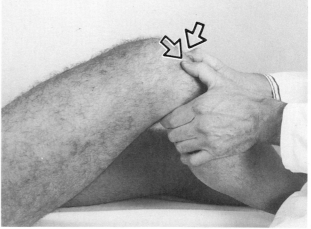

a

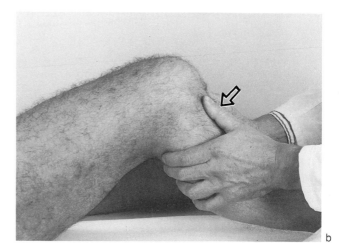

b

Joint: Knee

Examination: Traction

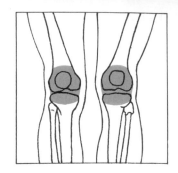

Performance

Patient supine. Knees on end of couch. Traction applied in approximately 45° flexion. Totally relaxed knee. Monitor joint line with fingertips, noting separation medially and laterally (Fig. 6.**22a**). *Three variations on technique.*

Slight medial (Fig. 6.**22b**) and lateral (Fig. 6.**22c**) rotations can be incorporated as well.

Possible Pathological Findings

Normally elastic end point. Reduced traction or hard stop, or both, may indicate osteoarthritis. Unstable knees are often painful upon stretching joint capsule.

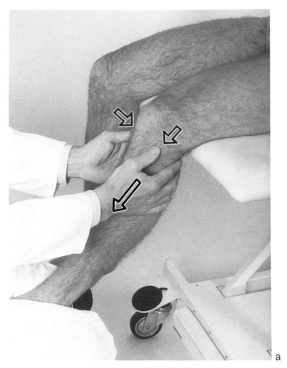

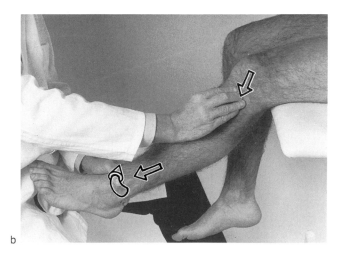

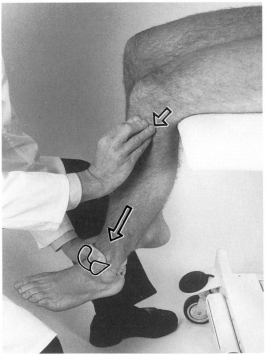

148

Joint: Knee

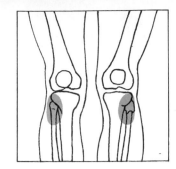

Examination: Translation proximal tibiofibula joint

Performance

Patient supine. Knees flexed and totally relaxed. Fixate tibia and translate fibula in anteroposterior direction (Fig. 6.**23**).

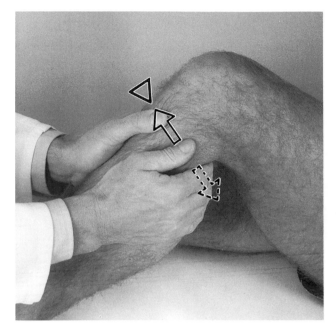

Possible Pathological Findings

Motion-induced pain with or without hard stop may indicate degeneration — good indication for mobilization therapy. Hypermobility.

Note

Peroneal nerve nearby can be compressed and painful.

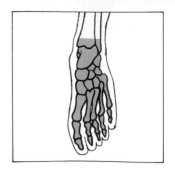

Examination: Inspection

Performance

Examine angulation at ankle joints and compare. Prominence of bony landmarks medial (Fig. 6.**24a, b**) and lateral (Fig. 6.**24c**) side. Observe gait — initiation and liftoff, pronation and heel strike.

Remarks

Inspection from behind: valgus angulation between foot and leg (Fig. 6.**24d, e**).

Inspection from below: look for body weight impression on skin (Fig. 6.**24f, g**). With body weight moved to forefoot, changes in subcutaneous pressure by blanching may be obvious (Fig. 6.**24h**).

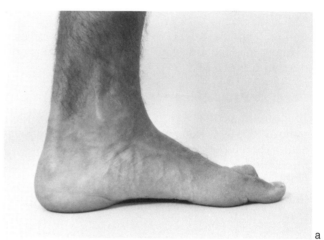

a

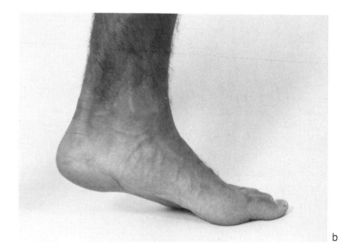

b

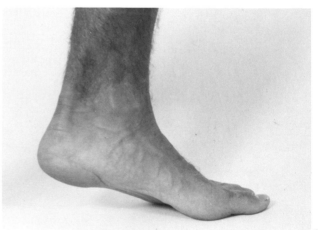

c

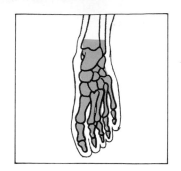

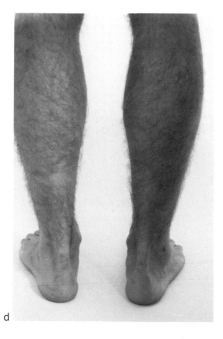

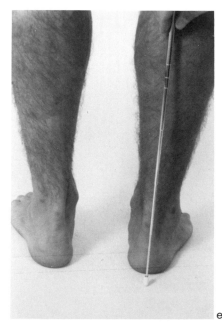

Fig. 6.**24**   d   e

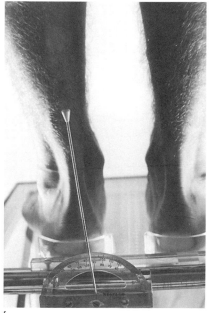

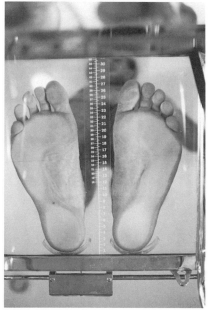

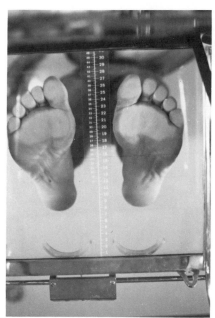

f   g   h

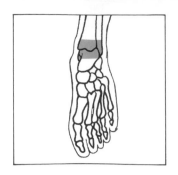

Examination: **Passive extension and flexion**

Performance

Heel is grasped with one hand, and foot passively moved in extension (dorsiflexion) (Fig. 6.**25a**) and flexion (plantar flexion) (Fig. 6.**25b**). The angles and quality of movement are observed.

Remarks

Extension should be 20°.

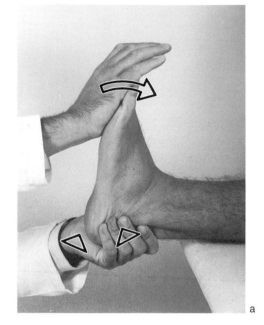

a

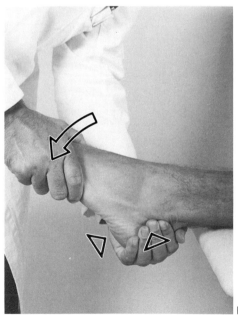

b

Examination: **Passive inversion and eversion (internal and external rotation) of foot**

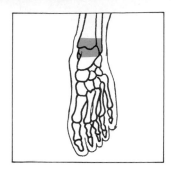

Performance

Subtalar joint and midtarsal joints all involved. Inversion (Fig. 6.**26a**) and eversion (Fig. 6.**26b**) movements performed with ankle and foot in neutral position.

Remarks

Midtarsal bones allow rotation and motion. Can be monitored. Patient can walk on sides of feet to demonstrate *active, internal, and external rotation.* Subtalar joint frequently involved in rheumatoid arthritis.

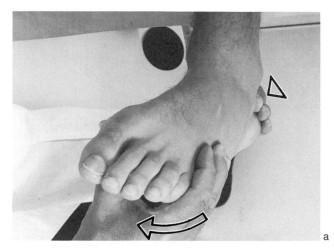

a

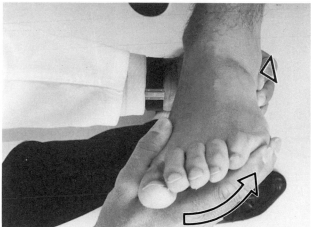

b

Joint: Ankle and Foot

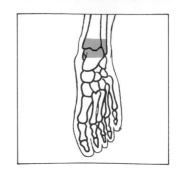

Examination: Anteroposterior translation of talus on tibia

Performance
Simple gliding action (Fig. 6.**27**)

Remarks
Anterior instability in case of fibulo-talar ligament insufficiency.

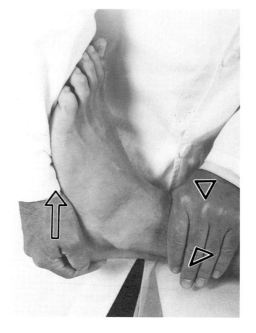

Joint: Ankle and Foot

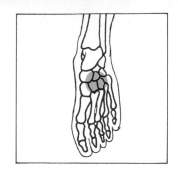

Examination: Identify and test extensor digitorum brevis

Performance

Dorsiflex (extend) actively and identify body mass of extensor digitorum brevis (EDB) (Fig. 6.**28**).

Remarks

Extensor digitorum brevis is the only muscle in the foot innervated by L5 nerve root. In nerve root compression of L5, this muscle becomes weak and atrophies earlier than tibialis anterior.

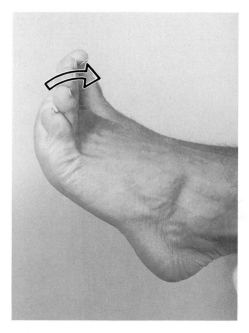

Examination: Dorsoplantar translation of midtarsal joints — navicular on talus

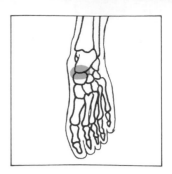

Performance

Fixate talus and ankle, then translate navicular backward and forward in a dorsoplantar direction (Fig. 6.**29**).

Remarks

Hard stop and pain in osteoarthritis. Usually reduced motion in arthritic conditions.

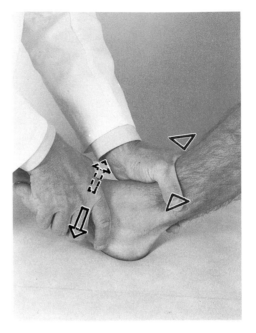

Examination: **Anteroposterior translation of midtarsal joints — cuneiform on navicular**

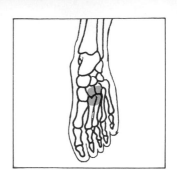

Performance

Fixate the talus and calcaneum, as well as navicular, between finger tips. Translate the cuboid backward and forward in dorsoplantar direction (Fig. 6.**30**).

Remarks

Hard stop and pain in osteoarthritis, usually with reduced motion.

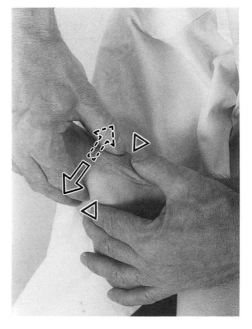

Examination: **Translation and angulation of cuneiform-metatarsal joints**

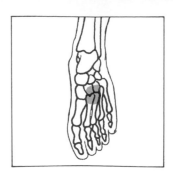

Performance

Two maneuvers:

1. The tarso-metatarsal (TMT) joint between the cuneiform and the first metatarsal is moved in dorsoplantar translation with slight traction (Fig. 6.**31a**).

2. Flexion and extension angulation movements are performed across the same joint with the same grip. Fix the proximal midtarsus and move the distal part (Fig. 6.**31b**).

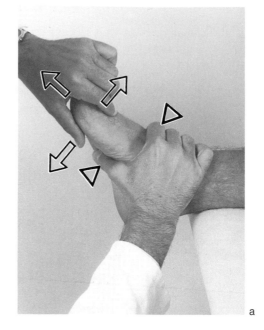

a

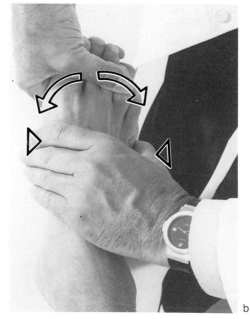

b

Joint: Foot

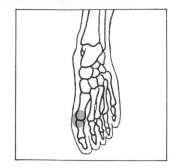

Examination: Angulation of first metatarsophalangeal joint

Performance

Fixate metatarsals between thumb and fingers. Angulate hallux with other hand (Fig. 6.**32a, b**).

Possible Pathological Findings

The "gout joint." Osteoarthritis common.

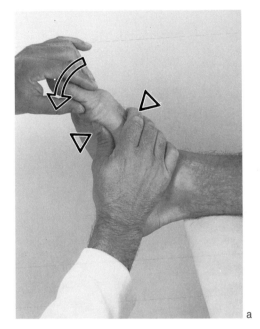

a

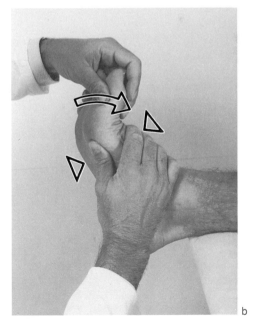

b

Joint: **Foot**

Examination: **Angulation of first phalangeal-interphalangeal joint**

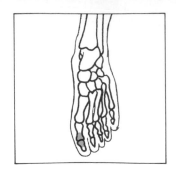

Performance

Fixate metatarsals and proximal phalanx with thumb and fingers. Angulate distal phalanx. Slight traction (Fig. 6.**33a, b**).

Possible Pathological Findings

Osteoarthritis common

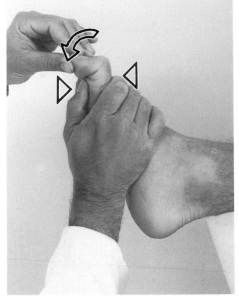

a

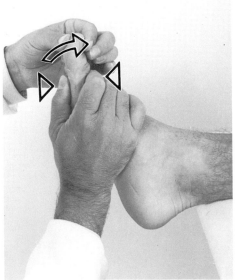

b

Joint: Ankle and Foot

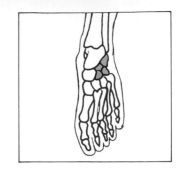

Examination: Dorsoplantar translation — cuboid on calcaneum

Performance

The joint line between calcaneum and cuboid is identified. The bones are firmly grasped as accurately as possible and moved relative to each other in dorsal and plantar directions (Fig. 6.**34**).

Possible Pathological Findings

Frequently dysfunctional following prolonged immobilization of ankle or foot, or both (e.g., ankle and lower limb fractures and plaster cast). Reduced range of motion and hard end feel usually felt with degenerative changes.

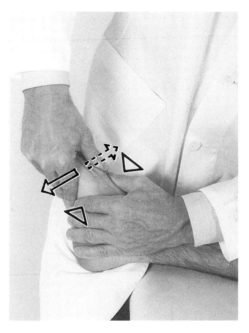

Examination: Dorsoplantar translation of cuboid and fifth metatarsal

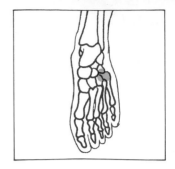

Performance

The cuboid and base of the fifth metatarsal are firmly grasped between thumb and fingers. The joint line between is identified. Dorsoplantar translation movements with some traction are carried out (Fig. 6.**35**).

Possible Pathological Findings

Reduced motion and hard end feel indicates probable degenerative change (usually late), or post-traumatic changes.

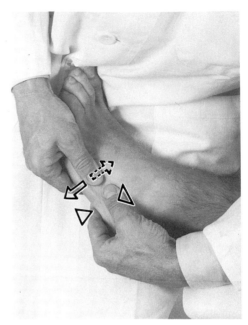

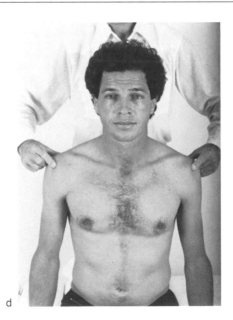

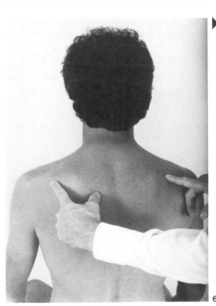

Fig. 6.**36**   **a**   Neutral position

b   Trapezius muscle palpation
c   Acromioclavicular joint palpation
d   Palpation of edge of acromion
e   Palpation of the scapula
f   Palpation of angulus scapulae
g   Passive abduction

d

e

Examination: **Surface anatomy**
Bony landmarks

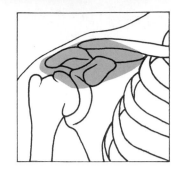

Performance

The patient is inspected from front and back. Landmarks are identified and compared bilaterally for symmetry and abnormality (Figs. 6.**36a–g**).

Remarks

Relate landmarks to vertebral segments.

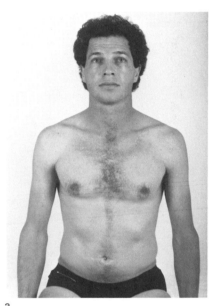

a

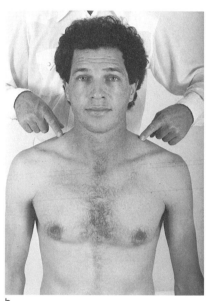

b

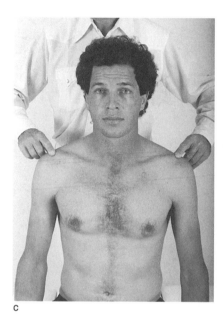

c

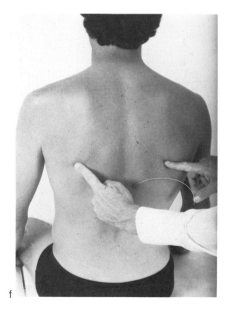

f

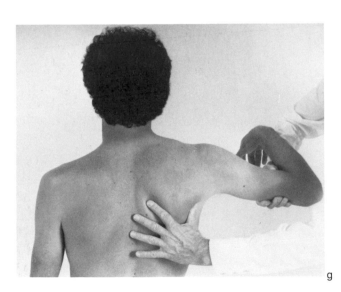

g

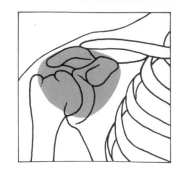

Examination: **Functional examination to give a rough evaluation of normality or pathology in the upper extremity within 1 minute**

Performance

Sequence of maneuvers from above to below (Figs. 6.**37a–f**) is efficient for patient and doctor. Differences in movements and surface contours are observed.

Remarks

All important shoulder, elbow, and finger movements are performed in these maneuvers. Pathology affecting a movement or movements is quickly identified. Restriction and asymmetry of mobility are visualized at once.

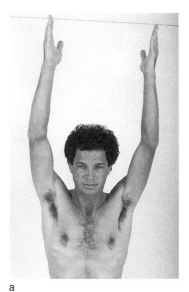

a

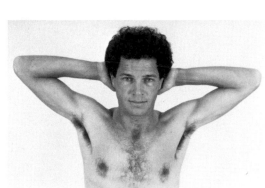

b

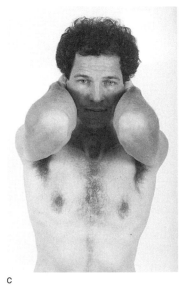

c

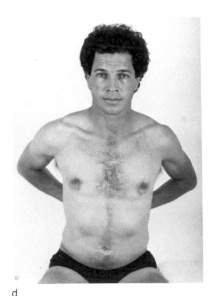

d

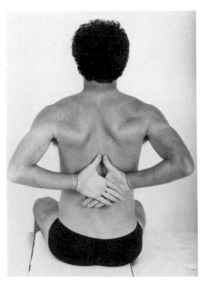

e

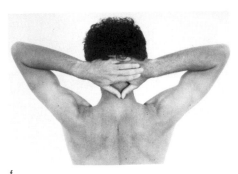

f

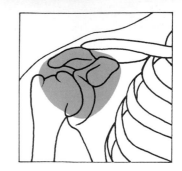

Examination: **Functional examination (continued)**

Performance

Figures 6.**38 a**—**e**.

Remarks

Neurological or primary muscular causes of abnormal movement are considered as well.

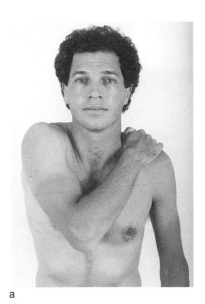

a

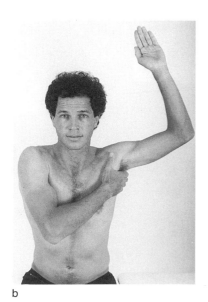

b

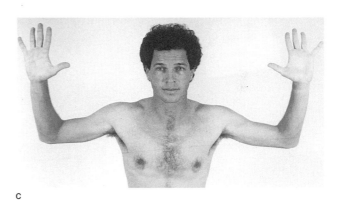

c

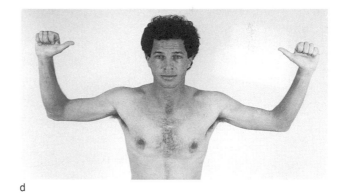

d

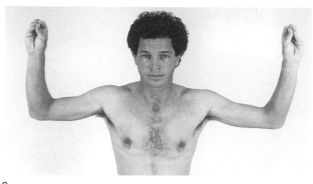

e

Examination: Passive internal and external rotation

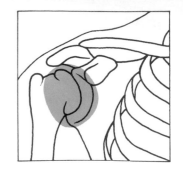

Performance

Examination of amount of passive external (Fig. 6.**39a**) and internal (Fig. 6.**39b**) rotation should preferably be tested in supine position.

Remarks

Most useful maneuver. "Throwing injuries" detected by examining in this position. While passively initiating throwing action, examiner suddenly resists the action to provoke pain response.

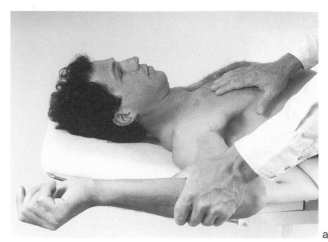

a

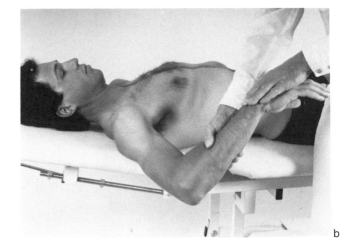

b

Joint: Shoulder

Examination: Passive internal and external rotation of glenohumeral joint

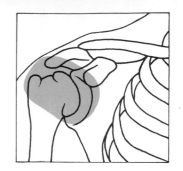

Performance

With the patient in a sitting position, the elbow is flexed and passive internal (Fig. 6.**40a**) and external rotation of the glenohumeral joint (Fig. 6.**40b**) are performed in maximum adduction. Monitor the range, quality, and end feel of movement with pincer fingertip palpation over the humeral head.

Remarks

Restricted motion, and pain, crepitus, and defects in the rotator cuff (in maximum adduction) may be felt. Hypermobility and apprehension if anterior joint structures are lax.

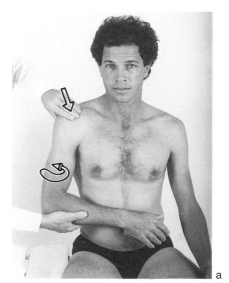

a

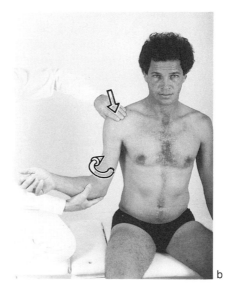

b

Joint: Shoulder

Examination: Painful arc for impingement

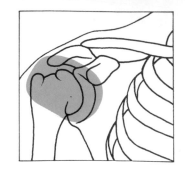

Performance

Active and passive abduction in the plane of the scapula (30−40° anteversion) is performed. Abduct the shoulder with elbow flexed to 90° (prevents rotation). Examiner monitors arc of painful movement and relates to muscles involved for that particular range of motion (Fig. 6.**41**).

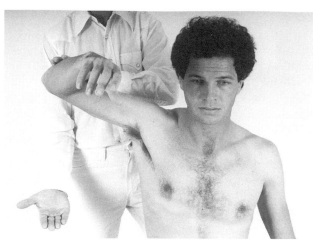

Remarks

Abduction 0°−60°: supraspinatus and deltoid mainly responsible. Abduction 60°−120°: deltoid, infraspinatus, and supraspinatus mainly responsible.

Painful arc between 60−120°: suspicion for subacromial impingement (calcific deposits, rotator cuff tear).

Note

The supraspinatus tendon and musculoteninous junction has to move under the arch formed by the acromion, coracoid process (defilé) during abduction to 120°. Impingement and compression causing a painful arc may occur. Superior translocation of the humeral head due to a more extensive rotator cuff defect where supraspinatus and infraspinatus are involved will predispose to this.

For the supraspinatus tendon, the Tobe test is more specific.

Examination: Upper painful arc

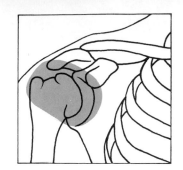

Performance

To achieve full elevation, the elbow is extended (Figs. 6.**42 a, b**). The lever arm becomes larger, and functional disturbances such as rotary cuff rupture become obvious.

Remarks

Serratus anterior mainly responsible for arm elevation 120°–180°.

Painful arc between 120–180°: upper painful arc; suspicion for AC joint involvement.

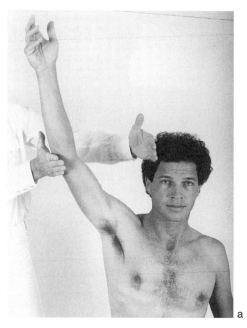

a

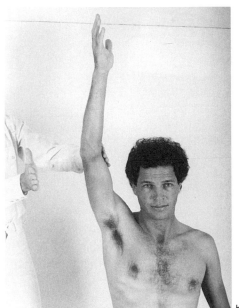

b

Joint: Shoulder

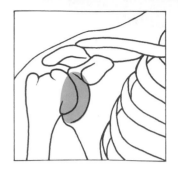

Examination: Strength test for rotatory cuff

Performance

Isometric contraction of each muscle group is symptomatically performed.

Test of external rotation strength against resistance possible for infraspinatus tear (Fig. 6.**43a**).

This is a more specific test for the infraspinatus muscle, in the plane of the scapula (abduction to 70°, arm flexed to 30°), with the elbow flexed to 90°. Isometric contraction in external rotation against resistance.

Abductor strength tested against resistance for weakness of rotator cuff (Fig. 6.**43b**); nonspecific—more muscles are involved.

Remarks

For more precise information, unilateral testing follows.

At the initiation of abduction, EMG confirms motor activity in the deltoid and supraspinatous from the beginning.

Possible Pathological Findings

– Rupture of tendon (infraspinatus)
– Neurogenic changes without inflammation
– Lesion of suprascapular nerve

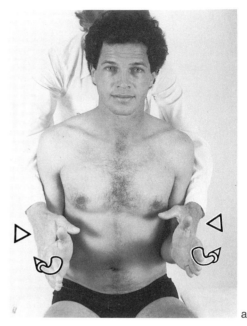

a

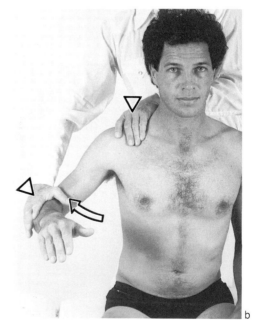

b

170

Examination: **Resisted internal rotation, bilateral and unilateral**

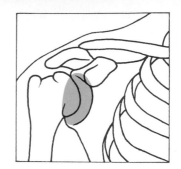

Performance

Elbow flexed 90°. Patient seated. Elbow stabilized by pincer fingertip grip. Internal rotation resisted (Fig. 6.**44**).

Remarks

Internal rotation equals function of anterior clavicular portion of deltoid, subscapularis, pectoralis major, latissimus dorsi, and teres major.

Internal rotation stronger than external rotation.

Resisting internal rotation provides more specific information on subscapularis muscle function.

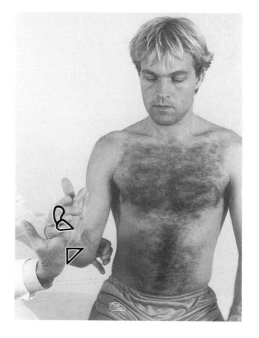

Joint: Shoulder

**Examination: Resisted flexion and supination at
elbow while palpating biceps tendon**

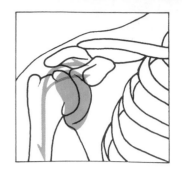

Performance

Patient seated. Elbow flexed 90°. Fingertip palpation
of biceps tendon at upper and bicipital groove.
Elbow flexion resisted (Fig. 6.**45**).

Remarks

Flexion and supination (palm up sign). Function of
biceps.

Irritation of the tendon is suspected if pain is evoked
during internal rotation under the palpating finger.

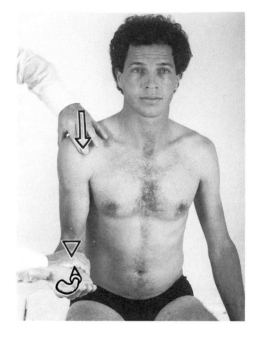

Examination: Instability apprehension test

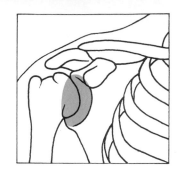

Performance

The arm is abducted to 60°. The monitoring fingers in the pincer "fingertip palpation technique" are placed over the rotating head of the humerus.

The thumb attempts to push the head of the humerus in an anterior direction while the index and middle fingers maintain a strong grip on the coracoid (Figs. 6.**46a**).

Passive external rotation of the arm is then carried out, with various degrees of abduction up to 120°−150° (Figs. 6.**46b, c**).

Remarks

This procedure can be performed with the patient supine.

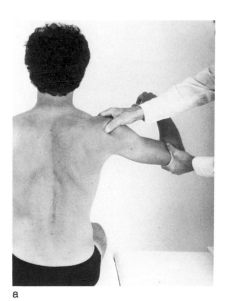

a

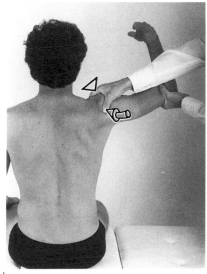

b

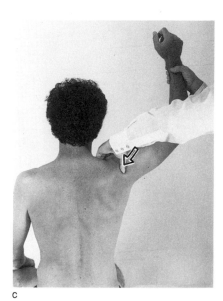

c

Examination: Glenohumeral instability

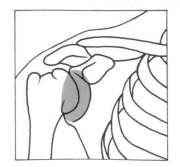

Performance

Patient supine. The examiner holds the upper arm (Fig. 6.**47a**) or forearm (Fig. 6.**47b**) with one hand. With the thumb and the other fingers, the humerus head is held firmly. Posterior and anterior translatory movement is performed.

Remarks

The anteroposterior stability is tested.

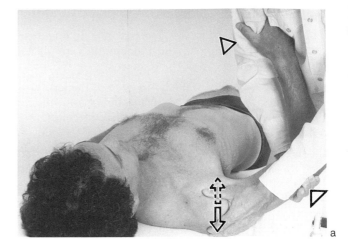

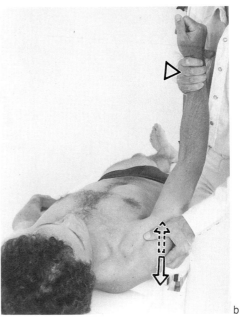

Joint: Shoulder

Examination: Glenohumeral instability

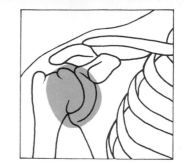

Performance

Patient prone. Holding the scapula, the humeral head is glided anteriorly over the articular surface (Fig. 6.**48**): apprehension? luxation?

Remarks

With anterior instability, the humeral head glides over the glenoid labrum.

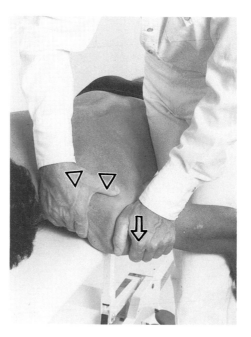

Joint: **Shoulder**

Examination: **Lateral traction**

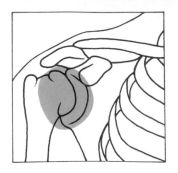

Performance

Approximately 30° abduction optimal. Elbow flexed to 90°. Fix scapula and clavicule. Axial traction: perpendicular to glenoid (Fig. 6.**49**). Avoid angulation (abduction).

Possible Pathological Findings

Distraction of 5 mm is normal. Hypermobility. Hypomobility. Restriction. Motion-induced pain.

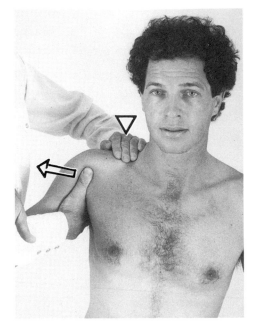

Joint: Shoulder

Examination: Translation in inferior direction

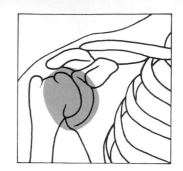

Performance

Seated position. Abduct to approximately 45° ("neutral zone") traction. Apply caudal glide using hypothenar (Fig. 6.**50**).

(Right hand pushing in inferior direction, left hand pushing back.)

Possible Pathological Findings

1. Crepitus and hard stop with pain indicates osteoarthritis.
2. Hard stop and decreased motion without pain indicates retraction and scarred capsule inferiorly.

Remarks

Attention to subacromial bursa and supraspinatus tendon. Hard grip may evoke pain.

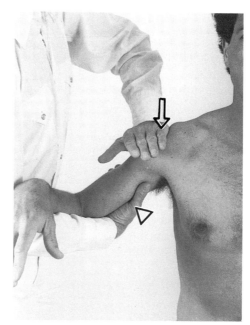

Examination: Translation in anterior – inferior direction

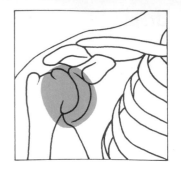

Performance

Two grips possible:

1. Anterior fixation with one hand. Axial traction (not easy to obtain). Try to get posterior hand under posterior border of deltoid. Glide forward. Fixing hand, medial aspect of axilla with extended fingers over pectoral tendons.
2. Posterior gliding hand grips humerus to translate, using thumb and patient's elbow close to examiner's body (pivot effect). More axial traction possible (Fig. 6.**51**).

Right hand with thumb in axilla for palpation of the head of humerus and its shifting downwards.

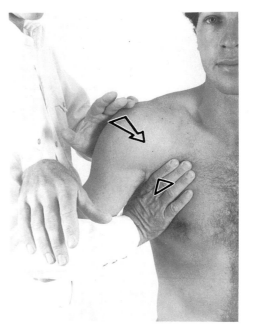

Possible Pathological Findings

Inferior instability (most common).
Hard stop and pain: osteoarthritis, osteophytes.

Examination: **Translation in posterior direction**

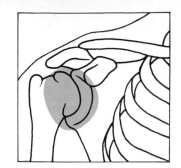

Performance

Two grips possible:

1. Seated or supine position. Some slight axial traction perpendicular to glenoid. Abduct to 35°−40° (greater abduction causes tuberosity to impinge under acromion). Apply gliding translation posteriorly using thumb along bicipital groove. Place thumb of posterior hand on the spina scapulae (Fig. 6.**52a**).
2. Alternative grip: apply translation force over anterior aspect of tuberosity using hypothenar (Fig. 6.**52b**).

Support flexed forearm to ensure relaxation.

Possible Pathological Findings

Posterior instability (less common than anterior instability). Trauma affecting posterior element. Osteoarthritis affecting posterior element. Pain and crepitus.

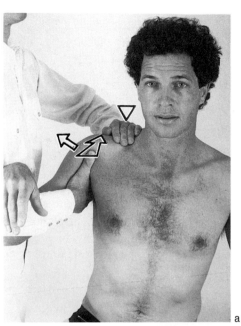

a

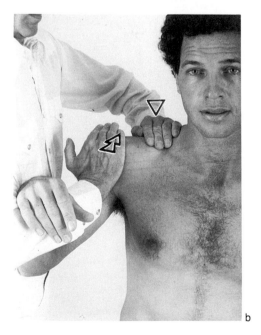

b

Joint: Shoulder

Examination: Translation of sternoclavicular joint

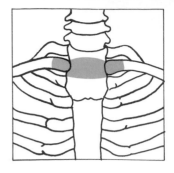

Performance

Cranial gliding achieved by thenar upwards under medial clavicle (Fig. 6.**53**).

Possible Pathological Findings

Motion-induced pain.

Note

Consideration is usually given to first rib following this procedure.

1. Identified by sidebending neck and monitoring first rib elevation.
2. Monitor first rib elevation during inspiration.
3. Palpate scaleni and monitor during inspiration. Scalenus medius is the strongest of the group.

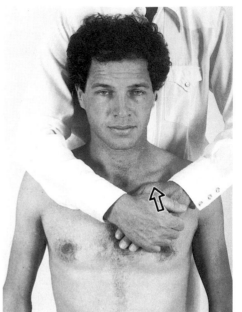

Joint: **Shoulder**

Examination: **Translation of sternoclavicular joint**

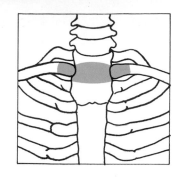

Performance

1. Try to avoid digging fingertips behind clavicle. Do not squeeze sternocleidomastoid muscle into bone. Place fingers behind the edge of the clavicle (Fig. 6.**54**).
2. Alternative: use the thenar across the medial aspect of clavicle, directing the gliding movement caudaly across the joint.

Possible Pathological Findings

Look for motion-induced pain. If painful, palpate for local tenderness.

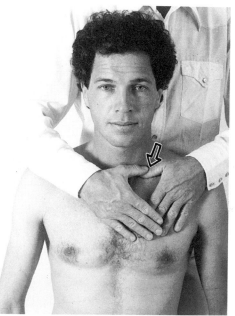

Examination: Translation of a acromioclavicular joint

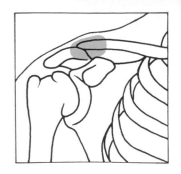

Performance

Hold (fix) the humerus head between fingers and thumb and perform anteroposterior gliding between thumb and the index finger of the other hand (Fig. 6.**55**).

Possible Pathological Findings

Evaluate motion, end feel, and motion-induced pain. Good fixation of the shoulder girdle is important for accurate information. Either clavicle or acromion may be fixed.

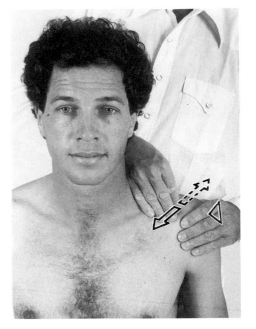

Joint: Elbow

Examination: Inspection

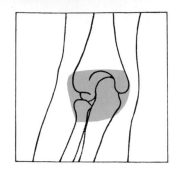

Performance

Both arms extended and supinated (Fig. 6.**56**). Degree of valgus 5°−10°.

Remarks

Observe carring angle: limitation to extension.

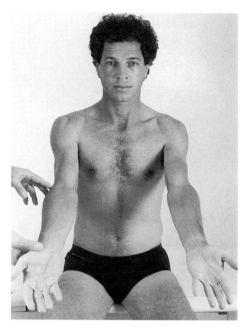

Joint: Elbow

Examination: Active flexion and extension

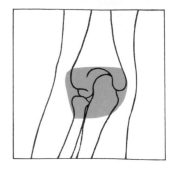

Performance
Move slowly.

Remarks
Observe range of motion. Look for hypermobility or motion restriction. Active extension 0° according to 0-Neutral Method (Fig. 6.**57a**). During flexion, the patient should be able to touch the acromioclavicular joint (Fig. 6.**57b**).

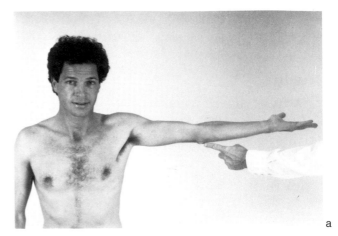

a

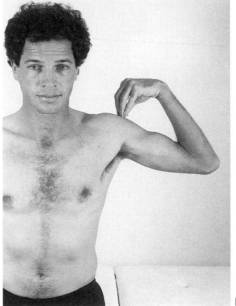

b

Joint: Elbow

Examination: Passive flexion and extension

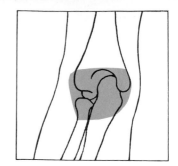

Performance

Passively move elbow slowly (Fig. 6.**58a**). Monitor end feel. Monitor joint behavior by fingertip pincer grip (palpation of joint line) (Fig. 6.**58b**).

Remarks

An increase in the range of motion over the active range is observed. Motion-induced pain indicates a pathological condition.

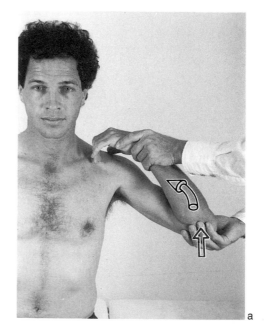

a

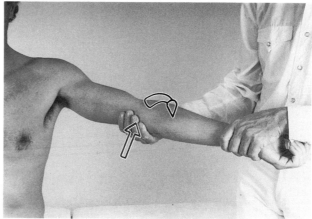

b

Joint: Elbow

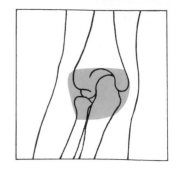

Examination: Varus and valgus stress to elbow joint

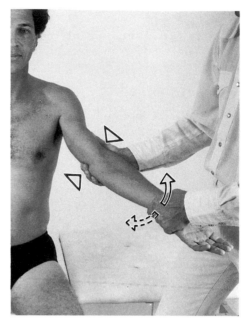

Performance

Fix distal end of humerus. Grasp wrist. Elbow in full extension. Gently stress (Fig. 6.**59**).

Remarks

Passive increase of valgus of 5° normal.

Examination: **Active and passive pronation and supination**

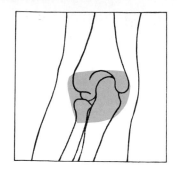

Performance

Can use pens grasped in both hands to measure pronation and supination.

Move arm slowly through pronation (Fig. 6.**60a**) and supination (Fig. 6.**60b**) in slightly flexed position (90°), monitoring radiohumeral joint with pincer fingertip palpation.

Remarks

Elbow in 90° flexion!

Range of motion normally 160°−180°. Look for motion-induced pain. Note when and where the pain is located. Innervate isometric contraction to provoke pain.

A slight increase in range of motion beyond the active range is normal.

Note

Hold isometric contraction against resistance for 30 seconds to try to provoke compression of the radial nerve in the supinator muscle. The forearm is held in pronation while the patient tries to supinate it against the resistance. This procedure causes pain in the proximal forearm (supinator muscle).

Isometric pronation may provoke compression of the deep branch of the median nerve. Less common (pronator teres muscle).

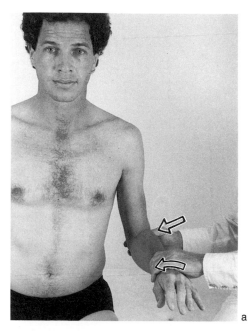

a

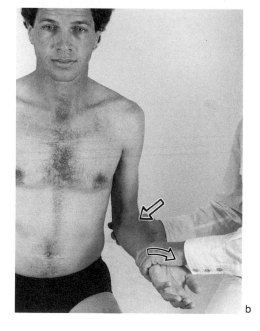

b

Joint: Elbow

Examination: **Passive pronation and supination**
Palpation of proximal radioulnar and
humeroradial joint

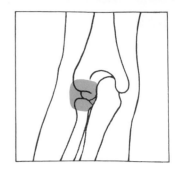

Performance

Arm slightly flexed. Passive movements (pronation/
supination) slowly from hand grasping wrist. Monitor
humeroradial joint (Fig. 6.**61**).

Remarks

Observe smooth rotatory movement at joint.
Restricted movement? Crepitus due to osteoarthritis.

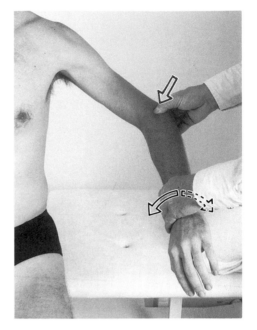

Joint: Elbow

Examination: Isometric contraction of wrist extensors against resistance

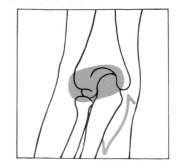

Performance

Monitor radial head with pincer fingertip palpation. Stretch extensors by wrist flexion (Fig. 6.**62a**). Isometric contraction of extensors (Fig. 6.**62b**). Gradually extend elbow, maintaining maximal wrist flexion (Fig. 6.**62c**).

Remarks

Should be painless. Radial head should rotate slightly. Pain may be provoked: myotendinosis?

Arthritic change of radioulnar or humeroradial joint.

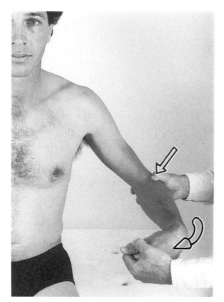

a

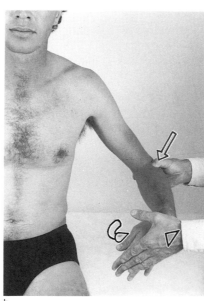

b

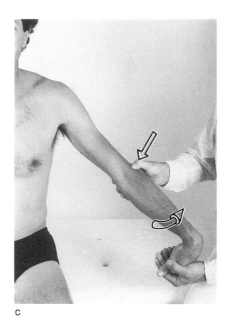

c

Examination: **Screening technique for humeroradial joint**
Monitor rotation of radial head

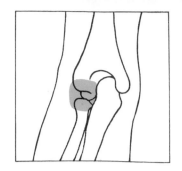

Performance

Elbows in 40° flexion. Both hands on examiner's hips (Fig. 6.**63a**). Examiner passively lifts elbows out and monitors radiohumeral joint between thumb and index finger (Fig. 6.**63b**).

Remarks

May vary the degree of elbow flexion (changes the degree of radial rotation: blocked when fully extended).

Note

No radiohumeral rotation is possible when the elbow is fully extended. Rotation takes place at the shoulder joint.

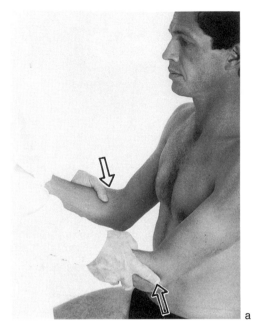

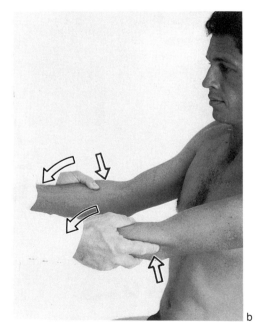

Joint: Elbow

Examination: Translation of proximal radioulnar joint

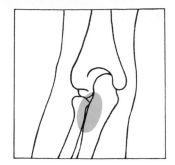

Performance

Patient supine. Examiner's thumbs on extensor aspect of elbow. Fix ulnar and move radius relative to it (Fig. 6.**64**).

Possible Pathological Findings

Pain in translation motion may be due to osteoarthritis. Look for restriction or increase in the motion range. Crepitus.

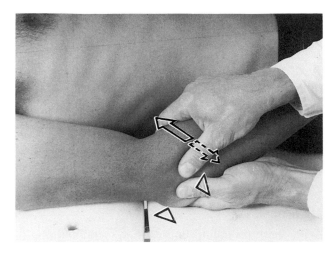

Joint: Elbow

Examination: Axial traction

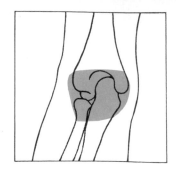

Performance

Patient supine. Elbow in the neutral position (approximately 30° flexion; 40° shoulder abduction). Axial traction using body weight, especially at humeroulnar joint. Monitor translation and motion-induced pain (Fig. 6.**65**).

Possible Pathological Findings

Look for hard end feel. Traction may diagnose pathology at humeroulnar joint by translation of the olecranon relative to the trochlea.

Note

With slight pronation and change of pulling grip to mainly over the distal radius, some additional movement is obtained at the proximal radioulnar joint.

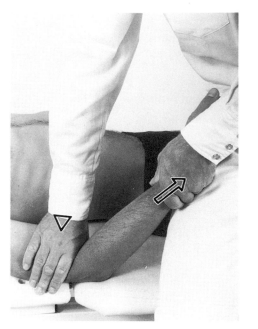

Examination: Palpation of elbow joint structures

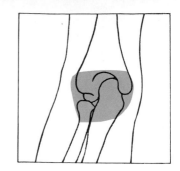

Performance

Palpation of ulnar nerve (Fig. 6.**66**).

Remarks

Thickening of nerve and lack of mobility. Subluxation/luxation of nerve out of sulcus with elbow flexion. Lateral displacement of the ulnar nerve by the triceps muscle in flexion.

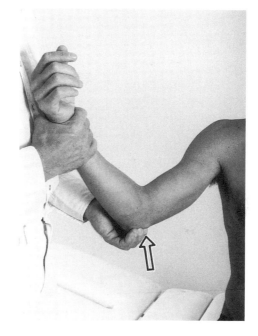

Joint: Wrist and Hand

Examination: General screening

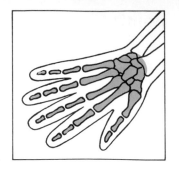

Performance
Make fist slowly (Fig. 6.**67**).

Remarks
Obtain information concerning proximal inter-phalangeal (PIP) joints and metacarpophalangeal (MP) joints. Observe and measure any inability to flex or extend wrist or isolated fingers. Fingers should touch the midpalm (distal crease of palm).

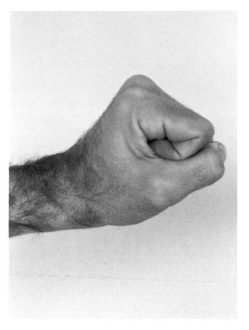

Joint: **Wrist and Hand**

Examination: **General screening movements**

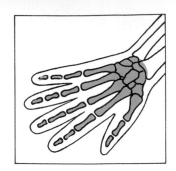

Performance

Approximate dorsal surfaces of hand and fingers as closely as possible with both wrists at maximal flexion (Fig. 6.**68**).

Remarks

Flexion of 90° at the wrists.

May diagnose posttraumatic degenerative changes of carpus and distal radius (i.e., fractures, nonunion of scaphoid, fracture of radius, ligamentous carpal lesions, aseptic necrosis).

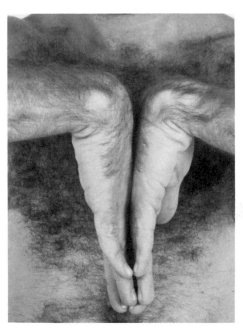

Examination: Tests for neurological integrity

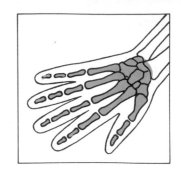

Performance

Various precise movements are performed as illustrated (Fig. 6.**69 a–h**).

Remarks

Peripheral nerve compression syndromes and other neurological causes of muscle weaknesses detected by lack of activity, often with atrophy of the affected muscle or muscles. Ulnar nerve usually implicated.

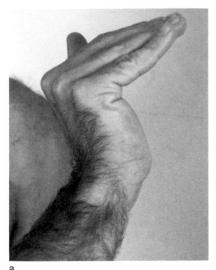

a

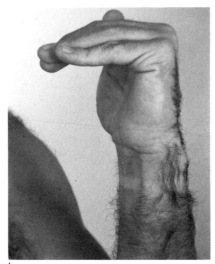

b

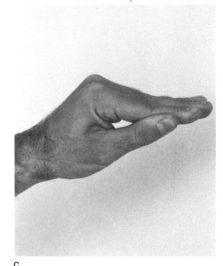

c

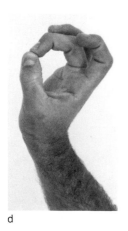

d

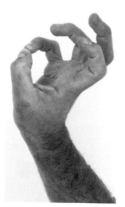

e

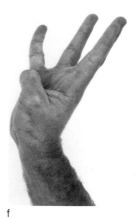

f

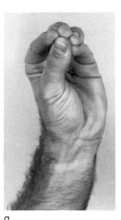

g

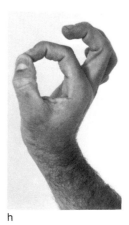

h

Examination: **Median nerve function to thumb (bottle sign)**

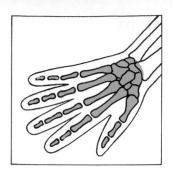

Performance
Should be able to grasp and hold a one liter bottle (or object of similar circumference) (Fig. 6.**70**).

Remarks
Bottle sign is mainly a test for the flexor digitorum profundus, superficialis for II and III fingers, as well as flexor pollicis longus muscle. Those muscles are innervated by medianus branches having the nerve trunk proximal to the carpal tunnel (pronator teres syndrome). For adduction of the thumb, both muscles, that is, interosseus dorsalis II (ulnar nerve) and adductor pollicis, are of importance.

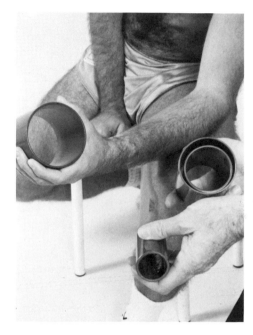

Examination: **Active and passive extension**
Extensor tendon palpation

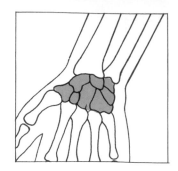

Performance

The patient should actively flex the finger and extend it slowly. Fingertip monitoring of the extensor tendons at the wrist ist carried out. This follows passive extension of the wrist (Fig. 6.**71**).

Remarks

Look for motion-induced pain, range of motion, and the presence of tenderness or crepitus, or both, over the tendons.

Nodules in the extensor tendons can be palpated with active flexion and extension of the wrist.

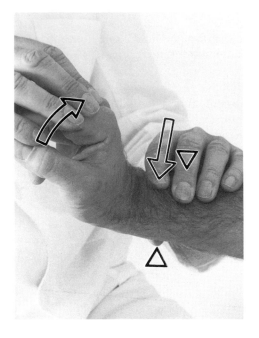

Examination: **Maximal flexion movements while palpating over carpal bones**

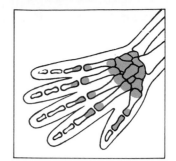

Performance

Isolated and increasing flexion movements are made at wrist, metacarpophalangeal joints, and interphalangeal joints. Fingertip monitoring of extensor tendons over wrist (Fig. 6.**72a, b**).

Remarks

Symmetry of metacarpophalangeal (MCP) joints in maximum passive flexion are observed. Pain or crepitus, or both, are noted over tendons.

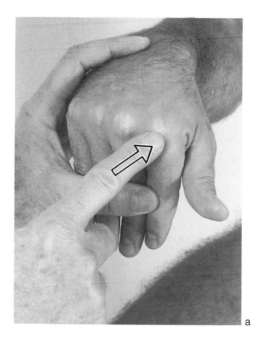

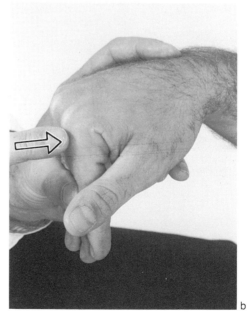

Examination: Passive flexion and extension of wrist

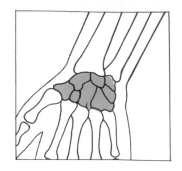

Performance

Holding the radius and ulna, passive movements are slowly induced. The radiocarpal (Fig. 6.**73a**) and ulnocarpal (Fig. 6.**73b**) joint are monitored.

Remarks

Motion-induced pain and motion restriction may indicate degeneration.

Carpal instability itself can seldom be detected; secondary degeneration must be looked for. Pain is typical of Kienböck's disease.

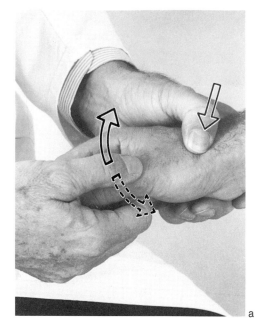

a

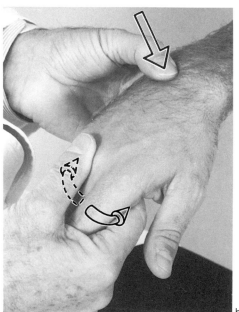

b

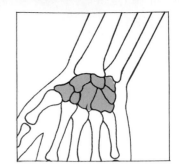

Examination: **Palpation flexor tendons**

Performance

The flexor tendons in the palm (Fig. 6.**74a**) and the flexor tendons at the wrist (Fig. 6.**74b**) are palpated in extension.

Remarks

Move the finger joints carefully and slowly to its maximal range.

This test is useful for the examination of tendovaginitis. During active and passive flexion and extension of fingers, crepitation (and pain at the annular ligament) may be evoked.

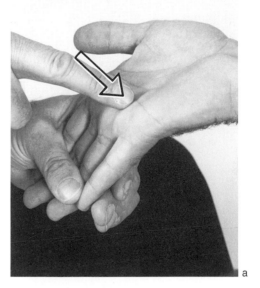

a

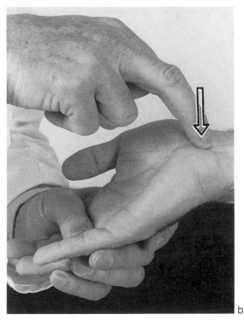

b

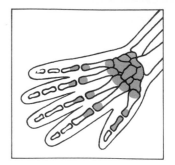

Examination: Selective extension of fingers with adjacent fingers fully flexed

Performance

Some wrist flexion facilitates finger movements (Fig. 6.**75a, b**).

Remarks

Inability to extend may indicate rupture or partial rupture of tendon, or a neurological cause. The index finger and the small finger have separate extensors in addition to the extensor digitorum communis.

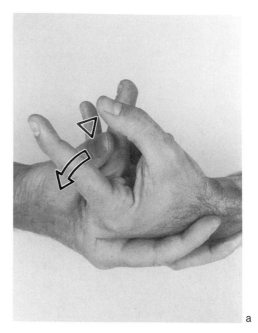

a

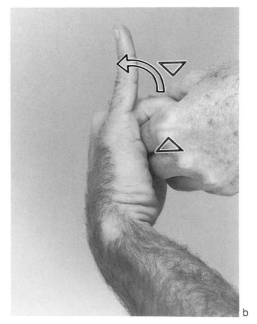

b

Joint: **Wrist and Hand**

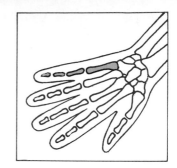

Examination: **Test ulnar nerve**
Abduction and adduction of fifth finger

Performance

Isometric abduction of little finger against examiner's fingertip (Fig. 6.**76**).

Active adduction of the little finger against resistance from the examiner.

Adduction (interosseus III muscle) is a more sensitive test for ulnar compression.

Remarks

Ulnar nerve integrity and function of abductor and interossei (especially of the third finger) observed.

Note

The third interosseus muscle gets weak *sooner* than the small abductor of the fifth finger. *First sign* in compression of C8 nerve root and consequent weakness of ulnar-innervated structures.

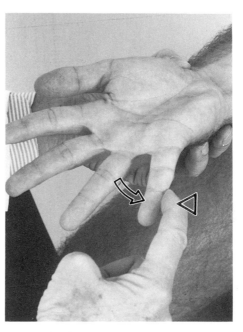

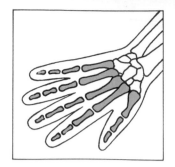

Examination: Test ulnar nerve (Froment sign)

Performance

Paper is grasped between each extended digit in turn, with the wrist in neutral position (Fig. 6.**77**).

Remarks

Test for ulnar nerve integrity. Hold the paper between fingers of both hands to compare relative strengths. Watch for compensating flexion of thumb on the weak side.

Note

Ulnar nerve pathology causing isolated muscle weakness in the hand is common in cobblers and users of short screwdrivers. "Loge de Guyon" syndrome.

With the Froment sign, the force of the adductor pollicis muscle is tested. If the force is reduced, compensation occurs due to flexor pollicis longus (median nerve) (flexion of interphalangeal joint).

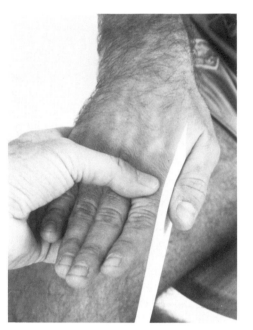

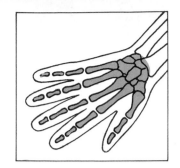

Examination: **Ulnar and median nerve compression**
                 Two-point discrimination
                 Phalen test

Performance

Various means of applying pressure from two discreet points are possible (Fig. 6.**78**).

Passive flexion of the wrist, held for at least one minute (Phalen test).

Remarks

Should be able to detect two points on the fingertips that are 5 mm or more apart. When the instrument is moved (moving two-point-discrimination), two points 3 mm apart should be detected.

A positive Phalen test provokes paresthesia in fingers I–III.

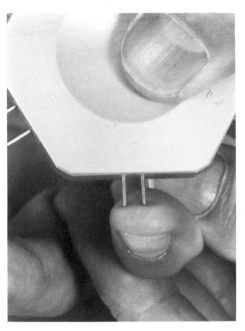

Examination: Measure passive motion at metacarpophalangeal and interphalangeal joints

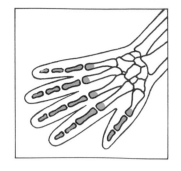

Performance

Passive flexion (Figs. 6.**79a–c**) and extension (Fig.
6.**79d**) movements performed and measured.

Remarks

Movements reduced in arthritis or posttraumatic conditions. Opposing tendon may be shortened (old
injury?).

Compare to active range of motion.

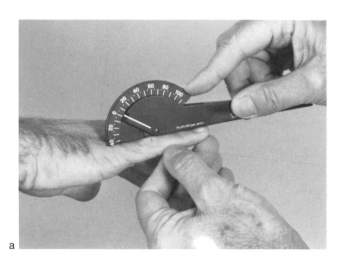

a

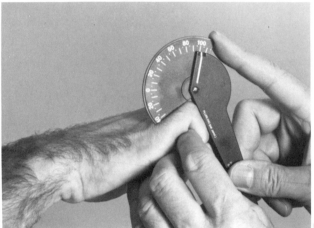

b

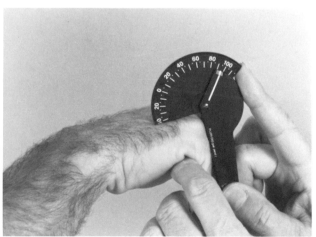

c

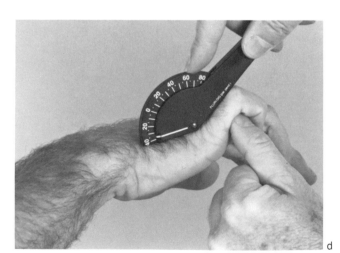

d

Examination: **Screening of finger power**

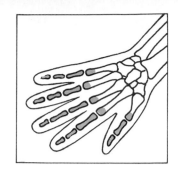

Performance

Various means can be employed to measure finger strength. Compare both hands. For closing the fist, the JAMAR meter should preferably be used (Figs. 6.**80a—c**).

Remarks

Suitable for monitoring, increasing, or decreasing weakness of follow-up after surgery.

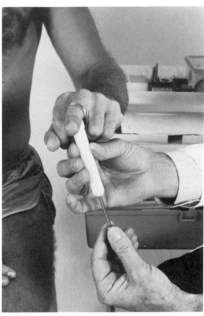

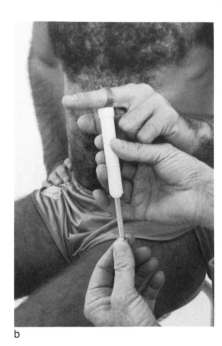

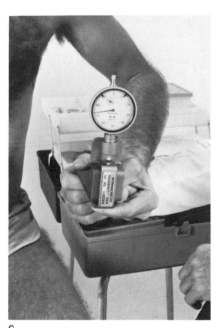

a

b

c

Joint: Wrist

Examination: Passive ulnar and radial deviation

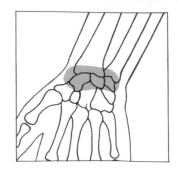

Performance

Passive movement slowly performed while monitoring scaphoid and triquetrum under fingertips. Each bone becomes more prominent on the convex side (Fig. 6.**81a, b**).

Possible Pathological Findings

A great amount of motion is possible. Motion-induced pain and restriction of motion may indicate degenerative changes and arthritis.

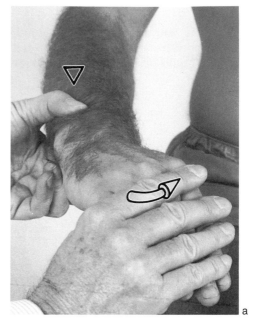

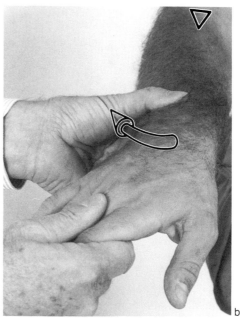

Joint: Wrist

Examination: Dorsopalmar translation of distal radioulnar joint

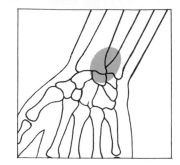

Performance

The ulna is fixed between the thumb and index finger while the radius is translated in palmar and dorsal directions (Fig. 6.**82**).

Possible Pathological Findings

Crepitus may indicate pathology in the ulnar triangular fibrocartilage complex region.

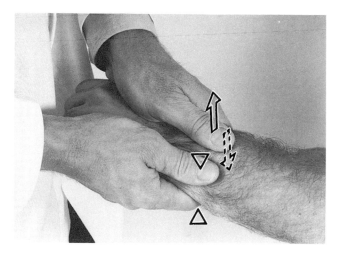

Joint: Wrist

Examination: Dorsopalmar translation at radiocarpal joint

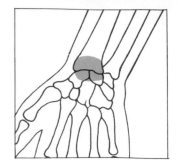

Performance

Examiner holds patient's wrist close to body. Wrist and hand are grasped firmly, keeping the hands as close together as possible. Wrist angulation easily occurs if examiner's hands are too far apart. Slight axial traction and slow translation in dorsal and palmar directions is performed (Fig. 6.**83**).

Possible Pathological Findings

Dorsal movement is less than palmar. Look for pathology (pain and crepitus) in the joint line between the radius proximally, and the scaphoid, lunate, and triquetrum distally.

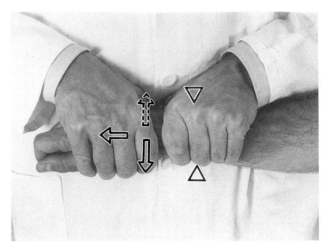

Joint: Wrist

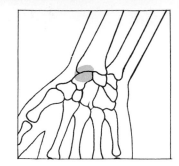

Examination: Dorsopalmar translation of scaphoid and radius

Performance

Hold radius firmly against body. Fix distal end of radius and translate scaphoid dorsopalmarly using slight traction (Fig. 6.**84**).

Remarks

Palmar movement normally greater than dorsal. Degeneration, posttraumatic change, and arthritis will reduce movement and cause pain. Note presence of crepitus.

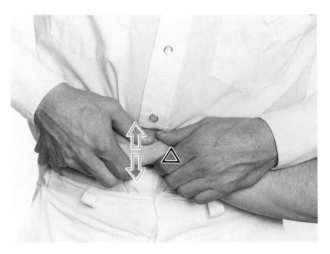

Joint: Wrist

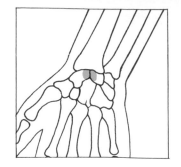

Examination: Dorsopalmar translation of scaphoid and lunate

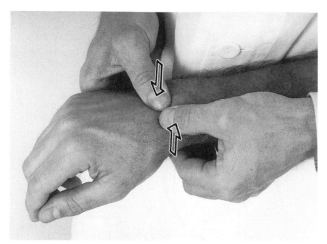

Performance

Fix scaphoid between thumb and index finger, and lunate with the same digits of the other hand. Gently translate bones relative to each other (Fig. 6.**85**).

Remarks

To distinguish scaphoid from lunate, flex wrist passively: lunate moves dorsally and can be felt more prominently. Note the presence or absence of pain and crepitus. Where instability or congenital looseness are present, there is increased mobility.

Joint: **Wrist**

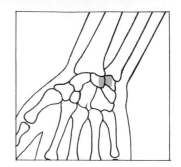

Examination: **Dorsopalmar translation of lunate and triquetrum**

Performance

Isolate bones and fix as accurately as possible between thumb and index finger. Translate relative to each other (Fig. 6.**86**). Triquetrum more difficult to isolate.

Remarks

Translation in palmar direction usually greater than in dorsal direction. Arthritis, especially osteoarthritis, common.

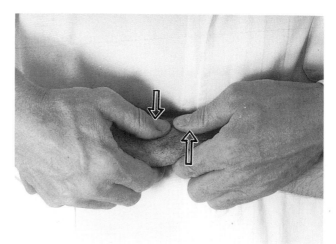

Joint: Wrist

Examination: **Dorsopalmar translation of trapezium and trapezoid against capitate**

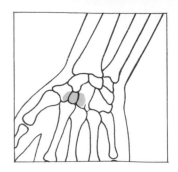

Performance

Trapezoid is difficult to isolate from trapezium. Fixate between thumb and index finger. Slight traction. Dorsopalmar translation.

Possible Pathological Findings

Reduced movement, pain, or crepitus. In the presence of instability, increased mobility may be palpated.

Joint: Wrist

Examination: **Dorsopalmar translation of capitate against hamate**

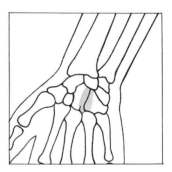

Performance

As for other wrist bones.

Remarks

Reduced movement, pain, crepitus. In the presence of instability, increased mobility may be palpated.

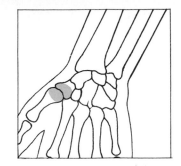

Examination: **Palpation of first carpometacarpal joint and translation in dorsopalmar and radioulnar directions**

Performance

Examiner holds patient's arm close to body. Fix trapezium and first metacarpal base between thumb and fingers of both hands. Slight traction, then slow translation in dorsopalmar and radioulnar directions (Fig. 6.**87**).

Possible Pathological Findings

Laxity of carpometacarpal joint I is a predisposing factor for basal joint arthritis and can be seen very often in cases of existing osteoarthritis.

Should be differentiated from traumatic subluxation or ulnar collateral instability of metacarpophalangeal joint (ski thumb).

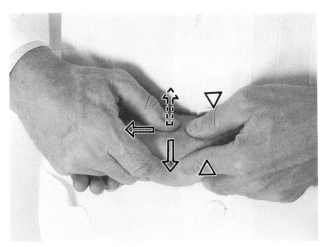

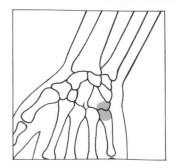

Examination: **Dorsopalmar translation at fifth carpometacarpal joint**

Performance

The joint between the fifth metacarpal and the hamate and capitate are examined. Grasp between thumb and fingers. Slight traction, then dorsal and palmar translation (Fig. 6.**88**).

Possible Pathological Findings

Look for motion-induced pain.

Note

1. Motion at 5th carpometacarpal joint normally greater than at the others.
2. Translation motion *between* metacarpals is minimal.
3. Same translation method is used between the 4th metacarpal and the capitate.
4. The 4th and 5th carpometacarpal joints are with the hamate and capitate.

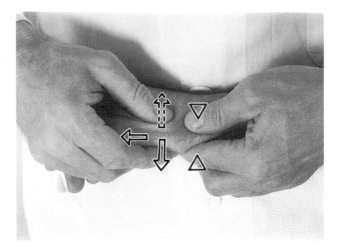

Examination: **Translation of metacarpophalangeal joints**

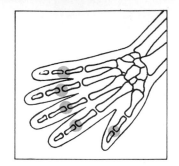

Performance

Hold hand close to body. Metacarpophalangeal joints in extension. Fix bones on either side of joint between thumb and fingers. Slight traction. Perform slow dorsopalmar and radioulnar translations on each joint (Fig. 6.**89**).

Possible Pathological Findings

Motion-induced pain, restricted motion, hypermobility consistent with trauma or arthritis. The 3rd metacarpophalangeal joint is commonly involved in osteoarthritis.

Joint locked in full flexion.

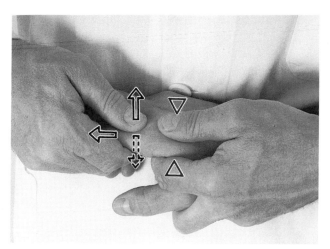

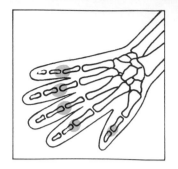

Examination: **Selective translation of all proximal interphalangeal joints**

Performance

Hold hand close to body. Fixate bones firmly on either side of joint. Slight traction. Slow dorsopalmar and radioulnar translations.

Possible Pathological Findings

Restricted movement, hypermobility, motion-induced pain, crepitus.

7 Zones of Irritation

The nature of the zone of irritation has been discussed in Chapter 3. Since the functionally abnormal position (segmental dysfunction) of a skeletal part cannot be visualized as such, it must be diagnosed by using its clinical presentation as well as its improvement after spontaneous or manual and therapeutic correction of the basic disturbance.

Therefore the zone of irritation acquires an important, as yet unmentioned property. Being an indicator for the spatially and functionally abnormal position of an axial skeletal part, the zone of irritation reacts by either increased or decreased intensity when the abnormal position is altered by specifically changing the relationship of the actual skeletal parts to each other. This process is also an important differential diagnostic technique for the latent zone (compare Chapter 3) that can be provoked and thus is called the test of provocation. The actual procedure is not the same for all zones of irritation and, for didactic reasons, is described along with the palpatory technique of the individual zones of irritation.

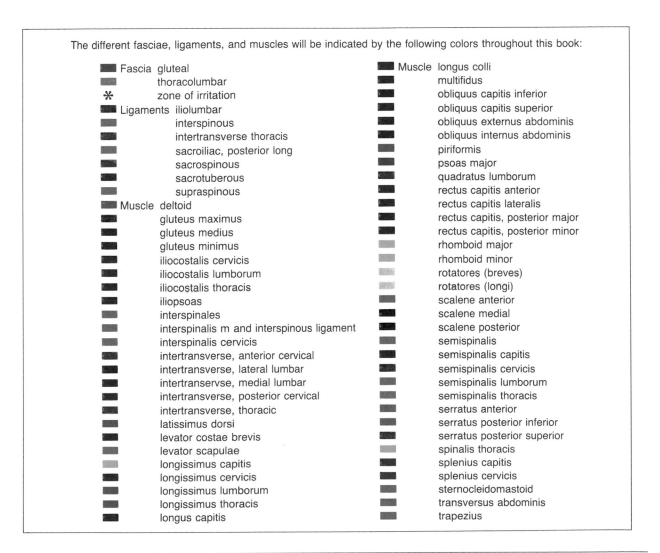

The different fasciae, ligaments, and muscles will be indicated by the following colors throughout this book:

Fascia gluteal
    thoracolumbar
    zone of irritation
Ligaments iliolumbar
    interspinous
    intertransverse thoracis
    sacroiliac, posterior long
    sacrospinous
    sacrotuberous
    supraspinous
Muscle deltoid
    gluteus maximus
    gluteus medius
    gluteus minimus
    iliocostalis cervicis
    iliocostalis lumborum
    iliocostalis thoracis
    iliopsoas
    interspinales
    interspinalis m and interspinous ligament
    interspinalis cervicis
    intertransverse, anterior cervical
    intertransverse, lateral lumbar
    intertranservse, medial lumbar
    intertransverse, posterior cervical
    intertransverse, thoracic
    latissimus dorsi
    levator costae brevis
    levator scapulae
    longissimus capitis
    longissimus cervicis
    longissimus lumborum
    longissimus thoracis
    longus capitis

Muscle longus colli
    multifidus
    obliquus capitis inferior
    obliquus capitis superior
    obliquus externus abdominis
    obliquus internus abdominis
    piriformis
    psoas major
    quadratus lumborum
    rectus capitis anterior
    rectus capitis lateralis
    rectus capitis, posterior major
    rectus capitis, posterior minor
    rhomboid major
    rhomboid minor
    rotatores (breves)
    rotatores (longi)
    scalene anterior
    scalene medial
    scalene posterior
    semispinalis
    semispinalis capitis
    semispinalis cervicis
    semispinalis lumborum
    semispinalis thoracis
    serratus anterior
    serratus posterior inferior
    serratus posterior superior
    spinalis thoracis
    splenius capitis
    splenius cervicis
    sternocleidomastoid
    transversus abdominis
    trapezius

In addition to the differential diagnostic significance, knowledge of the zone of irritation and of its reaction upon provocational testing is of decisive therapeutic consequence. With a well-planned manipulative strategy, the vertebrae in question are acted upon in such a direction as to achieve the decrease of the zone of irritation.

7.1 Zones of Irritation in the Cervical Spine Region
(Figs. 7.**3**, 7.**4**)

C0–C1

These two zones of irritation, situated in the occipital region, are related to the positional arrangement of the occiput and the atlas. They are located as follows.

C0 is lateral and superior to, and C1 is medial and inferior to the superior end of the mastoid notch (the bony part without muscles between the splenius capitis muscle and the obliquus capitis superior muscle).

When the atlantooccipital joint is in an abnormal position, these two zones of irritation are always present. Differentiation from other surrounding tendinoses is only possible with the help of provocative examination (see below).

The C1-zone of irritation can also be palpated at the lateral aspect of the transverse process of the atlas. The differentiation, however, from tendinoses of the numerous other muscles originating at this location is very difficult.

C2–C6

The zone of irritation located at the superior articular process is of practical importance. Since the muscular insertions at the transverse processes are often painful, the irritation zones in that region are only of theoretical significance.

For palpation, four fingers of the hand are placed over the spinous processes of C2–C6 and then reach in a hooklike manner for the strong semispinalis capitis muscle. A groove formed by the semispinalis capitis muscle and the longissimus capitis muscle is perceived (Figs. 7.**1**, 7.**4**). The fingers should be in as close contact with the bony structures as possible and should be able to feel the slight protuberance of the superior articular process (Fig. 7.**2**). In the neutral position, the superior articular process of C2 is one finger width below the occiput and about one finger width superior to the inferior edge of the spinous process of C2. The superior articular processes of C3 and C4 are each one finger width below. With maximal extension of the head, the zone of irritation of C4 is located at the lowest point of the concave cervical spine, whereas that of C5 is one and a half finger widths below that of C4 and two finger widths superior to the spinous process. The zone of irritation of C6 is one finger width below that of C5.

Since the head of the seated and totally relaxed patient can be moved in any direction with the nonpalpating hand (examiner is positioned behind the patient), fine joint play of the intervertebral joints can easily be examined with the finger, further facilitating orientation.

C7

The zone of irritation is more difficult to palpate, mainly due to the strong fibers of the trapezius muscle (descending portion) and the long, strong back muscles.

The transverse and the spinous processes of C7 (vertebra prominens) are located first. The zone of irritation is situated two finger widths above the spinous process and about one finger width medial to the tip of the transverse process.

Provocative Testing

All zones of irritation in the cervical spine region react upon provocative testing. A decrease of pain perception or any tissue change indicates the appropriate therapeutic direction for the segment being examined. It is to be noticed that most of the abnormal positions in the cervical region take place in the posterior direction. For instance, the zone of irritation increases posteriorly upon provocative testing and decreases anteriorly (Fig. 7.**6**).

Procedure: The index or middle finger rests over the zone of irritation, applying constant pressure. The pressure is such that the patient can barely feel the pain. The other hand embraces the parietal region of the head and introduces rotation to the left and right at the individual segments (Figs. 7.**7**, 7.**8**).

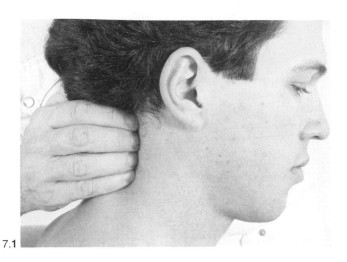
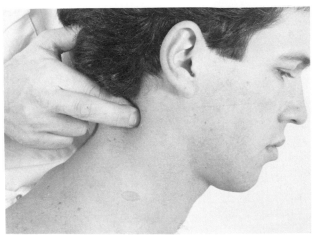

7.1

7.2

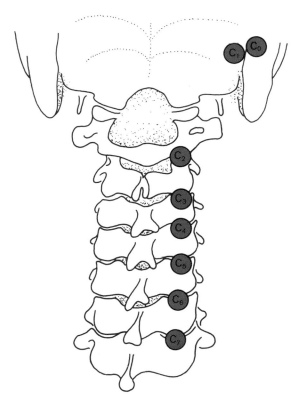

Fig. 7.3 Zones of irritation in the cervical spine region

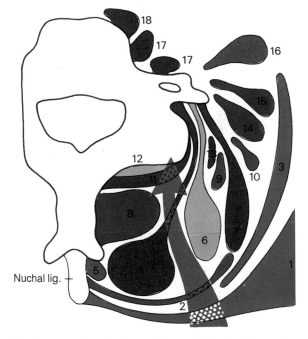

Nuchal lig.

Fig. 7.4 Cross-section of the central cervical spine. The arrow indicates the access to the zone of irritation (after Sutter)

1	Trapezius m	10	Splenius cervicis m
2	Splenius capitis m	11	Multifidus m
3	Sternocleidomastoid m	12	Rotatores muscles
4	Semispinalis capitis m	13	Iliocostalis cervicis m
5	Interspinalis cervicis m	14	Scalene posterior m
6	Longissimus capitis m	15	Scalene medius m
7	Levator scapulae m	16	Scalene anterior m
8	Semispinalis cervicis m	17	Longus capitis m
9	Longissimus cervicis m	18	Longus colli m

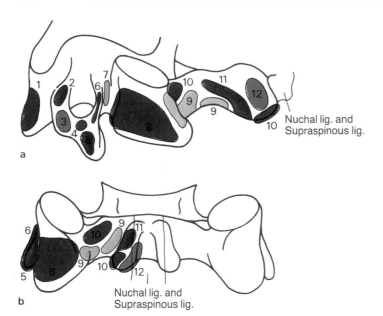

a

b

Nuchal lig. and
Supraspinous lig.

Nuchal lig. and
Supraspinous lig.

Fig. 7.**5**   Muscle origins and insertions at the midcervical vertebra

1 Longus colli m (inferior portion)
2 Anterior cervical intertransverse m
3 Scalene anterior m
4 Posterior cervical intertransverse m (lateral portion)
5 Scalene medius m
   Levator scapulae m
   Splenius cervicis m
   Iliocostalis cervicis m
   Longissimus cervicis and capitis m
6 Posterior cervical intertransverse m (medial portion)
7 Longissimus capitis m
8 Semispinalis capitis m
9 Rotatores muscles
10 Multifidus m
11 Semispinalis cervicis m
12 Interspinalis cervicis m

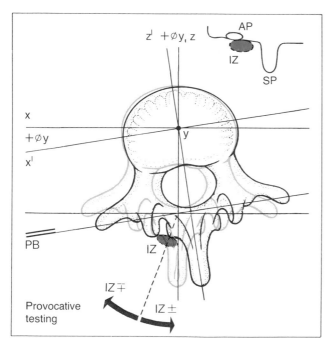

Fig. 7.**6**   Provocative testing for quantitative changes in the zone of irritation

IZ   Irritation zone
SP   Spinous process
AP   Articular process
PB   Pathologic limit to movement
$Z–Z' = +\emptyset y$
$X–X' = +\emptyset y$

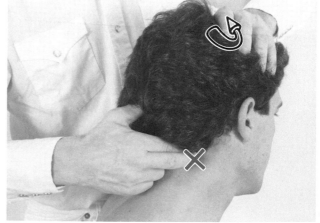

7.7

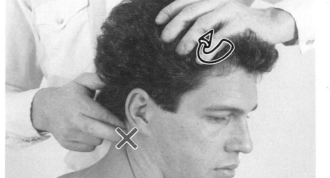

7.8

7.2 Zones of Irritation in the Region of the Thoracic Spine, Ribs, and Sternum

The relaxed patient is in the prone position. For better control, the thoracic kyphosis is accentuated by adjusting the examination table. The patient's arms hang either freely over the edge of the table or the elbows are spread so that the shoulder blades draw somewhat apart from the midline.

Thoracic Spine

In the thoracic spine, the irritational zone at the transverse process is of practical importance (Fig. 7.**12**). It can be located as follows: the thumb moves laterally along the rib toward the transverse process of the thoracic vertebra (Fig. 7.**9**). Two to three finger widths lateral to the spinous process it meets the massive muscle structure of the longissimus system, which is gently pushed medially (Fig. 7.**10**).

During this procedure, the thumb reaches a region where the rib disappears below the transverse process (Figs. 7.**12**, 7.**14**). The zone of irritation (1 to 2 cm long) located here presents itself as a nonmoveable, painful threshold. It should be noted that the palpatory pressure is applied in the lateral direction in order to avoid confusion with tendinoses of the longissimus thoracis muscle.

To determine the correct level, orientation is at the spinous processes. In the central thoracic spine region, the distance between the inferior margin of the spinous process and the superior margin of the transverse process of the same vertebra measures three finger widths and decreases to two finger widths when moving either superiorly or inferiorly (verify on a skeleton).

Provocative Testing

The palpating thumb remains over the zone of irritation, while the hypothenar of the other hand presses on the spinous process from the opposite side. If the zone of irritation does not decrease, pressure from either a superior or inferior direction is applied. Consequently, the behavior of the zone of irritation allows differentiation between an abnormal rotatory position and a possible ventralization of the vertebra.

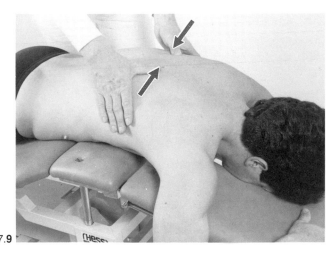

7.9

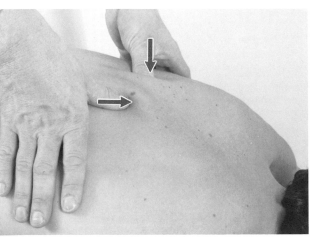

.10

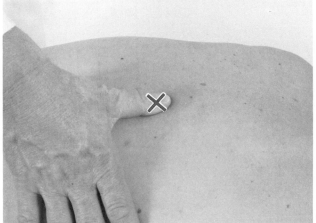

7.11

Ribs

The zones of irritation at the ribs lie in the region of the costal angle between the longissimus thoracis muscle and the iliocostalis thoracis muscle (Fig. 7.**12**).

The position of the patient for this examination is the same as for that of the thoracic spine.

About two finger widths lateral to the transverse process, the thumb presses vertically trying to get between both muscles to establish as close a contact with the bony structures as possible; the direction is posteroinferior. If a zone of irritation is present, little pressure is sufficient to cause pain (Fig. 7.**11**).

Provocative Testing

The thumb rests over the zone of irritation, exerting constant minimal pressure sufficient to cause pain.

The index finger of the other hand is placed with its whole surface over the corresponding rib, with the palpatory pressure in the sternal direction. If the zone of irritation does not decrease, pressure is changed toward the transverse process.

Sternum

When examining the zones of irritation of the ribs, the sternal zones of irritation should also be inspected. They are situated on the midline between the jugular notch and the xiphoid process (Fig. 7.**13**). Objective palpatory perception is often impossible, and thus the patient's specification about pain must be relied upon.

These zones of irritation also react upon provocative testing. The procedure is similar to that performed for the ribs.

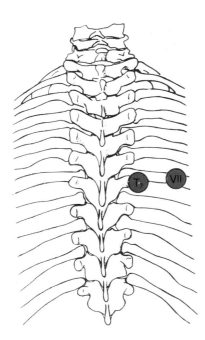

Fig. 7.**12** Zones of irritation in the region of the thorax and ribs (example: T7)

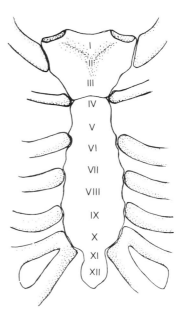

Fig. 7.**13** Regions of the individual zones of irritation of the ribs at the sternum

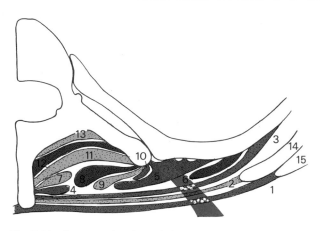

1 Trapezius m
2 Rhomboid minor and major m
3 Serratus posterior superior m
4 Splenius cervicis m
5 Longissimus thoracis m
6 Iliocostalis thoracis m
7 Spinalis m
8 Semispinalis capitis m
9 Longissimus capitis m
10 Longissimus cervicis m
11 Semispinalis thoracis m
12 Multifidus m
13 Rotatores muscles
14 Body of scapula
15 Spine of scapula

Fig. 7.14 Cross-section through the upper central thoracic spine. Arrow indicates access to the zone of irritation (after Sutter)

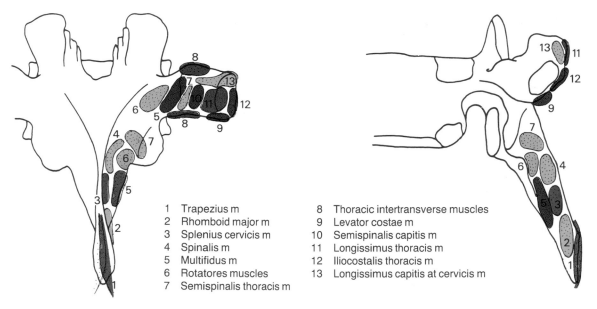

1 Trapezius m	8 Thoracic intertransverse muscles
2 Rhomboid major m	9 Levator costae m
3 Splenius cervicis m	10 Semispinalis capitis m
4 Spinalis m	11 Longissimus thoracis m
5 Multifidus m	12 Iliocostalis thoracis m
6 Rotatores muscles	13 Longissimus capitis at cervicis m
7 Semispinalis thoracis m	

Fig. 7.15 Muscle origin and insertions at the central thoracic vertebra

7.3 Zones of Irritation in the Lumbar Spine Region

L1–L4

In the L1–L4 region, the zones of irritation located at the costal processes are of practical significance. The relaxed patient rests in the prone position on the examination table. The palpating finger reaches and follows the iliocostalis muscle laterally, including the whole sacrospinal system, and continues between this muscle and the inferior abdominal muscles, finally terminating at the tip of the transverse process (Figs. 7.**16**, 7.**17**, 7.**19**). If the patient is not obese, good contact with the bone is possible, and the examiner searches for pathological painful resistance. With muscular or obese patients, the examiner relies rather on provocative testing and the consequent manifestation and alteration of pain.

The transverse process of L4 is normally located at the level of the iliac crest. The transverse processes of L3, L2 and L1 each lie two finger widths superior to the vertebra below, respectively. In other words, they can be found at the level of the lower pole of the spinous process of the vertebra immediately above. Due to its anatomical position, the costal process of L5 cannot be palpated easily (Fig. 7.**15**).

It is often impossible to make a distinction between the numerous tendinoses of the lateral lumbar inter-transverse muscles and the quadratus lumborum muscle. Thus, the examiner should look either for spondylogenically correlated tendinoses, for instance in the gluteus medius and gluteus maximus muscles, or for the mirror image tendinoses at the opposing poles of the involved muscles.

The zones of irritation are localized at the lateral aspect of the inferior pole of the spinous processes. The differentiation between tendinoses of the latissimus dorsi muscle and the posterior inferior serratus muscle is only possible with provocative testing. The zones of irritation at the superior articular processes are mentioned here for completeness and are only of theoretical value due to their proximity to the mamillary processes and the corresponding origins of the transversospinal and sacrospinal musculature.

L5

The zone of irritation of L5 is located above the flat, posterior inferior iliac spine, which can barely be palpated. It is found one finger width lateral and inferior to the prominent PSIS (Fig. 7.**18**).

Provocative Testing

The thumb remains with constant pressure over the zone of irritation while the other hand rests at the thoracolumbar junction and slowly increases the pressure in an anteroinferior direction. As a result, the abnormal position of the posteriorly displaced vertebra is corrected in part; the zone of irritation decreases.

If neither pain nor palpatory manifestation decrease, it is assumed that the abnormal vertebral position is in the anterior direction. This situation is often seen as the result of the static configuration of the lumbar spine and the influence of the psoas major muscle. Diagnostically to identify this abnormal position correctly, the prone patient is positioned over a rubber ball and is asked to relax totally; the zone of irritation should decrease.

The therapeutic correction for the anteriorly displaced thoracic vertebra is achieved with the hand of an assistant, which exerts a constant pressure transabdominally on the vertebra during manipulation.

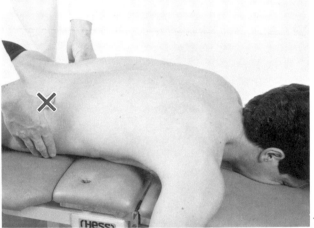

7.16

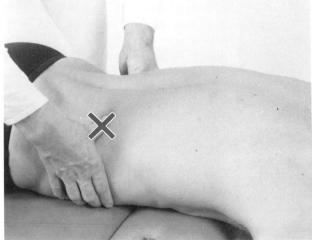

7.17

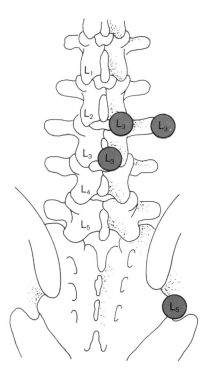

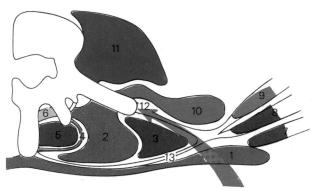

Fig. 7.**19**   Cross-section through the lumbar spine. Arrow indicates access to the zone of irritation (after Sutter)

1   Latissimus dorsi m
2   Longissimus thoracis m
3   Iliocostalis lumborum m
4   Semispinalis lumborum m
5   Multifidus m
6   Rotatores muscles
7   External abdominal oblique m
8   Internal abdominal oblique m
9   Transversus abdominis m
10   Quadratus lumborum m
11   Psoas major m
12   Thoracolumbar fascia (deep layer)
13   Thoracolumbar fascia (superficial layer)

Fig. 7.**18**   Zones of irritation in the lumbar spine region (example: L3)

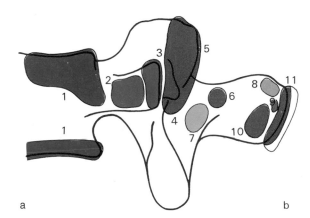

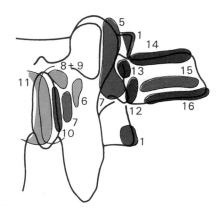

Fig. 7.**20**   Muscle origins and insertions at a lumbar vertebra

1   Psoas major m
2   Quadratus lumborum m (deep, anterior, layer)
3   Quadratus lumborum m (superficial, posterior layer)
4   Longissimus lumborum m (medial line of insertion)
5   Longissimus thoracis m
    Semispinalis lumborum m
    Multifidus m
    Rotatores muscles (origin)
6   Rotator m (insertion)
7   Multifidus m

8   Spinalis m
9   Interspinalis lumborum m
10   Longissimus thoracis m
11   Latissimus dorsi m
12   Medial lumbar intertransverse m (origin)
13   Medial lumbar intertransverse m (insertion)
14   Lateral lumbar intertransverse m (origin)
15   Longissimus lumborum m (lateral insertions)
16   Lateral lumbar intertransverse m (insertion)

7.4 Zones of Irritation of the Sacrum (Sacroiliac Joint) and the Pelvis

The zones of irritation of S1—S3 can easily be palpated by the beginner due to their anatomical location and relationship to the surrounding musculature. They react impressively upon provocative testing ("ventral-testing" according to Sutter).

The zones of irritation are localized in the region of the articulating tubercle of the sacrum, between the posterior inferior iliac spine and the cornu of the sacrum. The S1 zone of irritation lies about 1 cm medial to the posterior inferior iliac spine, the irritation zone of S3 proximally to the sacral horn, and the irritation zone of S2 between these two (Fig. 7.**21**).

The relaxed patient rests in the prone position on the examination table. Before palpation is started, the bony structures, such as the iliac crest, the posterior superior iliac spine, the free lateral angle of the sacrum, and the spinous processes of L5 and S1 are located exactly and are marked on the skin with a pen for better orientation (Fig. 7.**22**).

After the free lateral angle of the sacrum has been identified, the thumb that is used for palpation presses down vertically onto the amuscular, bony part, right between the erector spinae and the gluteus maximus muscles (Fig. 7.**23**). These muscles are incased in separate fasciae, almost forming a groove. This provides a close bony contact for palpation (Fig. 7.**25**). Multiple zones of irritation are seldom found at the sacrum, simultaneously. Since each irritational zone pattern calls for an appropriate therapeutic procedure, this region must be examined very carefully.

Provocative Testing for the Sacral Irritational Zones (Sacroiliac Region)

The zone of irritation in the SIJ region presents itself as a distinctly doughy, painful swelling that disappears when the hypothenar of the nonpalpating hand exerts pressure on the sacrum in the anterior direction. When the hand is removed, it reappears, concomitant with stabbing pain.

During this ventralization maneuver, the thumb that is used for palpation must remain at the irritational zone exerting constant pressure (Fig. 7.**24**).

When examining the SIJ, the symphyseal irritational zones should be located as well (Fig. 7.**26**). They are situated at the junction of the symphyseal cartilage and the pubic bone. Constructing a line paramedially to the symphysis, the zone of irritation of S1 lies at the superior pole, the zone of irritation of S2 lies in the center, and the S3 irritation zone lies at the inferior pole of the symphysis.

Provocative Testing for the Symphyseal Zones of Irritation

The finger rests over the zone of irritation. The ipsilaterally flexed thigh of the patient is first abducted then adducted. Since the examiner will not be able to palpate any abnormality, the patient's information concerning pain must be relied upon. If the zones of irritation are confined to the sacrum only, the disturbance is very likely limited to the SIJ. However, if symphyseal irritational zones exist, a disturbance in the pelvic region is indicated (hip bones and sacrum).

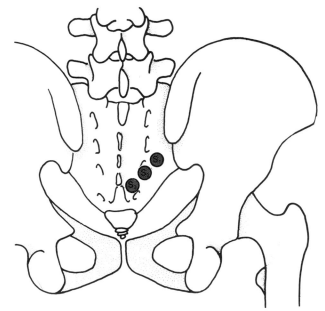

Fig. 7.**21** Zones of irritation at the sacrum

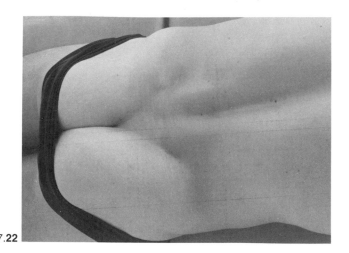

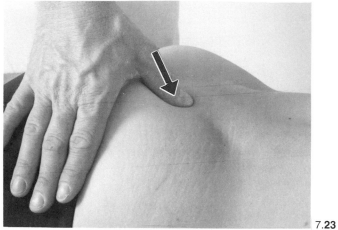

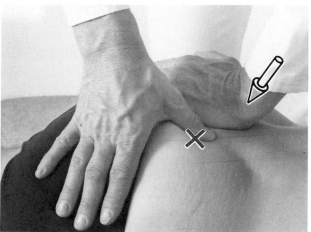

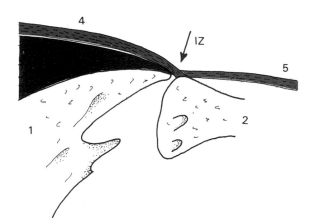

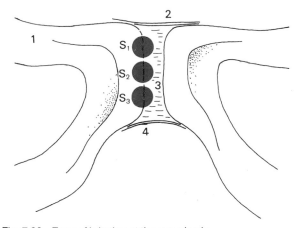

Fig. 7.**25** Cross-section of the sacrum and hip bones at the level of the zone of irritation S1 (IZ)

1 Hip bone
2 Sacrum
3 Gluteus maximus m (superficial layer)
4 Gluteal fascia
5 Thoracolumbar fascia

Fig. 7.**26** Zone of irritation at the symphysis

1 Ramus of the pubis
2 Superior pubic ligament
3 Interpubic disk
4 Arcuate ligament of the pubis

7.5 Overview of Important Tendinoses and Zones of Irritation in the Lumbar–Pelvic Region

(Fig. 7.27)

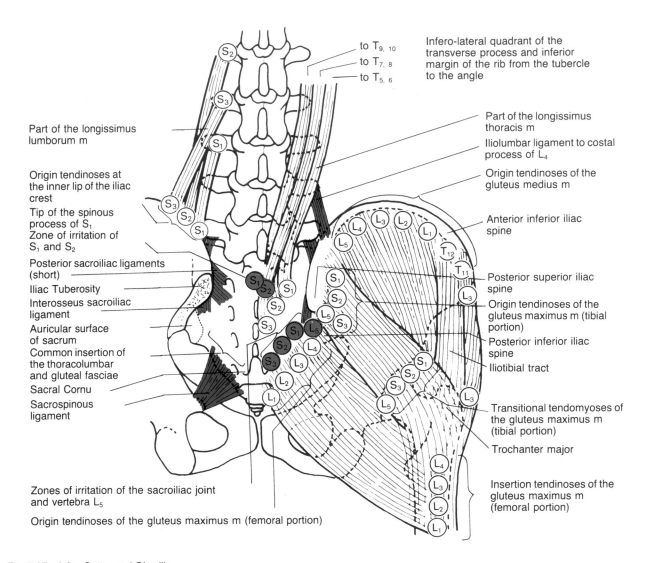

to $T_{9, 10}$
to $T_{7, 8}$
to $T_{5, 6}$

Infero-lateral quadrant of the transverse process and inferior margin of the rib from the tubercle to the angle

Part of the longissimus lumborum m

Origin tendinoses at the inner lip of the iliac crest

Tip of the spinous process of S_1
Zone of irritation of S_1 and S_2

Posterior sacroiliac ligaments (short)

Iliac Tuberosity

Interosseus sacroiliac ligament

Auricular surface of sacrum

Common insertion of the thoracolumbar and gluteal fasciae

Sacral Cornu

Sacrospinous ligament

Part of the longissimus thoracis m

Iliolumbar ligament to costal process of L_4

Origin tendinoses of the gluteus medius m

Anterior inferior iliac spine

Posterior superior iliac spine

Origin tendinoses of the gluteus maximus m (tibial portion)

Posterior inferior iliac spine

Iliotibial tract

Transitional tendomyoses of the gluteus maximus m (tibial portion)

Trochanter major

Insertion tendinoses of the gluteus maximus m (femoral portion)

Zones of irritation of the sacroiliac joint and vertebra L_5

Origin tendinoses of the gluteus maximus m (femoral portion)

Fig. 7.27   (after Sutter and Oberli).

8   Examination of the Muscles

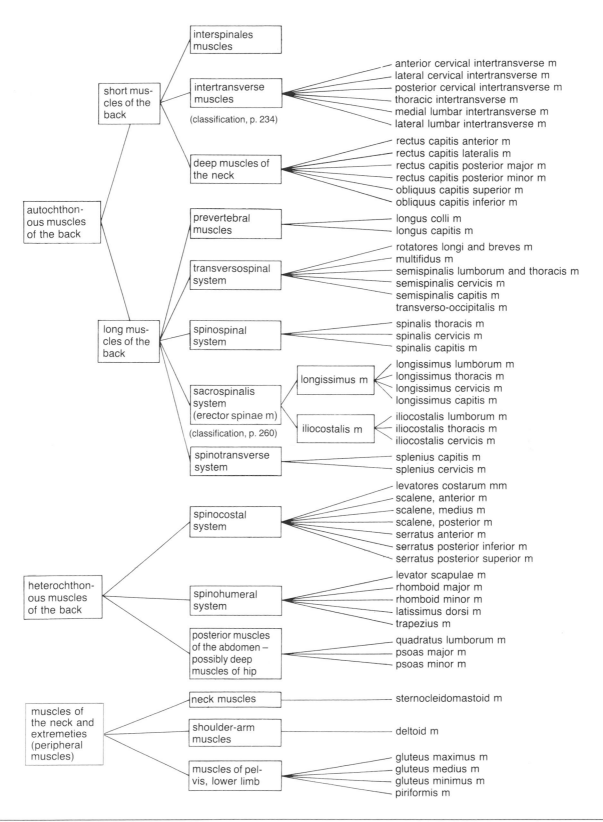

interspinales muscles

intertransverse muscles
(classification, p. 234)
- anterior cervical intertransverse m
- lateral cervical intertransverse m
- posterior cervical intertransverse m
- thoracic intertransverse m
- medial lumbar intertransverse m
- lateral lumbar intertransverse m

deep muscles of the neck
- rectus capitis anterior m
- rectus capitis lateralis m
- rectus capitis posterior major m
- rectus capitis posterior minor m
- obliquus capitis superior m
- obliquus capitis inferior m

short muscles of the back

prevertebral muscles
- longus colli m
- longus capitis m

transversospinal system
- rotatores longi and breves m
- multifidus m
- semispinalis lumborum and thoracis m
- semispinalis cervicis m
- semispinalis capitis m
- transverso-occipitalis m

spinospinal system
- spinalis thoracis m
- spinalis cervicis m
- spinalis capitis m

sacrospinalis system (erector spinae m)
(classification, p. 260)

longissimus m
- longissimus lumborum m
- longissimus thoracis m
- longissimus cervicis m
- longissimus capitis m

iliocostalis m
- iliocostalis lumborum m
- iliocostalis thoracis m
- iliocostalis cervicis m

spinotransverse system
- splenius capitis m
- splenius cervicis m

long muscles of the back

autochthonous muscles of the back

spinocostal system
- levatores costarum mm
- scalene, anterior m
- scalene, medius m
- scalene, posterior m
- serratus anterior m
- serratus posterior inferior m
- serratus posterior superior m

spinohumeral system
- levator scapulae m
- rhomboid major m
- rhomboid minor m
- latissimus dorsi m
- trapezius m

posterior muscles of the abdomen – possibly deep muscles of hip
- quadratus lumborum m
- psoas major m
- psoas minor m

heterochthonous muscles of the back

neck muscles
- sternocleidomastoid m

shoulder-arm muscles
- deltoid m

muscles of pelvis, lower limb
- gluteus maximus m
- gluteus medius m
- gluteus minimus m
- piriformis m

muscles of the neck and extremeties (peripheral muscles)

8.1   Interspinales Muscles

These short muscles are completely present only in the cervical and lumbar spine region. In the thoracic region, these muscles exist only to T4 and then again inferior to T11. Between T4 and T10, there are normally no interspinales muscles, but there are interspinous ligaments that are, however, of the same importance for the spondylogenic event as the muscles themselves (compare the SRS correlation).

Origin

Inferior surface of the spinous processes of C2−T3 and T11−S1.

Insertion

Superior surface of the spinous process directly below the respective origin-vertebra, C3−T4, T12−S2.

Course and Relations

Practically longitudinal; in the cervical region in pairs according to the bifurcated spinous processes (Fig. 8.**1**).

Innervation

Dorsal rami of the respective spinal nerves.

Function

Extension of the individual vertebrae.

Palpatory Technique

In the cervical region, the muscles provide easy access when the head is slightly flexed. Generally, the origins are palpated lateroinferiorly and the insertions, latero-superiorly (Fig. 8.**2**).

Supraspinous Ligament

The supraspinous ligament stretches superficially over the spinous processes from C3 to S3 (Fig. 8.**2**).

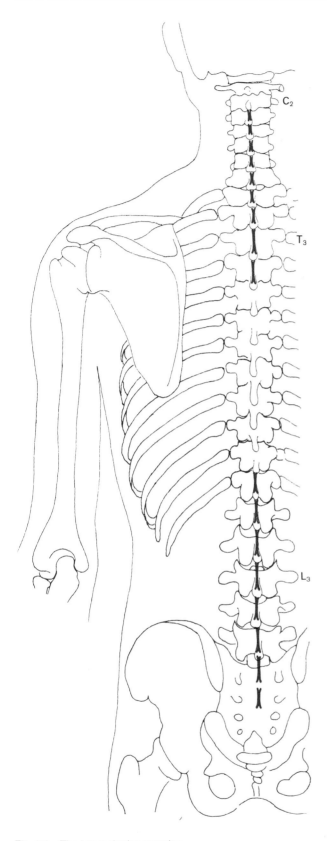

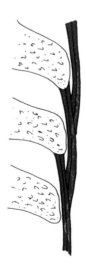

Fig. 8.1   The interspinales muscles

Fig. 8.2   Position of the supraspinous ligament

8.2   Intertransverse Muscles
(Fig. 8.**3**)

Classification

Intertransverse Muscles of the Cervical Region

The anterior cervical intertransverse muscles: located anterior to the ventral ramus of the spinal nerves; together with the anterior rectus capitis muscle.

The posterior cervical intertransverse muscles (lateral part): posterior to the ventral ramus of the spinal nerves; together with the lateral rectus capitis muscle.

The posterior cervical intertransverse muscles (medial part): together with the obliquus capitis superior muscle.

The anterior rectus capitis, lateral rectus capitis, and obliquus capitis superior muscles belong systematically to the deep neck muscles, that ist to the anterior part of the suboccipital musculature. Anatomically, however, they have to be considered as the continuation of the intertransverse muscles to the occiput, which again is supported by clinical experience with the SRS. Embryonically, the occiput represents a group of fused occipital vertebrae. Because of this, these three short suboccipital muscles are treated together with their corresponding intertransverse muscles. Thus, spondylogenically abbreviated, the myotenones C0−C1 are dealt with.

Intertransverse Muscles of the Thoracic Region

They exist between T2 and T10, probably as the intertransverse ligament only.

Intertransverse Muscles of the Lumbar Region

The medial lumbar intertransverse muscles and the lateral lumbar intertransverse muscles.

The posterior cervical intertransverse muscles, the thoracic intertransverse muscles, and the medial lumbar intertransverse muscles are considered one continuous and anatomical unit, which has been divided into the three muscle groups only as a result of their course through different anatomical regions with their respective local characteristics. In the cervical region they are found to overlap into the thoracic region, where, however, they are present mostly as ligaments. They are found as muscles again in the lumbar region. As a consequence of their division into the three distinct groups, these muscles are presented in three different tables even though they belong systematically together. This is similar to the multifidus muscle, which also consists of different segments.

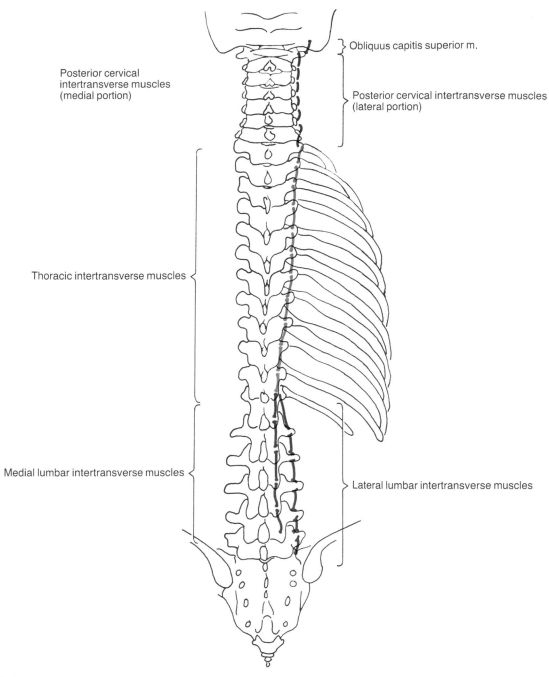

Posterior cervical intertransverse muscles (medial portion)

Obliquus capitis superior m.

Posterior cervical intertransverse muscles (lateral portion)

Thoracic intertransverse muscles

Medial lumbar intertransverse muscles

Lateral lumbar intertransverse muscles

Fig. 8.3   The intertransverse muscles

8.2.1 Anterior Cervical Intertransverse Muscles

Origins and Insertions

These short muscles are positioned between the anterior tubercles of the transverse processes of the cervical vertebrae. The most superior muscle lies between C1 and C2, the most inferior one lies between C6 and C7 (Fig. 8.**4**).

Course and Relations

With the exception of the first, all anterior cervical intertransverse muscles are covered at the anterior cervical spine by the longus colli and longus capitis muscle. Posteriorly, they are in proximity to the vertebral vessels. Anteriorly, they are close to the carotid artery.

Innervation

Anterior rami of the corresponding spinal nerves.

Function

Lateral flexion of the cervical spine, which is more of static than dynamic importance.

Palpatory Technique

The anterior cervical intertransverse muscles lie practically behind the carotid artery. The anterior tubercles can be palpated anteriorly with the finger used for palpation pressing deeply at the medial margin of the sternocleidomastoid muscle and pushing the carotid artery medially. The palpatory direction for the origins and insertions is the same as the muscle direction. Caution is necessary with the carotid sinus at the C4 level (see Fig. 7.**4**, the cross-section of the cervical spine).

When the fingertip is placed between the two respective anterior tubercles, increased tenderness is evident. When changing the direction of the palpatory force appropriately, the tendinosis pain appears very distinctly.

8.2.2 Rectus Capitis Anterior Muscle

Origin

As a thin tendon from the lateral mass of the atlas (Fig. 8.**4**).

Insertion

The basilar part of the occipital bone; starting about 6 to 8 mm distant from the pharyngeal tubercle and ending in front of the hypoglossal canal (Fig. 8.**5**).

Course and Relations

The rectus capitis anterior muscle lies in the immediate superior continuation of the first anterior cervical intertransverse muscle. The internal carotid artery, ascending pharyngeal artery, and the superior cervical (thyroid) ganglion of the sympathetic nervous system cross the anterior surface of the muscle laterally. At the lateral margin, the hypoglossal nerve appears superiorly. The posterior surface of the muscle lies next to the atlanto-occipital joint.

Innervation

Ventral rami of C1.

Function

Bilateral contraction results in flexion of the head, and unilateral contraction results in lateral bending of the head to the side of the contracted muscle.

Palpatory Technique

Due to its location, palpation is practically impossible.

SRS Correlation

The anterior cervical intertransverse muscles, along with the anterior rectus capitis muscle, belong spondylogenically to C1−C7 in opposite sequence, however. They frequently are involved in the spondylogenic event and can cause persistent unyielding relapse tendencies, especially in the midcervical spine, where the myotendinosis and the corresponding irritational zone meet on almost the exact same level, which in turn can lead to new abnormal positions or to the maintenance of the former abnormal position.

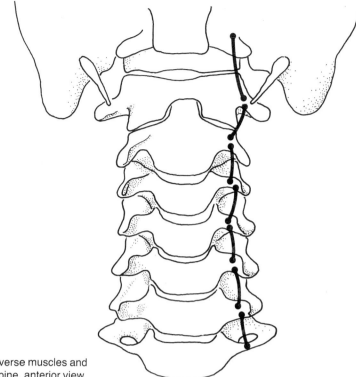

Fig. 8.4   The anterior cervical intertransverse muscles and
rectus capitis anterior muscle. Cervical spine, anterior view

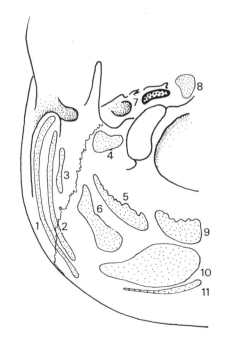

Fig. 8.5   Muscle origins and insertions at the occiput

1   Sternocleidomastoid m
2   Splenius capitis m
3   Longissimus capitis m
4   Rectus capitis lateralis m
5   Rectus capitis posterior major m
6   Obliquus capitis superior m
7   Rectus capitis anterior m
8   Longus capitis m
9   Rectus capitis posterior minor m
10 Semispinalis capitis m
11 Trapezius m

8.2.3 Posterior Cervical Intertransverse Muscles (Lateral Portion)

Origins and Insertions

The muscles are fixed between the posterior tubercles of the cervical transverse processes. The most superior muscle lies between C1 and C2, the one most inferior, between C6 and C7. Further inferior, these muscles turn into the first levator costae muscle, which extends from the posterior margin of the first rib (the center of the neck to the costal tuberosity) to the posterior tuberosity of the transverse process of C7 (Fig. 8.**6**).

Course and Relations

Posteriorly, they are almost fused with the medial portion of the posterior cervical intertransverse muscles. Posterolaterally, they lie next to the iliocostalis cervicis muscle, C3(4)–C6, and the longissimus cervicis muscle, C1(2)–C5.

Innervation

Ventral rami of the corresponding spinal nerves.

Function

Lateral flexion of the cervical vertebrae to the side of the contracted muscle.

Palpatory Technique

The fingers press behind the sternocleidomastoid muscle on the posterior tubercles of the transverse processes. Differential diagnosis distinguishing between other muscles that attach here is not simple. The origins and insertions are examined according to the fiber direction of the muscle (compare Fig. 7.**4**, the cross-section of the cervical spine). The procedure is analogous to that of the anterior cervical intertransverse muscles. Differentiation from the medial portion of the posterior cervical transverse muscles can prove to be difficult in this small area.

8.2.4 Rectus Capitis Lateralis Muscle

Origin

Superior surface of the transverse process of the atlas, not including its posterior tubercle (Fig. 8.**7**).

Insertion

Lateral portion of the occipital bone reaching the center of the jugular foramen.

Course and Relations

The rectus capitis lateralis muscle joints the posterior cervical intertransverse muscles (lateral portion), becoming their most superior member. Its medial surface borders on the ventral ramus of the first cervical nerve, while laterally the muscle adjoins to the posterior belly of the digastric muscle and the trunk of the facial nerve.

Innervation

Ventral rami of C1.

Function

Lateral bending (sidebending) of the head.

Palpatory Technique

The examiner palpates around the transverse process of the atlas from a posteroinferior direction. To obtain contact with the occiput, pressure is applied anteriorly. Consequently, the fingertip is between the atlas and the occiput and light pressure is exerted on the muscular insertions according to their directions.

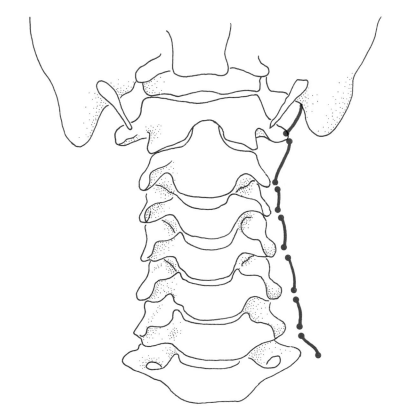

Fig. 8.6 Posterior cervical intertransverse muscles (lateral portion) and lateral rectus capitis muscle. Cervical spine, anterior view

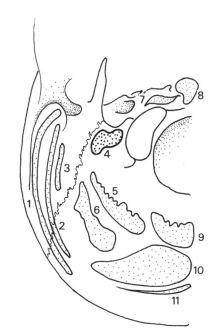

Fig. 8.7 Muscle attachments at the occiput

1 Sternocleidomastoid m
2 Splenius capitis m
3 Longissimus capitis m
4 Rectus capitis lateralis m
5 Rectus capitis posterior major m
6 Obliquus capitis superior m
7 Rectus capitis anterior m
8 Longus capitis m
9 Rectus capitis posterior minor m
10 Semispinalis capitis m
11 Trapezius m

8.2.5 Rectus Capitis Posterior Major Muscle

Origin

The rectus capitis posterior major muscle arises by a pointed tendinous origin from a narrow sagittal region on the lateral and superior half of the spinous process of the axis. The thick muscle belly takes on a triangular shape, with its muscle bundles spreading toward the skull. In this arrangement, the muscle fibers are twisted so that those bundles originating most anteriorly have their insertion medially (Fig. 8.**8**).

Insertion

Lateral half of the inferior nuchal line (Fig. 8.**9**).

Course and Relations

The rectus capitis posterior major muscle courses from its origin obliquely and superolaterally to the occiput and is primarily superimposed by the trapezius muscle (descending portion) and the semispinalis capitis muscle.

Innervation

Dorsal rami of the spinal nerves C1 and C2.

Function

Bilateral contraction results in extension of the head, and unilateral contraction results in lateral bending to the side of the contracted muscle.

Palpatory Technique

The muscle can easily be palpated. Starting from the mastoid process, the finger presses deeply under the semispinalis capitis muscle. The fleshy insertion presents itself in a region of 1×0.5 cm below the lateral third of inferior nuchal line. The lateral portion of the insertion is covered by the obliquus capitis superior muscle, and the medial portion is covered by the lateral part of the semispinalis capitis muscle. Palpation of the origin is according to the anatomical position. The palpatory direction is from superomedial to inferolateral.

SRS Correlation

The whole rectus capitis posterior major muscle represents a single myotenone and is correlated with the SIJ.

Remarks

Myotendinosis of the rectus capitis posterior major muscle may influence the mechanics of the occipital-atlanto-axial joints via its origin at the spinous process of C2.

8.2.6 Rectus Capitis Posterior Minor Muscle

Origin

Tuberosity on the posterior arch of the atlas (Fig. 8.**10**).

Insertion

Between the medial third of the lower nuchal line and the external margin of the occiput (Fig. 8.**11**).

Course and Relations

Superimposed mainly by the trapezius muscle (descending portion) and the semispinalis capitis muscle (medial portions).

Innervation

Dorsal rami of the spinal nerves C1 and C2.

Function

Bilateral contraction results in extension of the head, and unilateral contraction results in lateral bending to the side of the contracted muscle. Due to its short leverage, however, the function of this muscle is of theoretical value only. The main function of this muscle is that of posture and stabilization of the occipitocervical junction.

Palpatory Technique

About 2 cm below the external occipital protuberance, the finger used for palpation presses deeply between the two semispinalis capitis muscles. Palpatory direction is inferiorly, going from medial to lateral. Palpation of the origin at the posterior tuberosity of the atlas is according to its anatomic location.

SRS Correlation

This occipital muscle also represents one single myotenone, which is correlated with L5.

Remarks

Myotendinotic changes (i. e., palpable bands) in the rectus capitis posterior minor muscle can influence the normal physiologic motion in the atlanto-occipital joints.

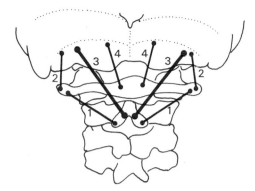

Fig. 8.**8**   Suboccipital musculature

1 Obliquus capitis inferior m
2 Obliquus capitis superior m
3 Rectus capitis posterior major m
4 Rectus capitis posterior minor m

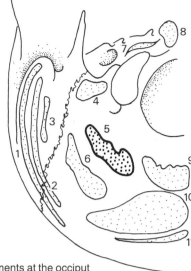

Fig. 8.**9**   Muscle attachments at the occiput

1   Sternocleidomastoid m
2   Splenius capitis m
3   Longissimus capitis m
4   Rectus capitis lateralis m
5   Rectus capitis posterior major m
6   Obliquus capitis superior m
7   Rectus capitis anterior m
8   Longus capitis m
9   Rectus capitis posterior minor m
10 Semispinalis capitis m
11 Trapezius m

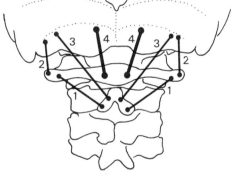

Fig. 8.**10**   Suboccipital musculature

1 Obliquus capitis inferior m
2 Obliquus capitis superior m
3 Rectus capitis posterior major m
4 Rectus capitis posterior minor m

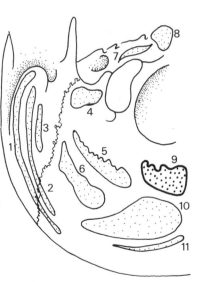

Fig. 8.**11**   Muscle attachments at the occiput

1   Sternocleidomastoid m
2   Splenius capitis m
3   Longissimus capitis m
4   Rectus capitis lateralis m
5   Rectus capitis posterior major m
6   Obliquus capitis superior m
7   Rectus capitis anterior m
8   Longus capitis m
9   Rectus capitis posterior minor m
10 Semispinalis capitis m
11 Trapezius m

8.2.7 Posterior Cervical Intertransverse Muscles (Medial Portion)

Origins and Insertions

The medial portion of the posterior cervical intertransverse muscles, like the lateral portion of the posterior cervical intertransverse muscles, extends between the posterior tuberosities of the spinous processes, although somewhat more posteriorly. The most superior segments are between C2 and C1 (at the transverse process of C1 between the obliquus capitis inferior muscle and the splenius cervicis muscle), and the most inferior portion is located between rib I and C7 (inferior surface of the posterior tubercle) (Figs. 8.**12**, 8.**13**).

Course and Relations

Practically the same as the lateral portion of the posterior cervical intertransverse muscles.

Innervation

Dorsal rami of the cervical nerves C2-C7.

Function

Lateral flexion of the vertebrae to the side of the contracted muscle.

Palpatory Technique

Palpation is the same as for the lateral portion of the posterior cervical intertransverse muscles. Palpatory differential diagnosis can be difficult in such a small region, but can become evident from the overall presentation of the SRS.

8.2.8 Obliquus Capitis Superior Muscle

Origin

This muscle arises by thick tendinous fibers from the posterior corner and the lateral segment of the transverse process of C1 (Fig. 8.**14**).

Insertion

Superior to the lateral third of the inferior nuchal line.

Innervation

Dorsal rami of C1.

Function

Bilateral contraction results in extension of the head, and unilateral contraction results in lateral bending of the head to the side of the contracted muscle.

Palpatory technique

The origin is palpated inferiorly below the most lateral insertion of the semispinalis capitis muscle (about 3 cm lateral to the external occipital protuberance). The origin is palpated superoposteriorly in the direction of the tip of the transverse process of the atlas.

SRS Correlation

The posterior cervical intertransverse muscles and the obliquus capitis superior muscle play an important role in the spondylogenic event. The correlation can be seen from the table. Even though the obliquus capitis superior muscle belongs anatomically to the posterior cervical intertransverse muscle group, it is spondylogenically and reflexogenically correlated with the SIJ.

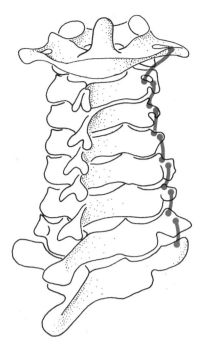

Fig. 8.**12** Posterior cervical intertransverse muscles (medial portion)

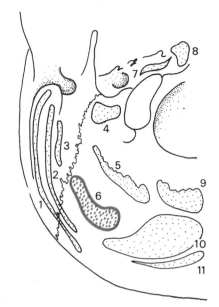

Fig. 8.**13** Muscle attachments at the occiput

Fig. 8.**14** Suboccipital muscles

1 Sternocleidomastoid m
2 Splenius capitis m
3 Longissimus capitis m
4 Rectus capitis lateralis m
5 Rectus capitis posterior major m
6 Obliquus capitis superior m
7 Rectus capitis anterior m
8 Longus capitis m
9 Rectus capitis posterior minor m
10 Semispinalis capitis m
11 Trapezius m
12 Obliquus capitis inferior m

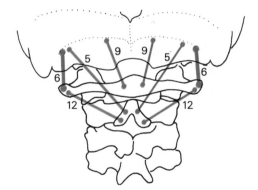

8.2.9 Obliquus Capitis Inferior Muscle

Origin

Anteriorly between the apex of the spinous process of the axis, the arch.

Insertion

Inferior and posterior surface of the transverse process of the atlas reaching the root of its posterior part.

Course and Relations

See Figure 8.15.

Innervation

Dorsal rami of the spinal nerves C1 and C2.

Function

Rotation of the head to the side of the contracted muscle.

Palpatory Technique

The origin is palpated laterally at the spinous process of C2 according to the direction of the muscle fibers. The insertion, at the transverse process of the atlas, is palpated medioinferiorly. The correct palpatory depth has to be assured for both the origin and the insertion. It is very difficult to distinguish the insertion tendinosis from the zone of irritation. Myotendinotic changes in the muscle belly (i. e., hard, palpable band) appear in the suboccipital soft tissue as a perpendicular, laterosuperiorly directed spindle.

SRS Correlation

The whole muscle is correlated as one single myotenone with the SIJ.

8.2.10 Length Testing of the Suboccipital Muscles

(see sections 8.2.2–8.2.9)

Examination Procedure

The patient is in the supine position. The examiner cradles the patient's head by placing one palm over the patient's occiput while the other embraces the forehead. The examiner then carefully introduces flexion to the upper cervical spine, that is specifically inclination to the upper cervical spinal segments, while at the same time applying traction. The axis of rotation is hypothetically placed through both mastoid processes (Fig. 8.16).

Possible Pathological Findings

1. Loss of inclination motion with soft endfeel indicates shortening of the suboccipital muscles.
2. Loss of inclination motion with hard endfeel indicates degenerative joint changes.

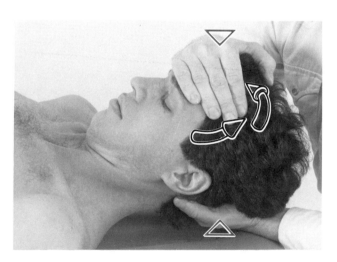

Fig. 8.16   The intertransverse muscles

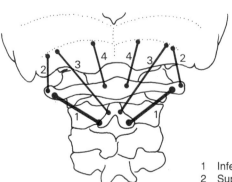

Fig. 8.15   Suboccipital muscles

1   Inferior obliquus capitis m
2   Superior obliquus capitis m
3   Rectus capitis posterior major m
4   Rectus capitis posterior minor m

8.2.11 Thoracic Intertransverse Muscles

Three pairs of these muscles are normally present, the rest being either ligamentous or absorbed in the long musculature, mainly the longissimus muscle.

Origin and Insertion

These are short muscles, which are principally located between the individual transverse processes, from the inferior margin of the superior thoracic transverse process to the superior border of the inferior thoracic transverse process. The last muscle often divides into two portions, arising from the inferior surface of the transverse process of T11 and reaching the mamillary and accessory processes of T12 (Fig. 8.**17**).

This bifurcation can sometimes continue into the lumbar spinal region. Thus, the continuation of the thoracic intertransverse muscles into the lumbar spinal region is formed by the medial lumbar intertransverse muscles, which in turn are divided into a medial and lateral portion. This is of no relevance to the diagnosis, however.

Course and Relations

These muscles belong to the deep and short autochthonous musculature and therefore, lie beneath the rest of the muscles. At the last thoracic and lumbar vertebrae, they nestle between the longissimus muscle (lateral) and the multifidus muscle (medioposterior).

Innervation

Dorsal rami of the segmental nerves.

Function

Lateral bending of the corresponding vertebrae.

Palpatory Technique

Palpation of these small and deep spondylogenic units in the thoracic region and especially the differentiation from neighboring tendinoses is very difficult. The fingertip is placed over the origin and insertion on the skeleton and then the halfway point is determined, from which only the direction of the palpatory pressure is changed: along the muscle belly in the direction of the origin tendinosis and in the opposite direction to the insertion tendinosis!

SRS Correlation

From clinical experience it is also known that in the area of the so-called nondeveloped posterior thoracic intertransverse muscles, a regular myotendinosis can be found. This shows that the phenomenon of myotendinosis with its clinical correlation does not necessarily require the presence of real muscle tissue.

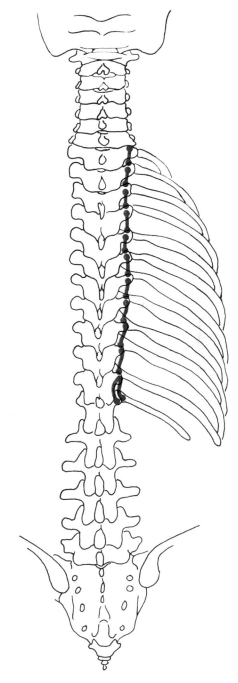

Fig. 8.**17** The thoracic intertransverse muscles

8.2.12 Medial Lumbar Intertransverse Muscles

The medial lumbar intertransverse muscles can exist as one single unit or they can be divided into a medial and lateral portion, starting from their insertions (compare thoracic intertransverse muscles) (Figs. 8.**19**, 8.**20**).

Origin

Inferior margin of the accessory process, tendinous arch to the inferior border of the mamillary process (nerve exit, dorsal ramus of the spinal nerves; Fig. 8.**20**).

Insertion

Between the superior edge of the adjoining mamillary process anteriorly and the root of the costal process and the superior edge of the accessory process. It normally does not reach below L5.

Course and Relations

The sagittally oriented muscle belly lies in the deep muscle layer between the longissimus muscle (lateral) and the multifidus muscle (medioposterior and dorsal).

Innervation

Dorsal rami of the spinal nerves.

Palpatory Technique

Palpation of this muscle is difficult due to its close proximity to the transversospinal system and is thus only possible in isolated circumstances. The muscle often causes paravertebral lumbar pain. Considering the anatomical arrangement, the general principles of the palpatory technique apply here as well (8.**18**).

8.2.13 Lateral Lumbar Intertransverse Muscles

Origin

The superior margin of the costal process, from the tip to its root, with exit of the dorsal ramus of the spinal nerves. The most inferior muscle originates at the lateral mass of S1 (Fig. 8.**21**).

Insertion

The muscle located most superiorly inserts at the lateral tubercle of T12 and the lumbocostal ligament; all others insert at the inferior border, reaching to the tip of the costal process.

Innervation

Dorsal rami of the spinal nerves.

Function

Lateral flexion of the vertebra involved to the side of the contracted muscle.

Palpatory Technique

Myotendinosis of the lateral lumbar intertransverse muscles must be distinguished from the corresponding segmental zones of irritation by provocative testing (compare page 226).

It is best to palpate from both sides simultaneously, whereby both thumbs reach around and below the sacrospinal system and do not press directly on the tip of the costal processes, but rather between the two costal processes in order to palpate them inferiorly and superiorly.

SRS Correlation

The lateral lumbar intertransverse muscles are associated with the upper thoracic spine. They are often involved in the SRS event and palpatory access is usually easy. Thus, they are of practical importance for the beginner both for the diagnosis and therapy.

Remarks

The quadratus lumbar muscle and the longissimus lumbar muscle must be diagnostically differentiated from each other.

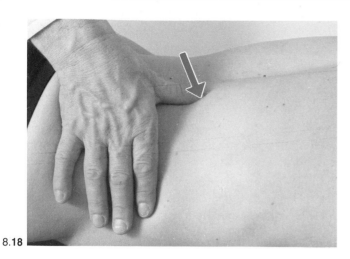

8.**18**

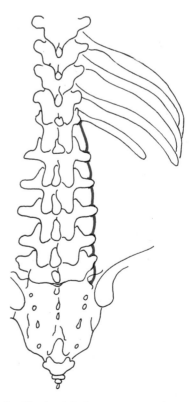

Fig. 8.**19** The medial lumbar intertransverse muscles

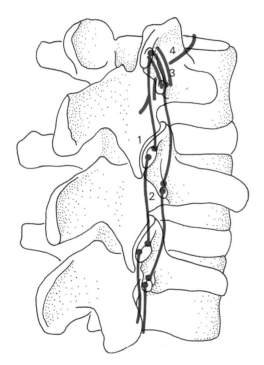

Fig. 8.**20** Detail of the origins and insertions of the medial lumbar intertransverse muscles

1 Mamillary process
2 Accessory process
3 Connective tissue bridge
4 Dorsal ramus of the spinal nerve

Fig. 8.**21** The lateral lumbar intertransverse muscles

8.3   Longus Colli Muscle

Origin

See Figures 8.23 and 8.24. **Superior portion:** the anterior tubercle and anterior surface of the transverse processes. **Inferior portion:** lateral side of the vertebral bodies of C5−C7 and the anterolateral portion of the vertebral bodies of T1−T3 (always strong).

Insertion

Superior portion: the tubercle on the anterior arch of the atlas and vertebral bodies of C2−C4, immediately next to the longitudinal ligament. **Inferior portion:** the most inferior side on the anterior surface of the transverse processes of C5−C7.

Function

Bilateral contraction results in flexion of the cervical spine, and unilateral contraction results in lateral bending of the head to the side of the contracted muscle.

Innervation

Ventral rami of the spinal nerves C2−C6.

Palpatory Technique

Origin tendinosis can be palpated superomedially after having moved the sternocleidomastoid muscle aside.

The origins of the inferior portion cannot be palpated due to the position and course of the scalene muscles. The insertion at C1 can be palpated inferiorly. This may be confused with the zone of irritation of C1. To reach the insertions at C2−C4, the finger presses deeply between the sternocleidomastoid muscle and the pharynx (Fig. 8.22). Because of the anatomical location and relation to the pharynx, palpation is difficult and therefore, not always useful for diagnosis.

SRS Correlation

Due to its reflexogenic correlation to the upper thoracic spine, the longus colli muscle takes part in the spondylogenic event and can cause an anteriorly abnormal position of a cervical vertebra. The examiner should observe the response of the zone of irritation upon provocative testing of the cervical spine.

8.4   Longus Colli and Longus Capitis Muscles

Origin

With four projections from the anterior tubercles of the transverse processes of C3−C6, between the origins of the longus colli muscle and anterior scalene muscle.

Insertion

At the pharyngeal tubercle, about onehalf of a finger width from the anterior condyle at the occiput, the basilar part of the occipital bone.

Innervation

Ventral rami of C1−C3.

Function

Flexion of the head.

Palpatory Technique

Similar to the longus colli muscle, the origins are palpated from a superior direction. The insertion at the occiput cannot be easily palpated. To test for possible myotendinosis in the muscle belly, the orientation is best at the C3 level. The recognition of myotendinosis in the longus system is of therapeutic importance. Myotendinosis is responsible for the anterior component of the abnormal position, which, however iseldom (Fig. 8.24).

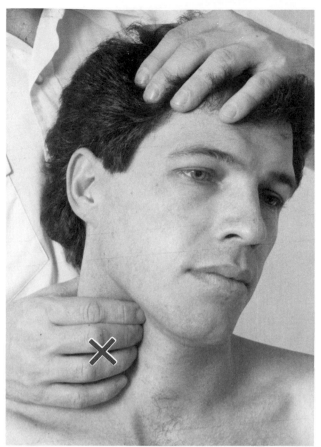

Fig. 8.**22**

Fig. 8.**23**   Longi colli and capitis muscles

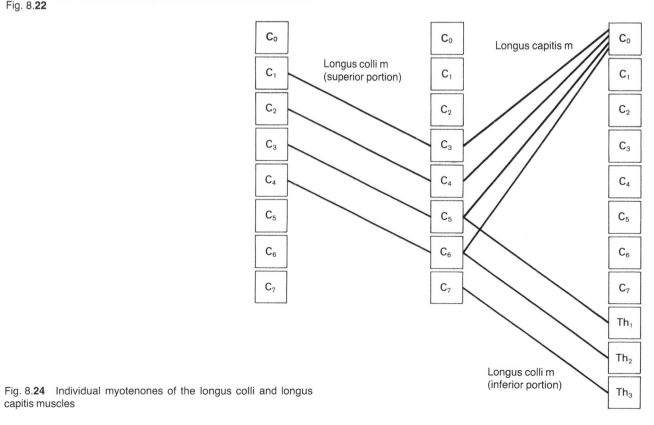

Fig. 8.**24**   Individual myotenones of the longus colli and longus capitis muscles

8.5   Rotatores Breves and Longi Muscles

Origin

Cervical region, from the posterior boundary of the superior articular process. Thoracic region, from the transverse process (medial portions, see diagram). Lumbar region, from the mamillary process.

Insertion

Cervical region at the inferolateral margin of the spinous processes of the next one or two vertebrae above. Thoracic and lumbar regions at the vertebral arch (Fig. 8.**25**).

Course and Relations

These muscles course above the posteromedial boundary of the upper apophyseal joints (cervical spine). The breves muscles are almost horizontal, whereas the longi muscles are angled superomedially (Fig. 8.**26**).

Innervation

Dorsal rami of the corresponding segmental nerves.

Function

Bilateral contraction results in extension of the superior vertebra, and unilateral contraction results in rotation of the superior vertebra to the other side.

Palpatory Technique

The insertions are palpated according to the fiber direction of the muscle, from lateral to medial, whereas the origins are palpated from the medial to the lateral. The muscle is palpated perpendicularly in the direction of the fibers. Even though of small size, the rotatores muscles can be detected palpatorily, since they lie directly above the hard skeleton with minimal amounts of soft tissue intervening. In order to determine whether myotendinosis is present, the fingertip must be introduced carefully and slowly into the spinotransverse vertebral groove in order to finally reach definite contrast with the bones of the articulating processes (cervical spine, thoracic spine) or the vertebral arches of the laminae (lumbar spine).

SRS Correlation

In contrast to the anatomical unit, the spondylogenic unit is represented as the myotenone depicted in Figure 8.**27**. In practice, with an abnormal position of L3 (zone of irritation), for instance, a myotendinosis or tendinosis (latent zone) is found in the spondylo-genically associated myotenone at the T7, T8 or T9 levels; at the T7 level, at the insertion at the vertebral arch; and at T8 and T9 levels, at the origin on the transverse process. The tendinoses at the transverse processes are accompanied by corresponding segmental zones of irritations, especially in the thoracic spine region.

Remarks

The distinction between the rotatores longi and breves muscles dates back to the nomenclature of Basle. Some books incorrectly correlate the rotatores longi and breves muscles with the multifidus muscle and designate them as its deepest layer.

Spine	SRS Correlation		
C_0	T_{10}	T_{11}	T_{12}
C_1	T_{11}	T_{12}	L_1
C_2	T_{12}	L_1	L_2
C_3	L_1	L_2	L_3
C_4	L_2	L_3	L_4
C_5	L_3	L_4	L_5
C_6	L_4	L_5	S_1
C_7	L_5	S_1	S_2
T_1		C_2	C_3
T_2	C_1	C_2	C_3
T_3	C_2	C_3	C_4
T_4	C_3	C_4	C_5
T_5	C_4	C_5	C_6
T_6	C_5	C_6	C_7
T_7	C_6	C_7	T_1
T_8	C_7	T_1	T_2
T_9	T_1	T_2	T_3
T_{10}	T_2	T_3	T_4
T_{11}	T_3	T_4	T_5
T_{12}	T_4	T_5	T_6
L_1	T_5	T_6	T_7
L_2	T_6	T_7	T_8
L_3	T_7	T_8	T_9
L_4	T_8	T_9	T_{10}
L_5	T_9	T_{10}	T_{11}
S_1	T_{10}	T_{11}	T_{12}
S_2	T_{11}	T_{12}	L_1
S_3	T_{12}	L_1	L_2

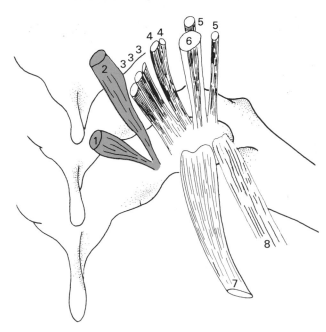

Fig. 8.**25** Muscle attachments at the transverse process of a thoracic vertebra

1 Rotator brevis m
2 Rotator longus m
3 Multifidus m
4 Semispinalis thoracis m
5 Longissimus capitis and longissimus cervicis m
6 Semispinalis capitis m
7 Longissimus thoracis m
8 Levator costae m

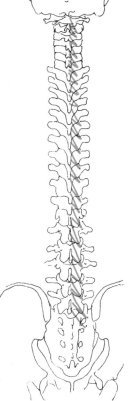

Fig. 8.**26** Rotatores breves and longi muscles

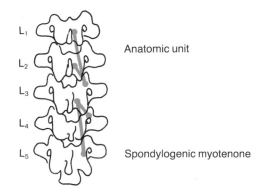

Anatomic unit

Spondylogenic myotenone

Fig. 8.**27** The individual units of the rotatores muscles

8.6 Multifidus Muscle

With the origins of the multifidus muscles extending from C4(5) to S4, and the insertions from C2 to L5, the multifidus muscle has a complicated structure. Yet, it is possible to anatomically divide this muscle into four different groups (Virchow): the cervical, the upper thoracic, the lower thoracic, and the lumbar (Fig. 8.**28**).

Cervical Group (from T1 to C2):

Origin

From the posterior border of the inferior articular process of the cervical spine, whereby the origins can reach the deep posterior surface of the vertebral arch. The origin at T1 is located at the superior border of the transverse process up to the root.

Insertion

In the ipsilateral tips of the bifurcated cervical spinous processes up to C2, where they occupy almost the entire inferior border.

Upper Thoracic Group (from T7 to T1):

Origin

Transverse processes of T2−T6 (Fig. 8.**25**).

Insertion

Inferior margins of the spinous processes up to C5.

Lower Thoracic Group (from L1 to T7):

Origin

Similar to the upper thoracic portion; the origins extend from the arch to the neck of the transverse process.

Insertion

Inferior margins of the spinous processes from the tip to the root.

Lumbar Group (from S4 to L1):

Origin

Very complicated, from the posterior sacrum to S4, from the median sacral crest at S3−S4 then laterally from the lateral sacral crest and the posterior sacroiliac ligaments to the posterior end of the iliac crest. In the lower lumbar region from the mamillary processes.

Insertion

Inferior margins of all lumbar and thoracic spinous processes to T7.

Course and Relations

The fasciculi of this muscle draw out from their origin in the mediosuperior direction to the spinous process. Its structure is very complicated in the cervical and lumbar spine regions. Its muscle mass fills the groove between the transverse and spinous processes. It covers the rotatores muscles and vertebral arches, is positioned laterally to the interspinales muscles, and is beneath the semispinalis muscle. In the lumbosacral region, it is covered by the muscle belly and the origin and aponeurosis of the longissimus thoracis muscle.

Innervation

The medial branches of the dorsal rami of the spinal nerves C3−L5.

Function

Bilateral contraction results in extension of the vertebral column, and unilateral contraction results in rotation of the vertebral column to the opposite side.

Palpatory Technique

Like the rotatores muscle, the multifidus muscle is difficult to palpate because of its deep location. In accordance with the direction of the muscle fibers, the origins are palpated in the mediosuperior direction and the insertion in the lateroinferior direction. To prevent confusion, the correct palpatory direction and palpatory depth must first be established and then sustained. In contrast to the anatomical arrangement, for palpation, the finger finds the insertion at the portion of the spinous process close to the arch. From the arrangement of the entire myotenone, it can be determined whether or not the muscle is a member of the multifidus group by using spondylogenic correlation with the appropriate zone of irritation four segments more superior than the uniform insertion area of tendinosis.

SRS Correlation

The multifidus muscle very often participates in the spondylogenic event. Despite its deep location, it can easily be palpated (see above). With an L4 abnormal position (zone of irritation), for instance, the examiner palpates an origin tendinosis at the transverse process of T12, and the insertion tendinoses according to the myotenone structure at the roots of the spinous processes of T7−T9 (Fig. 8.**29**).

Remarks

The muscle fibers generally fan out from their origin in three fasciculi, resulting in three insertions, and thus creating a functional and spondylogenic unit three to five vertebral levels higher (the so-called myotenone) (Fig. 8.29).

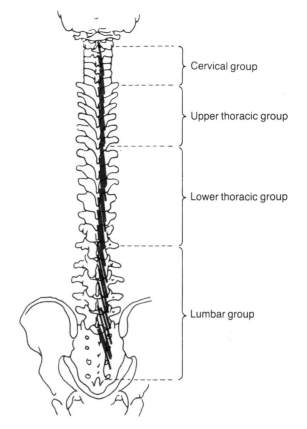

Cervical group

Upper thoracic group

Lower thoracic group

Lumbar group

Fig. 8.28   Multifidus muscle

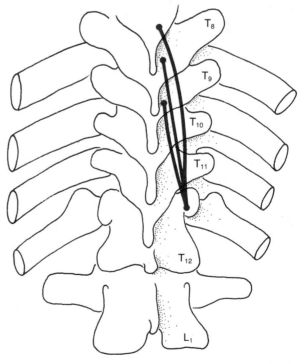

Fig. 8.29   The multifidus myotenone; it can be palpated with a segmental dysfunction of L4

8.7 Semispinalis Muscle

General Remarks

This muscle is a flat, nonuniform mass; a system consisting of many fasciculi. The muscular units overlap superoinferiorly in a tile-roof manner. This characteristic feature of the transversospinal system, starting from the axis going inferiorly, occurs because the muscle fibers arriving from the individual transverse processes cannot be associated with one single vertebra, but rather fan out into several portions. These individual portions then insert on different vertebrae, explaining the different lengths. For the long muscle segments (superficial), the direction of the fibers is almost vertical, whereas the short (deep) muscle portions run almost in a transverse direction (Fig. 8.**30**).

8.7.1 Semispinalis Lumborum Muscle

Origin

This muscle arises by a strong fascia from the mamillary processes of S1, L5 and L2; from the mamillary processes of L1 and T12, it arises directly.

Insertion

It inserts as long tendons at the inferior portions of those two spinous processes that are positioned six and seven segments superior to that vertebra from which the myotenone originates. The anatomical musculatur unit of the semispinalis muscle described here is identical to the spondylogenic unit, the myotenone.

8.7.2 Semispinalis Thoracis and Cervicis Muscles

Origin

From the superior edge of the transverse process, that is, the thoracic portion from T6−T10, and the cervical region from T2−T5 (Fig. 8.**31**).

Insertion

The structure of the myotenone remains the same, as described previously. The insertions are found at the spinous processes, which are six to seven segmental levels higher than the vertebra from which the myotenone originates. The insertion tendinosis is usually best developed in the medioposterior region (Fig. 8.**31**).

Course and Relations

All three semispinales muscles are positioned at the same level. The superior surface is covered by the longissimus muscle and the spinalis muscle, and partially by the semispinalis capitis muscle. A thin connective-tissue layer demarcates this muscle from the multifidus muscle below, which is important for palpation. Differentiation from the multifidus muscle is facilitated by keeping in mind that the longest portions of the multifidus muscle skip two fewer vertebrae than the semispinalis muscle.

Innervation

Dorsal rami of the spinal nerves.

Function

Bilateral contraction results in extension of the vertebral column, and unilateral contraction results in contralateral rotation of the vertebral column.

Palpatory Technique

Due to its frequent spondylogenic participation, exact palpation of the transversospinal system is extremely important. As a result of the close anatomical arrangement, it cannot be distinguished at the mamillary or transverse process whether the origin tendinosis belongs to the semispinalis muscle, the multifidus muscle, or the rotatores muscles. Only when the attachment tendinoses are present in both directions is differentiation possible. The rotators muscles pass from one vertebra to the first or the second above (be aware of the difference between the anatomical and spondylogenic units). The multifidus muscle passes from one vertebra to the third above and inserts via three fasciculi. The semispinalis muscle extends from one vertebra to the sixth above and inserts via two fasciculi. When a painful superior margin of the mamillary bodies is located, all seven spinous processes must be palpated from their lateral aspect to the root in order to eliminate the rotatores muscles and the multifidus muscle.

The origin tendinosis is determined to belong to the semispinalis muscle when the insertion is on opposite poles and lies six to seven levels superior at the roots of the spinous process. The myotendinosis of the individual muscle fibers can normally be palpated as a thin, matchlike band.

SRS Correlation

The spondylogenic unit, the myotenone, is represented in Figure 8.**32**. The 17 myotenones of the semispinalis muscle are correlated with segments C0−T9.

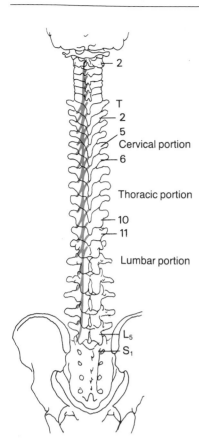

Fig. 8.**30** Semispinalis muscle

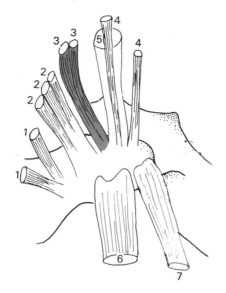

Fig. 8.**31** Muscle attachments at the transverse process of a thoracic vertebra

1 Rotatores muscles
2 Multifidus m
3 Semispinalis cervicis m
4 Longissimus cervicis and capitis m
5 Semispinalis capitis m
6 Longissimus thoracis m
7 Levator costae m

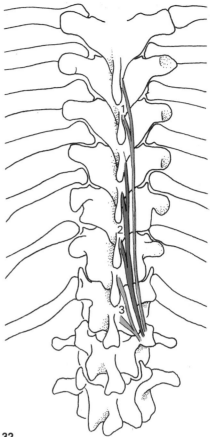

Fig. 8.**32**

1 Myotenone of the semispinalis thoracis muscle
2 Myotenone of the multifidus muscle
3 Rotatores longus and brevis muscles

8.7.3 Semispinalis Capitis Muscle

Origin

This muscle arises from the root of the transverse processes of C3–C6 (which is in close proximity to the insertions of the posterior scalene muscles, the levator scapulae muscle, the splenius cervicis muscle, the iliocostalis cervicis muscle, the longissimus cervicis muscle, the longissimus capitis muscle, and the posterior cervical intertransverse muscles). Further, it arises from the thick tip of the transverse processes of C7, T1–T8 and posterosuperiorly from the planum nuchale (Fig. 8.**33**).

Insertion

The semispinalis capitis muscle inserts in the planum nuchale of the occipital bone directly beside the midline. The insertion has a characteristic shape (see diagram) and lies between the superior and inferior nuchal lines. In the transverse direction it measures about 3 cm, in the sagittal direction, about 2 cm (Figs. 8.**35**, 8.**36**).

Course and Relations

The semispinalis capitis muscle, being lateral to the nuchal ligament, overlies the bifurcated spinous processes of the cervical spine, including C7. Further inferiorly, it is imbedded superficially in a bony and ligamentous groove formed by the spinous processes, vertebral arches, apophyseal joints, and transverse processes. In the thoracic region, it is situated lateral to the thoracic spinous processes. The muscle itself is flat and superficial in the medial neck portion. In the cervical region, it is covered by the splenius capitis muscle and the trapezius muscle only. The semispinalis capitis muscle covers the semispinalis cervicis muscle, as well as a portion of the semispinalis thoracis muscle. As a result, when palpating, the examiner perceives the semispinalis capitis muscle as a round bundle. It borders the longissimus capitis muscle laterally (Fig. 8.**34**).

Innervation

Dorsal rami of the cervical nerves C1–C4.

Function

Bilateral contraction results in extension of the head and the cervical spine, and unilateral contraction results in rotation of the head and the cervical spine contralaterally.

Palpatory Technique

The whole muscle mass is examined in the cervical region at the C3 level, where the muscle has a cylindrical appearance. By palpating from medial to lateral (i. e., perpendicular to the fiber direction), the examiner can detect possible myotendinosis. When the semispinalis capitis muscle is palpated following an arch, the examiner reaches the deep articular and transverse processes. The longissimus and cervicis muscles lie lateral to the finger being used for palpation. The tips of the transverse processes must be examined from the posterosuperior direction (if the direction of palpation is altered, the examiner can confuse them with other muscles). When palpating, the examiner should be aware of the close anatomical relationship between the tendinoses and the segmental zones of irritation. Thus, when the head is in a neutral position, the area of insertion is located at the inferior portion of the planum nuchale of the occipital bone. When the head is flexed, it rises and thus exposes its upper portions superiorly. This area of insertion is differentiated from other muscle insertions at the posterior occiput as a result of the cushioning effect of the soft tissue. The palpatory direction is from the inferior and can be followed to the lateral end (about 3.5 cm from the external occipital protuberance). At the thoracocervical junction, it is very difficult to palpate the myotenones that arise inferior to T3. Here, the muscle belly is simply a tendon in which the myotendinotic changes appear weakly.

SRS Correlation

1. Each origin of the semispinalis capitis muscle represents one individual myotenone.
2. Each of these myotendinoses is correlated with one particular SRS.
3. Each myotenone of the semispinalis capitis muscle belongs to that SRS, whose causative functional abnormal position (segmental dysfunction) is located eight vertebral levels more inferior ("rule of eight").

With an abnormal position of L3, for instance, (zone of irritation), myotendinoses are found in its spondylogenically related myotenone, in this case at the transverse processes of T7 and furthermore at its insertion area at the occiput (Fig. 8.**35**).

Remarks

The myotendinoses of T5–T6 demonstrate a special relationship to the greater occipital nerve. With myotendinosis, sensory disturbances in the field of innervation of the nerve can appear.

The semispinalis capitis muscle therefore represents to some degree a mirror image of the sacrospinal system and as such is often affected in the spondylogenic event.

Clinically, myotendinosis (e.g., a hard, palpable band) in the semispinalis capitis muscle can be associated with a persistent headache radiating from the occipital to the frontal areas.

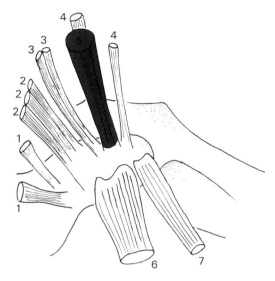

Fig. 8.33   Muscle attachment at the transverse process of a thoracic vertebra

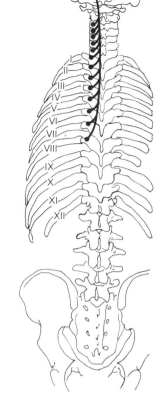

Fig. 8.34   Semispinalis capitis muscle

1	Rotatores m	
2	Multifidus m	
3	Myotenone of the semispinalis cervicis m	
4	Longissimus cervicis and longissimus capitis m	
5	Semispinalis capitis m	
6	Longissimus thoracis m	
7	Levator costae m	

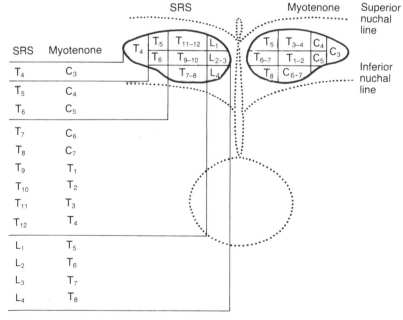

SRS	Myotenone
T_4	C_3
T_5	C_4
T_6	C_5
T_7	C_6
T_8	C_7
T_9	T_1
T_{10}	T_2
T_{11}	T_3
T_{12}	T_4
L_1	T_5
L_2	T_6
L_3	T_7
L_4	T_8

Fig. 8.35   SRS correlation (after Sutter)

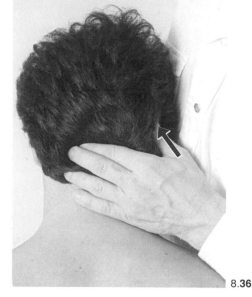

8.36

8.8 Spinalis Muscle

The spinospinal system is made up of three muscles: the spinalis capitis, spinalis cervicis, and spinalis thoracis muscles. They interconnect the spinous processes and show great variability in their distribution. If present, the spinalis capitis muscle is fused anatomically with the semispinalis muscle.

The discussion is restricted to the spinalis thoracis muscle, which is the only one of some importance to manual therapeutic diagnosis.

8.8.1 Spinalis Thoracis Muscle

Origin

Spinous processes of T11−L2 (3) (Fig. 8.**38**).

Insertion

Tips of the spinous processes of (C7) T1−T9 (Fig. 8.**39**).

Course

The longest fasciculi run from L3 to C7 and T1; the shortest, from T11 to T8 or T9. This arrangement results in the largest muscle profile in the lower thoracic region where the fibers can be palpated above the tips of the transverse processes (when myotendinosis — e.g., hard, palpable band — is present) (Fig. 8.**40**).

Innervation

Dorsal rami of the thoracic nerves T6−T8.

Function

Bilateral contraction results in extension of the vertebral column, and unilateral contraction results in lateral flexion of the vertebral column.

Palpatory Technique

The origin tendinosis of the spinalis thoracis muscle is palpated from a superior direction in order to reach the proximal pole of the spinous process. It must be differentiated from the adjoining origin tendinoses (such as that of the latissimus dorsi muscle in the lumbar region and serratus posterior inferior muscle in the upper thoracic and cervical region) (Fig. 8.**37**).

SRS Correlation

The spinalis muscle is spondylogenically and reflexogenically correlated with the lumbar spine.

Remarks

As already noted, the spinalis cervicis and capitis muscles are nonuniform and, for all purposes, spondylogenically and reflexogenically insignificant.

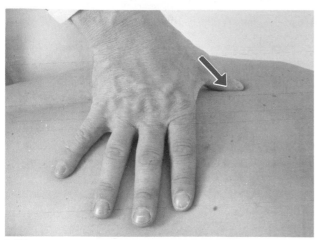

8.**37**

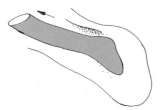

Fig. 8.**38**   Origin of the spinalis muscle

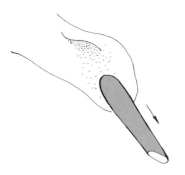

Fig. 8.**39**   Insertion of the spinalis muscle

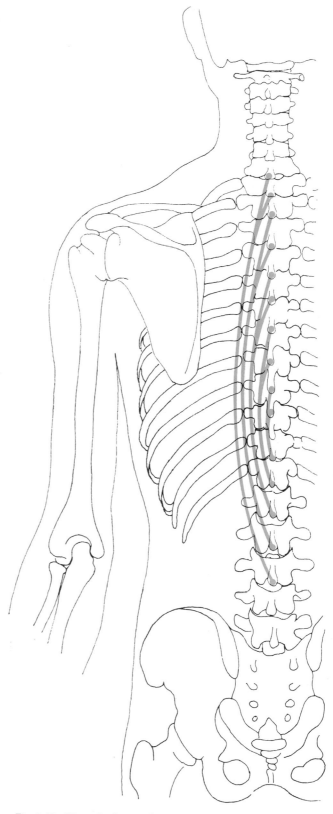

Fig. 8.**40**   The spinalis muscle

8.9 Erector Spinae (Sacrospinales) Muscles—Organization

Origin (General)

The longissimus and iliocostalis muscles are arranged anatomically in such a manner that their origins at the pelvis cannot be differentiated from one another. They share a common, remarkably broad origin, just like a two-headed muscle. Their origin extends from the spinous processes of all lumbar vertebrae via the median sacral crest, the posterior portion of the sacrum in the S3–S4 region, to the lateral sacral crest. They continue further to the medial and superior side of the iliac tuberosity, the short posterior sacroiliac ligaments, and the anterior side of the posterior part of the inner lip of the crest of the ilium (Fig. 8.**41**).

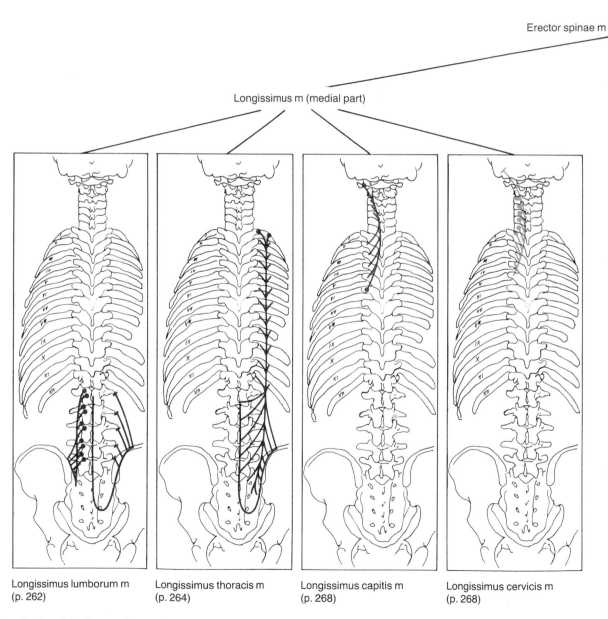

Erector spinae m

Longissimus m (medial part)

| Longissimus lumborum m (p. 262) | Longissimus thoracis m (p. 264) | Longissimus capitis m (p. 268) | Longissimus cervicis m (p. 268) |

Fig. 8.**41**   This division of the iliocostalis muscle into three portions is not complete, since it is usual for smaller or larger portions of this muscle to be continuous from one section of the abdomen to another

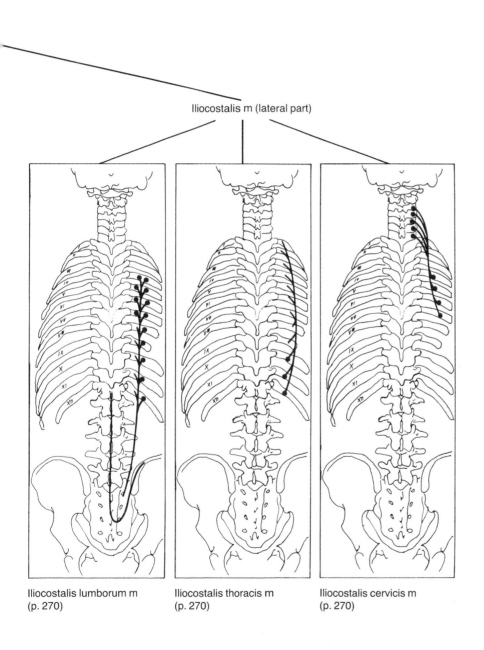

Iliocostalis m (lateral part)

Iliocostalis lumborum m
(p. 270)

Iliocostalis thoracis m
(p. 270)

Iliocostalis cervicis m
(p. 270)

8.9.1 Longissimus Lumborum Muscle

Origin

The longissimus lumborum muscle arises the examine from the broad sacrospinous ligament primarily at the superior and anterior portions of the iliac tuberosity (Fig. 8.**45**).

Insertion

It inserts via two tendons at all lumbar vertebrae. A lateral row of broad insertions attaches to the entire inferior edge and the whole length of the posterior surface of the transverse processes of the lumbar vertebrae. The insertion at L5 usually only reaches the iliolumbar ligament (Fig. 8.**45**).

The medial row overlies the lateral row and converges toward the ligamentous fascia, above the mamillary and accessory processes. The dorsal ramus of the spinal nerves is located below this fascia (Fig. 8.**45**).

Course and Relations

The longissimus lumborum muscle lies deep in relation to the iliocostalis muscle and the longissimus thoracis muscle. By way of its origin at the iliac tuberosity, it connects to the interosseous sacroiliac ligaments.

Innervation

Dorsal rami of the spinal nerve.

Function

Bilateral contraction results in extension of the vertebral column, and unilateral contraction results in lateral bending of the spine to the side of the contracted muscle.

Palpatory Technique

Except for very rare cases, it is almost impossible to distinctly palpate the origin tendinoses of the longissimus lumborum muscle. Thus, the examiner must rely on the reporting of pain by the patient. The *medial* insertion tendinoses are determined from the inferior direction at the mamillary process. A frequent mistake is the palpation from the posterior direction (or the origin of the transversospinal system).

The lateral portion is stronger than the medial, and is palpated from the lateroinferior direction (Fig. 8.**42**). The examiner must attempt palpatory differentiation between this muscle and the lateral lumbar inter-

transverse muscles, whereby it should be noted that these two muscles can develop myotendinosis (e.g., hard, palpable band) simultaneously.

SRS Correlation

The insertions at the lateral and medial rows have different spondylogenic correlations. The lateral row of insertion is correlated with the first three sacral vertebrae, the medial one with the last cervical and the first four thoracic vertebrae.

Remarks

The longissimus lumborum is a strong muscle. Myotendinosis of this muscle can cause a functionally abnormal position (segmental dysfunction) in a lumbar vertebra. In the case of the "functionally unstable pelvis" (according to Sutter), a functionally abnormal position of the segments L1, L2 and L3 can be caused by the lateral insertions that are correlated with S1, S2 and L3. Due to the crossover of the SRS of L1, L2 and L3, a complex clinical picture can arise in the axial skeleton, as well as in the extremities.

Length Testing

Examination Procedure

First, while the patient is sitting, the muscle contours are evaluated for symmetry. The patient is then examined in the lateral recumbent (side-lying) position, where both thighs are flexed passively in order to introduce flexion to the lower spine. In this way, the range of motion can be evaluated. Equally important is the evaluation of the end feel (Fig. 8.**43**). Clinical evaluation of the longissimus lumborum muscle is difficult, however, and has therefore proved to be of only limited value, especially when pain is elicited with the procedure.

A similar examination can be performed with the patient in the seated position (Fig. 8.**44**).

Possible Pathological Findings

1. Prominent erector spinae muscle contours in the lumbar region with readily apparent increased tension in the standing patient is an indication that the erector spinae muscle is shortened.
2. Significant loss of flexion motion in the lumbar spine with a soft endfeel. The likelihood that the lumbar erector spinae muscle is shortened increases proportionally with the degree of loss of flexion motion in the lumbar area, especially when sidebending and extension motion are more or less preserved.

3. Muscle tone increases significantly when length testing the rectus femoris muscles at the end range position. This is a reliable test for evaluation of the length of the erector spinae muscle. In the differential diagnosis, the examiner must include lumbar root irritation above L3 with reversed pathological Lasegue test.

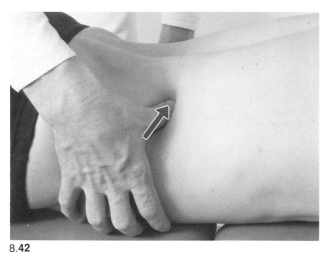

8.42

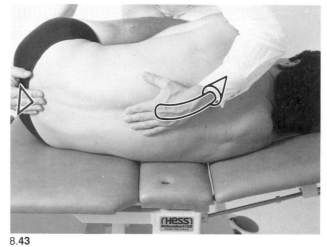

8.43

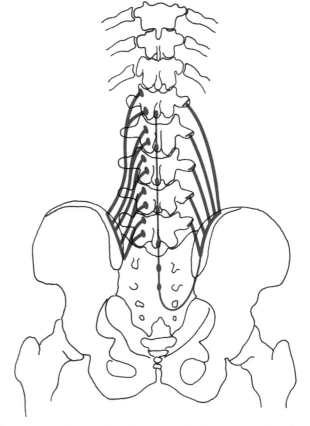

8.44

Fig. 8.45 Longissimus lumborum muscle. Depicted are on the left side, the medial line of insertions of the longissimus lumborum muscle, and on the right side, the lateral line of insertions

8.9.2 Longissimus Thoracis Muscle

Origin

See origin of the longissimus lumborum muscle.

Insertion

The insertions divide into two parts: the medial insertions (narrow) reach the tips of the transverse processes of the thoracic vertebrae (T1–T12) and the lateral insertions (broad) reach the ribs, in particular their inferior margin between the tubercle and costal angle (Fig. 8.**47**). Some of its superior portions are strengthened through other muscle segments originating from the mamillary processes of L1–L2 (see sector V).

Course and Relations

Muscle fibers originating at the iliac crest are destined for inferior insertions. The ones arriving from the lumbar spinous processes and the median sacral crest are directed toward the middle and upper thoracic spine (see sector division, Fig. 8.**48**). The longissimus thoracis muscle lies lateral to the spinalis muscle and medial to the iliocostalis muscle, thus being on the midline over the thoracic transverse processes and lying laterally on the levatores costarum muscles and the ribs, reaching the line of the costal angle (Fig. 8.**47**).

Innervation

Dorsal rami of the spinal nerves.

Function

Bilateral contraction results in extension of the vertebral column, and unilateral contraction results in lateral bending of the vertebral column to the side of the contracted muscle.

Spine	SRS Correlation				
C$_0$					
C$_1$					
C$_2$					
C$_3$					
C$_4$					
C$_5$					
C$_6$					
C$_7$					
T$_1$					
T$_2$					
T$_3$					
T$_4$					
	Sector V				
T$_5$	T$_1$	L$_1$			
T$_6$	T$_2$	L$_2$			
T$_7$	T$_3$	L$_1$			
T$_8$	T$_4$	L$_2$			
			Sector II		
T$_9$			T$_5$	S$_4$	
T$_{10}$			T$_6$	S$_4$	
T$_{11}$			T$_7$	S$_3$	
T$_{12}$			T$_8$	S$_3$	
	Sector III		Sector I		
L$_1$	T$_5$	L$_2$	L$_3$		T$_8$
L$_2$	T$_6$		L$_4$		T$_9$
L$_3$	T$_7$	L$_5$	S$_1$		T$_{10}$
L$_4$	T$_8$	S$_2$	S$_3$		T$_{11}$
L$_5$	T$_9$		S$_4$		T$_{12}$
	Sector IV				
S$_1$		T$_5$	T$_6$		
S$_2$		T$_9$	T$_{10}$		
S$_3$		T$_7$	T$_8$		

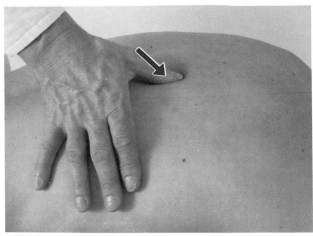

8.46

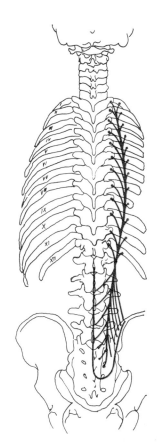

Fig. 8.47 Longissimus thoracis muscle (schematic representation)

Palpatory Technique

Origins (Compare sector division in Fig. 8.**48**).

Sector I: The origin of sector I arises between the origins of the longissimus lumborum muscle on one side and the iliocostalis muscle on the other. The tendinoses at the iliac tuberosity and the intermediate line of the iliac crest are 4 to 8 mm broad. They are palpated posterosuperiorly in the direction of the iliac crest (differential diagnosis of the short sacroiliac ligaments).

Sector II: The tendinoses at the lateral sacral crest are also palpated posterosuperiorly (differential diagnosis: the long dorsal sacroiliac ligaments).

Sector IV: The origin is at the posterior aspect of the sacrum (S3−S4). These tendinoses are also 4 to 8 mm broad and must be distinguished from the sacral zones of irritation (ventralization testing). The palpatory direction is posterosuperior, according to the muscle fiber direction.

Sectors III and V: The origins of these two sectors are located at the spinous processes of L1−L3 (at the median sacral crest). The palpatory direction is in accordance with the muscle fiber direction when performed at the correct palpatory level and with the proper pressure. At L1 and L2, the superior reinforcement (see above) of the mamillary processes must be considered. Palpatory technique is modified accordingly.

Insertion

The same for all sectors: slight lateroinferiorly from posterior in the direction of the inferior lateral margin of the transverse process (Fig. 8.**46**).

The insertion tendinosis of the longissimus thoracis muscle is almost always accompanied by an irritational zone of the corresponding thoracic vertebra (result of myotendinosis).

At the ribs, the insertions are palpated inferiorly, that is, between the tubercle and the costal angle at the inferior margin of the rib (comparison with the adjoining ribs is very important).

It is highly unlikely that the SRS correlation of these lateral lines of insertion is identical to that of the medial insertions. Since they have not been definitely categorized, they will not be treated here. The muscle overlying the hard surface of the ribs and the spinous processes can easily be palpated perpendicular to the fiber direction. This allows for the differential diagnosis of the adjoining muscle layers.

SRS Correlation

See the sector diagrams (Fig. 8.**48**). The longissimus thoracis muscle is one of the most important muscles for the SRS. It responds rapidly to a functional disturbance, and myotendinosis (e. g., hard, palpable band) usually results. It should not be difficult for persons with little palpatory experience to detect the myotendinosis of the longissimus thoracis muscle and to categorize it correctly.

Strength Testing (Mathiass Test)

Examination Procedure

The standing patient is requested to raise the arms 90° in front and subsequently rotate them externally. The patient should breathe freely without forcing respiration (Fig. 8.**49**).

Possible Pathological Findings

1. If the patient has difficulty maintaining this position (i. e., the patient is unsteady), it may be due to weak postural muscles.
2. If the patient drops the arms along with being unable to maintain a maximally erect posture, it is most likely the result of postural weakness.
3. The patient is either unable to maintain this position at all or only for a few seconds along with observable asymmetry. This is probably due to significant postural decompensation, but the possibility of neurogenic paralysis/paresis must always be kept in mind.

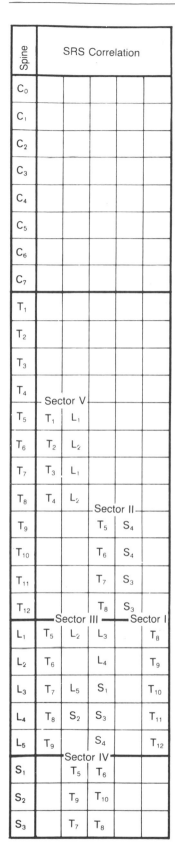

Spine	SRS Correlation				
C₀					
C₁					
C₂					
C₃					
C₄					
C₅					
C₆					
C₇					
T₁					
T₂					
T₃					
T₄	*Sector V*				
T₅	T₁	L₁			
T₆	T₂	L₂			
T₇	T₃	L₁			
T₈	T₄	L₂			
T₉			T₅	S₄	
T₁₀	*Sector II*		T₆	S₄	
T₁₁			T₇	S₃	
T₁₂			T₈	S₃	
L₁	*Sector III* T₅	L₂	L₃		*Sector I* T₈
L₂	T₆		L₄		T₉
L₃	T₇	L₅	S₁		T₁₀
L₄	T₈	S₂	S₃		T₁₁
L₅	T₉		S₄		T₁₂
S₁	*Sector IV* T₅	T₆			
S₂	T₉	T₁₀			
S₃	T₇	T₈			

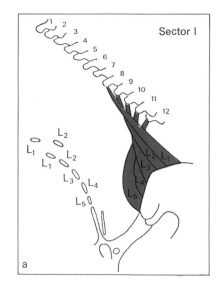

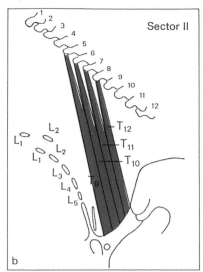

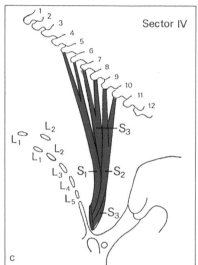

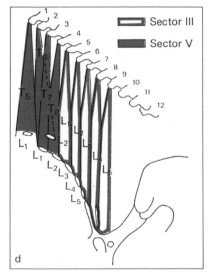

Fig. 8.**48** Myotendinoses of the longissimus thoracis muscle (for better demonstration, the thoracic spine is schematically presented as its mirror image) (after Sutter)

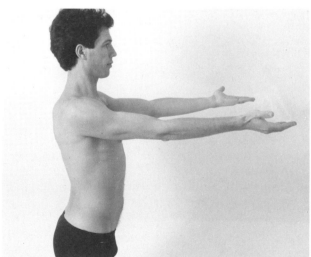

8.**49**

8.9.3 Longissimus Cervicis Muscle

Origin

The transverse processes of T(1)2−T6, close to the center of the superior surface of the tip. The muscle can reach T8 in some cases.

Insertion

The posterior surface and root of the transverse processes (posterior tubercles) of C(1)2−C5(6−7). It inserts practically together with the iliocostalis cervicis muscle, the splenius cervicis muscle, the levator scapulae muscle, the posterior scalene muscle, and the longissimus capitis muscle (Fig. 8.**50**).

Course and relations

This is a flat, weak muscle with its main surface in the sagittal direction. At the T4−T5 level, it is often connected to the belly of the longissimus thoracis muscle via a tendon. In its lower half, it runs medially to the longissimus thoracis muscle. The muscle belly in the lower cervical region runs deeply and laterally to the longissimus capitis muscle, which in turn is lateral to the semispinalis capitis muscle. The muscle fiber direction is almost perfectly longitudinal. The longissimus group and the semispinalis capitis muscle have their own muscular fascia and can therefore be easily distinguished from each other by palpation (Fig. 8.**51**).

Innervation

Dorsal rami of the spinal nerve, the cervical nerves, and the thoracic nerves C3−C2.

Function

Unilateral contraction results in lateral bending of the cervical spine to the side of the contracted muscle, and bilateral contraction results in extension of the cervical spine.

Palpatory Technique

The muscle belly is, as already described, easily palpable in the region of the lower cervical spine (perpendicular to the fiber direction).

The origins are palpated at the tip of the thoracic transverse processes from superior to inferior. It is very difficult to differentiate these origins from the semispinalis capitis and cervicis muscles (differential diagnosis at the insertion). The insertion at the posterior tubercle of the costal transverse processes are palpated from inferiorly to superiorly.

SRS Correlation

Each origin to insertion unit represents one myotenone (i.e., always the most superior insertion together with the most superior origin).

8.9.4 Longissimus Capitis Muscle

Origin

The transverse processes of C(3−4)5−C7 to T1−T3(5). It arises at the cervical spine medial to the insertions and at the thoracic spine medial to the origins of the longissimus cervicis muscle.

Insertion

The posterior margin of the mastoid process to its tip with a length of 1,5 cm (Fig. 8.**52**).

Course and Relations

The longissimus capitis muscle is a slender muscle oriented in the sagittal plane. The longitudinal muscle bundles are arranged in such a manner that the bundles originating most inferiorly lie at the anterior edge of the muscle belly. In the deep layer of the lower cervical region, the muscle can easily be palpated between the semispinalis capitis and the longissimus cervicis muscle. It is covered at its insertion by the splenius capitis muscle and the sternocleidomastoid muscle (Fig. 8.**53**).

Innervation

Dorsal rami of the cervical nerves C1−C3, possibly C4.

Function

Unilateral contraction results in lateral bending and rotation of the head to the side of the contracted muscle, and bilateral contraction results in extension of the head.

Palpatory Technique

The muscle belly can easily be palpated perpendicularly to the fiber direction in the deep layers of the lower cervical region between the semispinalis capitis muscle and the longissimus muscle (see Figs. 7.**4** and 7.**14** of the cervical spine and thoracic spine cross-sections).

The insertion at the mastoid is palpated from posteroinferior to superior under the splenius capitis muscle and the sternocleidomastoid muscle from which it must be differentiated (Fig. 8.**52**). The origins are palpated from superior to inferior in the direction of the root of the corresponding transverse processes.

SRS Correlation

For this muscle as well, the muscular unit arising from one vertebra represents one myotenone. Differentiation of the individual myotendinoses at the insertion at the mastoid is impossible due to the concentration of ten myotenoses in this small area. The examiner can only palpate a painful insertion. A differential diagnosis is established with the aid of the origin tendinoses and the correlating zones of irritation.

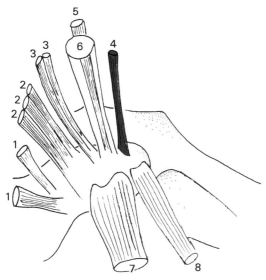

Fig. 8.**50** Muscle attachments at the tip of the thoracic transverse process

1	Rotatores m	5	Longissimus capitis m
2	Multifidus m	6	Semispinalis capitis m
3	Semispinalis cervicis m	7	Longissimus thoracis m
4	Longissimus cervicis m	8	Levator costae m

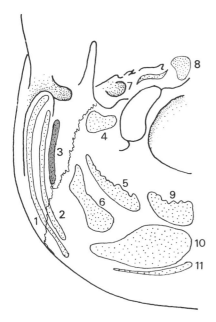

Fig. 8.**52** Muscle attachments at the occiput

1 Sternocleidomastoid m
2 Splenius capitis m
3 Longissimus capitis m
4 Rectus capitis lateralis m
5 Rectus capitis posterior major m
6 Obliquus capitis superior m
7 Rectus capitis anterior m
8 Longus capitis m
9 Rectus capitis posterior minor m
10 Semispinalis capitis m
11 Trapezius m

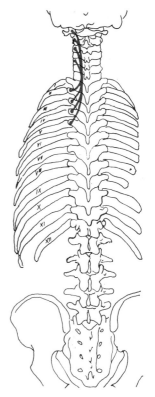

Fig. 8.**51** Longissimus cervicis m

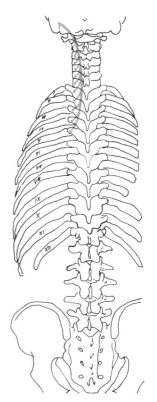

Fig. 8.**53** Longissimus capitis m

8.9.5 Iliocostalis Lumborum Muscle

Origin

The broad and thick sacrospinous ligament (see page 260), and the anterolateral surface of the iliac tuberosity.

Insertion

At the costal angle of ribs XII to IV (Fig. 8.55a).

8.9.6 Iliocostalis Thoracis Muscle

Origin

Medially at the costal angle of ribs XII to VII (Fig. 8.55b).

Insertion

Laterally at the costal angle of ribs VII to I (Fig. 8.55b).

8.9.7 Iliocostalis Cervicis Muscle

Origin

Directly medial to the costal angle of ribs VII to III (IV) (Fig. 8.55c).

Insertion

At the posterior tubercles of the transverse processes of C3(4)—C6 (refer to the insertion of the longissimus cervicis muscle) (Fig. 8.55c)

Course and Relations

The iliocostalis muscle shows a tilelike architecture. The iliocostalis lumborum muscle ascends from inferior, traverses the posterior surfaces of the ribs going superiorly, and runs lateral to the longissimus thoracis muscle. In the neck region, the iliocostalis cervicis muscle also lies lateral to the longissimus cervicis and capitis muscles and medial to the posterior and medial scalene muscles as well as the levator scapulae muscle. Its main plane is in the sagittal direction. The iliocostalis cervicis muscle can be isolated anatomically but must be seen as the direct continuation of the iliocostalis lumborum muscle (Fig. 8.55a—c).

Innervation

Dorsal rami of the spinal nerves.

Function

Bilateral contraction results in extension of the vertebral column, and unilateral contraction results in lateral bending of the vertebral column to the side of the contracted muscle.

Palpatory Technique

At its origin, the iliocostalis lumborum muscle cannot be distinguished from the tendon of the longissimus dorsi muscle. In its course, the iliocostalis muscle is found lateral to the longissimus dorsi muscle. Inferiorly, it is possible to palpate the insertion tendinoses at the inferior edge and the posterior surface of the costal angle (Fig. 8.54). To avoid the contact with the levator costae muscle, the direction must be perfectly inferior.

The iliocostalis cervicis muscle can also be palpated easily. Its origins are palpated from medial-superior to lateral-inferior in the direction of costal angles. The insertions are palpated from inferior to superior at the posterior tubercles of the cervical transverse processes. During this maneuver, the examiner has to differentiate between other muscles inserting at this location (longissimus cervicis muscle, levator scapulae muscle of C3—C4, scalene medial and posterior muscles, and the medial portion of the posterior cervical intertransverse muscles).

SRS Correlation

The spondylogenic correlation of the iliocostalis muscle is still undetermined. There are indications that the iliocostalis cervicis muscle is correlated with the myotenone L5.

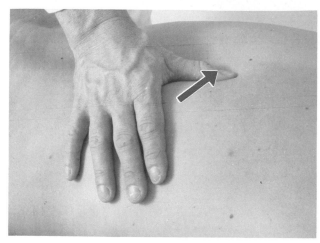

8.54

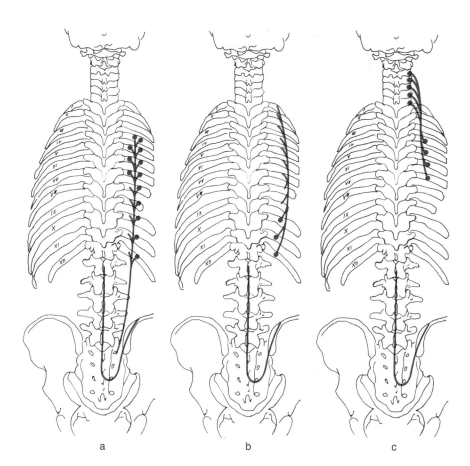

Fig. 8.55 a Iliocostalis lumborum m

b Iliocostalis thoracis m
c Iliocostalis cervicis m

a   b   c

8.10   Splenius Muscle

This is a flat muscle that typically divides at its insertion into the splenius capitis and splenius cervicis muscles.

8.10.1 Splenius Capitis Muscle

Origin

The nuchal ligament: inferior to and including C3. Further, from the spinous processes of C7 and T1–T3 and the supraspinous ligament (Fig. 8.**57**).

Insertion

At the lateral surface of the mastoid process, including its tip. This insertion forms a posterior arch reaching the lateral half of the superior nuchal line (Fig. 8.**56**).

8.10.2 Splenius Cervicis Muscle

Origin

The spinous processes and the supraspinous ligaments of T3–T10. The length of the tendons increases inferiorly. The parallel muscle bundles form a long, slender belly that is more vertical than that of the splenius capitis muscle and swings around the neck superolaterally.

Insertion

Via three tendons of disproportionate strength. The strongest fascicle inserts in the posteroinferior portion of the tip of the transverse process of the atlas, the second strongest, at the tip of the transverse process of the axis, and the third, at the posterior surface of the transverse process of C3 (Fig. 8.**57**).

Course and Relation

A broad section of the inferior and medial portions of the splenius muscle is covered by the trapezius muscle, the rhomboid muscle, and the serratus posterior superior muscle. The sternocleidomastoid and the levator scapulae muscles cover the splenius muscle superiorly and laterally. The splenius muscle overlies the semispinalis capitis muscle (see Fig. 7.**4**, the cervical spine cross-section). Many parts of the inserting tendons of the splenius cervicis muscles are fused with the tendons of the levator scapulae muscle and the longissimus cervicis muscle. The free medial border of the splenius capitis muscle forms together with the nuchal ligament and the medial end of the superior nuchal line, a triangular space through which the occipital vessels and the greater occipital nerve emerge.

Innervation

Dorsal rami of the cervical nerves C1–C5.

Function

Bilateral contraction results in extension of the head and the cervical spine, and unilateral contraction results in lateral bending and rotation of the head to the side of the contracted muscle.

Palpatory Technique

Due to the flat nature of these muscles, palpation is difficult. The spinous process of C3 is palpated first superolaterally. The examiner continues palpating inferiorly through C4–C5 to T5–T6, staying at the surface. The palpatory direction is almost vertical in the inferior segments. The inserting portion of the splenius capitis muscle is palpated inferiorly at the lateral surface of the mastoid process and is then followed in an arch to the superior nuchal line. The strongest insertion tendon of the splenius cervicis muscle is palpated posteroinferiorly in the direction of the tip of the transverse process of the atlas. The inserting tendons leading to C2 and C3 are substantially weaker and are palpated from a posteroinferior direction as well.

SRS Correlation

Both the splenius capitis and the splenius cervicis muscles are correlated with the vertebra of C7 as one single myotenone.

Remarks

The splenius cervicis muscle traverses the zone of irritation of C7, which can often lead to confusion with myotendinotic changes of the splenius capitis muscle. The examiner can avoid this situation, however, by flexing the head laterally (relaxation and displacement of the splenius cervicis muscle).

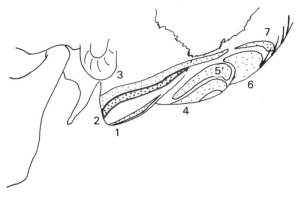

Fig. 8.**56** Muscle attachments at the mastoid process and the occiput

1 Longissimus capitis m
2 Splenius capitis m
3 Sternocleidomastoid m
4 Rectus capitis posterior major m
5 Obliquus capitis superior m
6 Semispinalis capitis m
7 Trapezius m

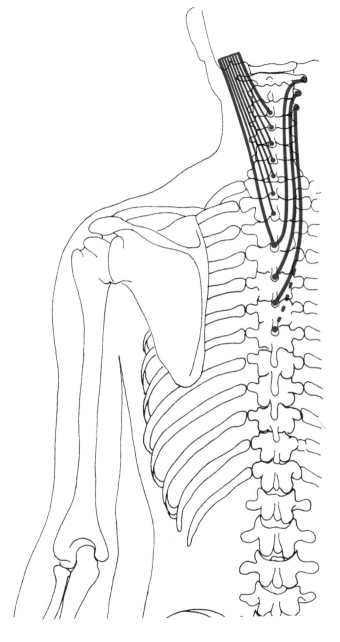

Fig. 8.**57** Splenius capitis muscle on the left, splenius cervicis muscle on the right

8.11 Levatores Costarum (Longi and Breves) Muscles

The levatores costarum muscles are short and strong and are only found alongside the thoracic spine. They owe their name to their action of lifting the ribs. There are 12 pairs of short levatores costarum muscles, and only four pairs of the long levatores costarum muscles are developed: that is, those for the four most inferior ribs. Here, they are discussed collectively, even though their SRS correlation is different.

Origin

The posterior tubercle of the transverse processes of C7 the inferior margin of the thick tip of the transverse processes of T1–T11, sometimes including its base.

Insertion

The levatores costarum muscles insert at the superoposterior surface of the ribs, that is, between the tubercle and the costal angle. The short levatores costarum muscles insert into the outer surface of the rib immediately below their respective origins. In contrast, the long levatores costarum muscles skip the rib immediately inferior and therefore insert two ribs below their respective origin.

Course and Relations

The levatores costarum muscles are found at the same level as the short deep muscles of the back (such as the intertransverse muscles and rotatores muscles). Thus, they lie under the muscle masses of the long and superficial back musculature (see Fig. 7.**14**, the cross-section of the thoracic spine).

The direction of the muscles from their origin to their insertion at the ribs is lateroinferior (Fig. 8.**58**).

Innervation

The intercostal nerves, T1–T11.

Function

Even though the levatores costarum muscles insert at the ribs, they belong functionally to the deep back muscles, rather than to the intercostales muscles. Bilateral contraction results in extension of the thoracic spine, and unilateral contraction results in rotation of the vertebral column to the opposite side and lateral bending of the vertebral column to the side of the contracted muscle.

Palpatory Technique

The close relationship to both the longissimus thoracis muscle at the origin and the iliocostalis thoracis muscle at the insertion, which cover these small muscles, for the most part, requires a precise palpatory direction. First the thumb locates the myotendinosis perpendicular to the direction of the fibers and then follows the muscle in order to determine the tendinoses.

SRS Correlation

These muscles, which have a very small diameter, are often responsible for certain vertebral and rib lesions, that is, the socalled blocked rib. This situation must be diagnosed via provocative testing. The pattern resulting from the zone of irritation dictates the adequate therapy both for the vertebra and the rib.

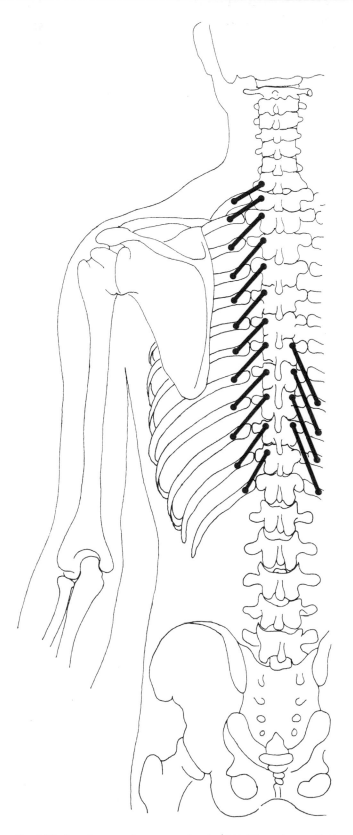

Fig. 8.**58** Levatores costarum muscles: longi (right) and breves (left)

8.12 Scalene Muscles

8.12.1 Anterior Scalene Muscle

Origin

This muscle arises as four tendons from the anterior tubercles of the transverse processes of C3−C6. The strongest, fleshy tendinous slip arises from the anterior tubercle (tuberculum caroticum) of C6.

Insertion

Tubercle of the anterior scalene muscle at the upper first rib (Figs. 8.**60**, 8.**61**).

8.12.2 Middle Scalene Muscle

Origin

Posterior margin of the groove for the spinal nerve and the posterior tubercles of the transverse processes of C3−C7 (Fig. 8.**60**).

Insertion

This muscle inserts along the entire width of the first rib, behind the subclavian roof, with tendinous insertion in the fascia of the first intercostal space (outer thoracic surface), and sometimes at the superior edge of the second rib (Fig. 8.**61**).

8.12.3 Posterior Scalene Muscle

Origin

The posterior tubercles of the transverse processes of C6 and C7.

Insertion

This muscle inserts as a thin aponeurosis at the outer surface of the second rib (next to the tuberosity for the serratus anterior muscle) (Fig. 8.**62**).

Course and Relations

The spatial arrangement of the scalene muscles can be deduced from their name. The anterior scalene muscle lies lateral to the inferior portion of the longus colli muscle. The middle scalene muscle lies posterolaterally to the scalene anterior muscle, and the posterior scalene muscle lies posteriorly to the middle scalene muscle.

The fiber direction of the three muscles is latero-inferior.

In contrast to the anterior and middle scalene muscles, the posterior scalene muscle traverses the first rib and inserts at the second rib.

When palpating, the examiner must be aware of the close relationship of the scalene muscles with the subclavian artery and the brachial plexus.

Innervation

The ventral rami of the cervical spinal nerves (C3−C8).

Function

Bilateral contraction results in flexion of the cervical spine, and unilateral contraction results in bending to the side of the contracted muscle, with opposite rotation of the cervical spine. When the cervical spine is fixed, the muscle raises the second rib.

Palpatory Technique

The origin tendinoses at the anterior and posterior tubercles are palpated anteroinferiorly. The origins can easily be reached with the finger used for palpation. The insertions at the first rib (anterior and middle scalene muscles) are palpated superiorly, behind the clavicles in the thoracic inlet. It should be noted that the patient finds this palpatory procedure extremely uncomfortable, which is primarily attributable to the brachial plexus. The insertion of the posterior scalene muscle is palpated at the second rib, from posterosuperior, about two finger widths lateral to the end of the transverse process of T2. Since palpation is through the trapezius muscle, the palpatory findings are not easily elicited.

SRS Correlation

The myotendinosis of the anterior scalene muscle may cause a "functionally abnormal position" (segmental dysfunction) at the cervical spine in the anterior direction, similar to the myotendinosis of the longus colli muscle (the more anterior the segmental dysfunction, the stronger the zone of irritation). The scalene muscle myotenones are correlated with the central portion of the thoracic spine.

Remarks

The so-called elevated rib is usually the result of myotendinosis (i. e., a hard, palpable band) in one part of the scalene muscles.

Length Testing of the Scalene Muscles

Examination Procedure

The shoulder girdle of the seated patient is fixed in two ways: anteriorly, by the examiner's flat hand and posteriorly, by the examiner's thigh. The anterior and medial scalene muscles are palpated by the examiner's index finger while the other hand introduces passive extension and rotation motion to the head in the opposite direction (Fig. 8.**6**).

Possible Pathological Findings

1. Soft endfeel at the motion barrier (extreme of movement). Perceivable increase in tissue tension immediately lateral to the sternocleidomastoid muscle. Musculatur imbalance with shortening of scalene muscles, often in combination with a shortened sternocleidomastoid muscle.
2. Localized pain in the region of the lateral triangle in the neck, occasionally radiating towards the arms. Pseudoradicular pain radiation may be present. This must be differentiated from the so-called thoracic outlet syndrome.

3. Slowly progressive vertigo may be present (please refer to the sternocleidomastoid muscle).
4. Immediate vertigo (please refer to the sternocleidomastoid muscle).

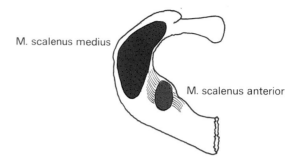

Fig. 8.**61**   Muscle attachments at the first rib

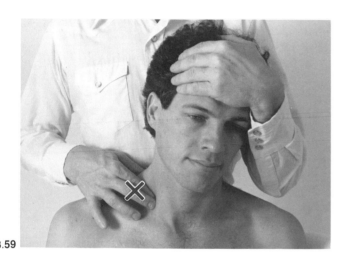

8.**59**

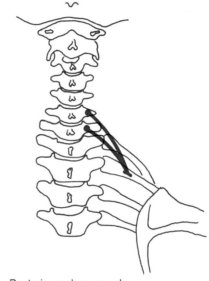

Fig. 8.**62**   Posterior scalene muscle

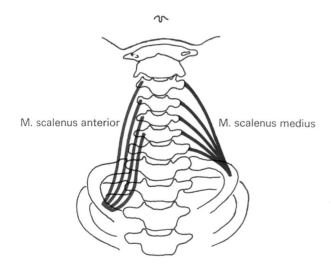

Fig. 8.**60**   Scalene muscles

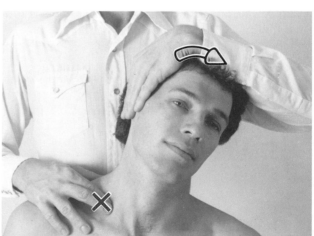

8.**63**

8.13 Muscles of the Serratus Group

8.13.1 Anterior Serratus Muscle

Origin

The anterior serratus muscle arises by nine, sometimes ten, strong fasciculi from the convex portion of the body ribs I to IX (X). The four most inferior fasciculi slide below the insertions of the external abdominal oblique muscle (Fig. 8.**66**).

Insertion

The muscle inserts at the costal surface of the medial margin of the scapula, between the superior and inferior angle. Fibers arising from the first and second rib insert at the superior angle, and those arising from the third and fourth rib insert at the center of the medial margin. The remaining muscle fibers, the strongest, arise from ribs V to X in a fan-shaped pattern. They insert at the inferior angle of the scapula (Fig. 8.**67**).

Innervation

Long thoracic nerve from C5−C7.

Function

The anterior serratus muscle draws the scapula forward, away from the vertebral column; primarily, the inferior portions rotate the scapula so that the glenoid cavity points in a superior direction (abduction of the arm beyond the horizontal).

Palpation

Starting with the fourth rib and below the origin fasciculi are easily palpated, even without pathological muscle changes. At the lateral thoracic wall, the fasciculi are palpated posteriorly (Fig. 8.**64**). In order to reach the insertion, the scapula must be elevated at the inferior angle. The finger follows along the costal surface of the medial margin as far as possible (Fig. 8.**65**).

SRS Correlation

Involved in the spondylogenic event are most often the myotenones arising from the sixth and seventh ribs; these myotenones are also responsible for the corresponding abnormal position of the ribs.

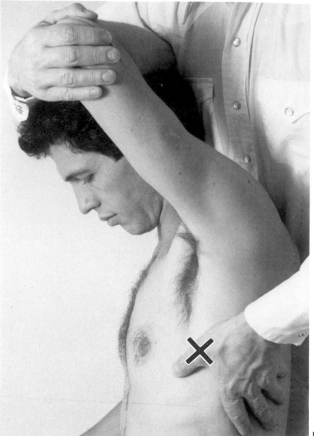

8.64

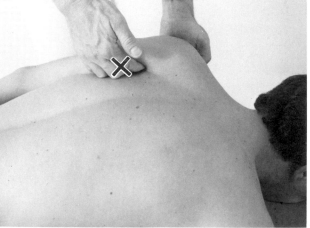

8.65

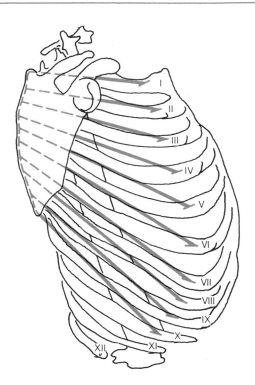

Fig. 8.**66**   Anterior serratus muscle

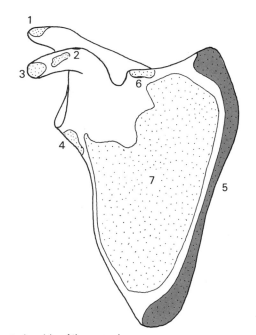

1   Deltoid m
2   Pectoralis minor m
3   Coracobrachialis m
    Biceps brachii m (short head)
4   Triceps brachii m (long head)
5   Serratus anterior m
6   Omohyoid m
7   Subscapularis m

Fig. 8.**67**   Muscle attachments at the anterior side of the scapula

8.13.2 Serratus Posterior Superior Muscle

Origin

The muscle arises from the nuchal ligament close to the spinous process of C6 and from the tips of the spinous processes of C7, T1, and T2.

Insertion

The muscle inserts by four fasciculi at ribs II to V, lateral to the costal angles.

Course and Relations

This deep muscle runs from the spinous processes to the ribs at an angle of about 30° and is primarily covered by the rhomboid and the trapezius muscles (Fig. 8.**68**).

Innervation

Intercostal nerves of T1−T4.

Function

Elevation of the ribs.

Palpation

This deep muscle can be palpated at the spinous processes only from an inferolateral direction, which in turn is only possible when the insertion tendinoses are localized and when differentiated from the spondylogenic correlation with the rhomboid muscle.

Strength Testing

See page 284.

8.13.3 Seratus Posterior Inferior Muscle

Origin

The spinous processes and the supraspinous ligament T11−L2(3). The tendon of the origin of the serratus posterior inferior muscle is practically identical with the superficial layer of the thoracolumbar fascia and the lumbar origin aponeurosis of the latissimus dorsi muscle (Fig. 8.**68**).

Insertion

The serratus posterior inferior muscle inserts by four fasciculi at the inferior margin of ribs IX to XII between the origins of the latissimus dorsi muscle and the iliocostalis muscle. The most lateral fibers travel to the ninth rib almost horizontally.

Course and Relations

This muscle, which shows an almost perfectly horizontal course, is only covered by the latissimus dorsi muscle. The tendon and muscle junction is located at the lateral edge of the iliocostalis muscle, where a painful myotendinosis can often be found.

Innervation

Intercostal nerves T9−T12.

Function

Fixation of the four most inferior ribs (resistance to diaphragm contraction), therefore considered to support inspiration.

Palpation

Even though the serratus posterior inferior muscle is completely covered by the latissimus dorsi muscle, a myotendinosis may be palpated very well.

The palpatory direction is perpendicular to the fiber direction, from inferior to superior. The insertion tendinoses are located at the ribs about four finger widths lateral to the spinous processes.

SRS Correlation

Both the serratus posterior superior muscle and the serratus posterior inferior muscle represent one individual myotenone. Segmental dysfunction of the first thoracic vertebra can cause a palpable band in the serratus posterior superior muscle. Segmental dysfunction of the first lumbar vertebra can cause a palpable band in the serratus posterior inferior muscle.

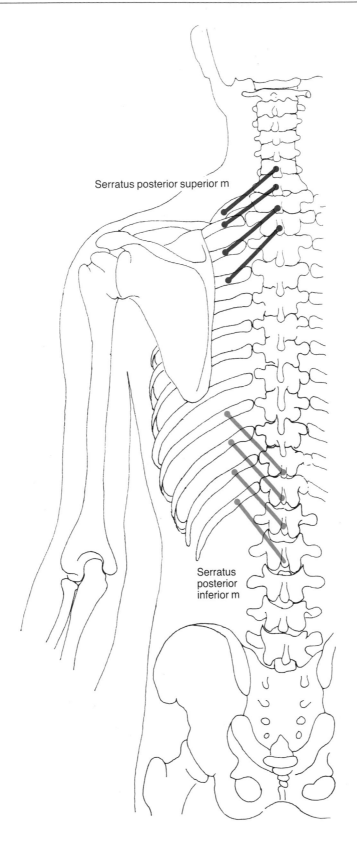

Serratus posterior superior m

Serratus
posterior
inferior m

Fig. 8.**68** Serrati muscles

8.14   Levator Scapulae Muscle

Origin

The levator scapulae muscle arises by four fasciculi from the transverse processes of the first four cervical vertebrae. The first, the strongest, origin tendon reaches around the transverse process of the atlas lateroanteriorly. The origin tendons from C2 to C4 arise from the posterior tubercles. The first two fasciculi are completely fused with the tendons of the splenius cervicis muscle, and the last two are commonly fused with the longissimus cervicis muscle (Fig. 8.**71**).

Insertion

The muscle inserts at the medial border of the scapula between the superior angle and the base of the scapular spine. The muscle bundles from C1 insert immediately below the superior angle of the scapula. The insertions of the muscle fibers originating from C2 to C4 reach the base of the spine of the scapula at an extremely sharp angle (Fig. 8.**72**).

Course and Relations

The levator scapulae muscle is located laterally at the neck between the anterior and posterior muscle mass, and from C5–C6 on is covered by fibers of the trapezius muscles.

Innervation

The cervical plexus and the nerve of the rhomboids (n. dorsalis scapulae C3–C5).

Function

Elevation of the scapula. When the scapula is fixed, it bends the neck laterally to the side of the contracted muscle.

Palpatory Technique

Palpation cannot differentiate between the origins of this muscle and other muscles originating in close proximity (see Fig. 7.**5** for a diagram of the cervical spine). The insertion tendinosis at the medial border of the scapula, however, can clearly be identified. Due to the steeply angled insertion, the palpatory direction is from the superior direction (Fig. 8.**69**).

SRS Correlation

Regional dysfunction of the upper thoracic spine can cause a palpable band (Table, p. 285).

Remarks

When myotendinotic changes affect both the levator scapulae muscle and the descending part of the trapezius muscle, an extremely painful "cross-myosis" at the T1 level often develops about three finger widths from the spinous process and thus complicates the correct manipulation of C3 and C4.

Length Testing of the Levator Scapulae Muscle

Examination Procedure

The arm of the supine patient is maximally abducted (elevated) at the shoulder. This causes the scapula to externally rotate. The patient's elbow comes to rest against the abdomen of the examiner, who is standing behind the patient. With one hand, the examiner fixates the patient's superior angle and the superior margin of the patient's shoulder (Fig. 8.**70**). The other hand introduces flexion and rotation of the head in the opposite direction. With this maneuver, the examiner evaluates whether pain is induced in addition to assessing range of motion and palpatory changes such as increased muscle tension in the levator scapulae muscle proximal to the superior angle.

Possible Pathological Findings

Loss of range of motion with soft endfeel accompanied by pain between the shoulder blades. Typically, when the levator scapulae is shortened, the origin tendinosis can be found at the medial margin of the scapula, and a hard, palpable band (myotendinosis) can be palpated above the superior angle of the scapula.

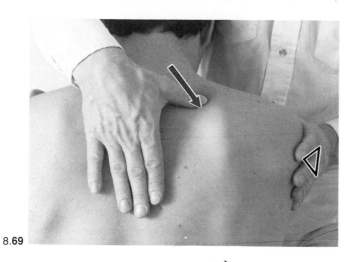

8.69

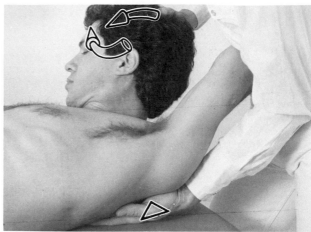

8.70

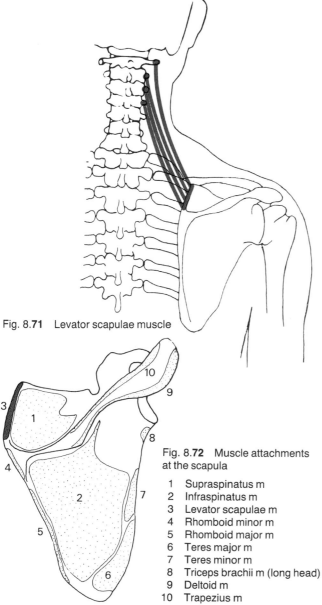

Fig. 8.71 Levator scapulae muscle

Fig. 8.72 Muscle attachments at the scapula

1 Supraspinatus m
2 Infraspinatus m
3 Levator scapulae m
4 Rhomboid minor m
5 Rhomboid major m
6 Teres major m
7 Teres minor m
8 Triceps brachii m (long head)
9 Deltoid m
10 Trapezius m

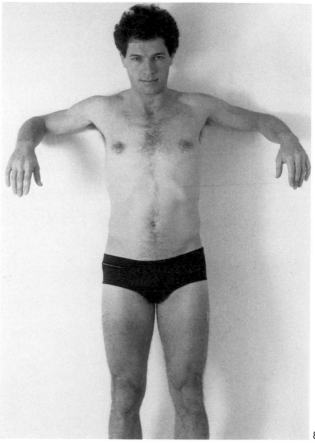

8.73

8.15 Rhomboid Major and Minor Muscles

Origin

The rhomboid minor muscle arises via a short aponeurosis from the nuchal ligament at the C6 level and from the spinous process of C7; the rhomboid major arises from the spinous processes of T1–T4, rudimentarily from T5 (Fig. 8.**75**).

Insertion

The medial border of the scapula: the rhomboid minor muscle inserts at the level of the spine of the scapula; the rhomboid major muscle inserts distally to the base of the spine of the scapula (Fig. 8.**76**).

Innervation

Nerve of the rhomboids (n. dorsalis scapulae C4, C5).

Function

Elevation and drawing of the scapula medially.

Palpatory Technique

The close relationship to the trapezius muscle (horizontal portion) requires that the finger presses deeply from the lateroinferior direction during palpation; a definitive differentiation is possible at the medial border of the scapula due to the insertion tendinoses, which are approached mediosuperiorly.

SRS Correlation

A palpable band can be observed as a result of regional dysfunction of the upper thoracic spine (Table, p. 285).

Remarks

Both rhomboid muscles often participate in the spondylogenic event; clinically, patients indicate pain between the shoulder blades.

Strength Testing of the Medial Shoulder Blade Fixator Muscles (Serratus superior muscle, and rhomboid and trapezius [horizontal portion] muscles)

Examination Procedure

The patient is in the standing position with the back against the wall and arms abducted to 90°. While keeping the trunk erect, the patient moves the feet two foot lengths in front of the wall. Subsequently, the patient is requested to push the trunk and thus the shoulder blades away from the wall (about 2 cm) and maintain this position for approximately 30 seconds. Healthy persons and persons who exercise regularly should have no difficulty in performing this maneuver (Fig. 8.**73**). In another maneuver, the arms of the prone patient are abducted at the shoulder. With the arms crossed, the examiner palpates the medial margin of the scapula. The patient is then requested to contract the muscles responsible for medial shoulder blade fixation, a maneuver performed by lifting the arms off the examination table (Fig. 8.**74**).

Possible Pathological Findings

1. The standing patient may start to recruit additional respiratory muscles causing forced respiration. This should make the examiner suspect weakness in the medial shoulder blade fixator muscles.
2. The patient in the prone position experiences difficulty in displacing the shoulder blades medially. This is usually due to prominent weakness of the medial shoulder blade fixator muscles.

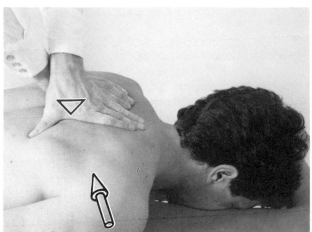

8.74

Spine	SRS Correlation		
C₀			
C₁			
C₂		Rhomboid minor/major muscle	
C₃			
C₄		C₇	
C₅			T₁
C₆			T₂
C₇			T₃
T₁	Levator scapulae m		T₄
T₂	C₁		T₅
T₃	C₂		
T₄	C₃		
T₅	C₄		
T₆			
T₇			
T₈			
T₉			
T₁₀			
T₁₁			
T₁₂			
L₁			
L₂			
L₃			
L₄			
L₅			
S₁			
S₂			
S₃			

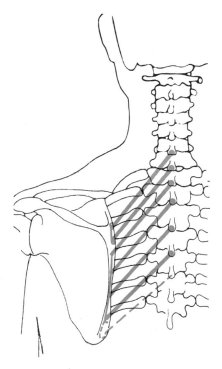
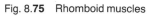

Fig. 8.75 Rhomboid muscles

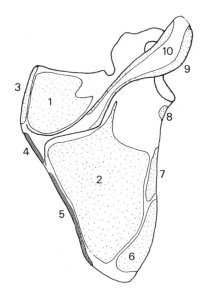

Fig. 8.76 Muscle attachments on the scapula

8.16 Latissimus Dorsi Muscle

Origin

1. **Vertebral region:** From the spinous processes and the supraspinous ligaments (T(7)8–L5, possibly from the median sacral crest (Fig. 8.**79**).
2. **Iliac region:** From the external lip of the iliac crest, at the junction of the iliac tuberosity and the iliac crest; about four finger widths broad.
3. **Costal region:** As thin fasciculi from the outer surfaces of ribs X to XII; between the origins of the obliquus externus abdominis muscle and the insertions of the serratus posterior inferior muscle.
4. **Thoracolumbar fascia**

Insertion

The proximal end of the crest of the lesser tuberosity, connecting distally to the insertion of the sub-scapularis muscle. The proximal portion of the insertion belongs to the distal vertebral, iliac, and costal myotenones, the distal portion to the proximal vertebral myotenones, causing the latissimus dorsi muscle to be somewhat twisted (Fig. 8.**80**).

Course and Relations

The superior bundles run horizontally above the inferior angle of the scapula and the origin of the teres major muscle. In the axilla, the muscle, which otherwise is flat, becomes considerably thick.

The lateral edge of the muscle descends from the axilla to the ilium vertically.

Innervation

Thoracodorsal nerves C6–C8.

Function: Adduction, extension, and medial rotation of the arm. The costal origins aid in inspiration.

Palpatory Technique

The iliac crest, the latissimus dorsi muscle, and the external abdominal oblique muscle form the lumbar triangle (Petiti). Due to the flat origin aponeurosis, myotendinosis in the lumbar region is almost impossible to palpate. Better information about the muscle is gained in the posterior axillary fold (Fig. 8.**77**). When investigating the condition of the latissimus dorsi muscle, the approach is similar to the descending portion of the trapezius muscle. The myotendinosis is palpated perpendicular to the muscle fiber orientation in both directions: superiorly to the insertion at the crest of the lesser tuberosity and inferiorly. At the spinous processes, the origin of the latissimus dorsi, which is often painful, must be distinguished from the longissimus thoracis muscle, which lies below (Fig. 8.**78**). The myotendinosis of this flat muscle can be palpated distinctly from rib to rib above its hard surface.

Remarks

The latissimus dorsi muscle is very often involved in the spondylogenic event. Patients indicate a rather fan-shaped, constant pain in the lumbar spine region.

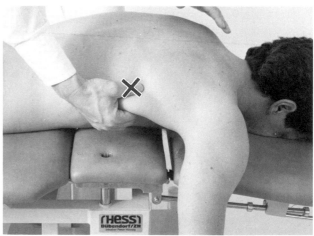

8.**77**

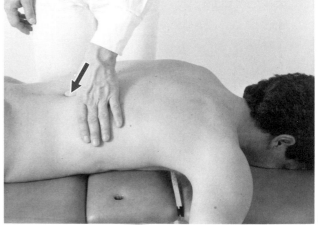

8.**78**

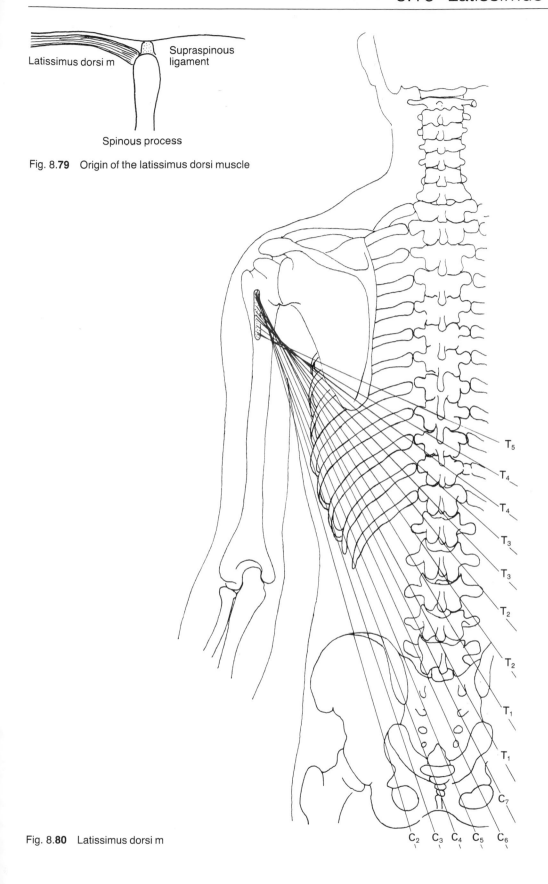

Latissimus dorsi m

Supraspinous
ligament

Spinous process

Fig. 8.**79** Origin of the latissimus dorsi muscle

T$_5$

T$_4$

T$_4$

T$_3$

T$_3$

T$_2$

T$_2$

T$_1$

T$_1$

C$_7$

C$_2$ C$_3$ C$_4$ C$_5$ C$_6$

Fig. 8.**80** Latissimus dorsi m

8.17 Trapezius Muscle

Origin

The origin of the trapezius muscle extends between the occipital bone and the twelfth thoracic vertebra. It is useful to anatomically and spondylogenically divide this muscle into three sections: the descending, horizontal, and ascending portions (Fig. 8.**83**).

Descending portion: the muscle arises from the superior nuchal line, 2 cm lateral to the external occipital protuberance; the nuchal ligament to the sixth cervical vertebra.

Horizontal portion: the spinous processes of C7−T3

Ascending portion: the spinous processes of T4−T12.

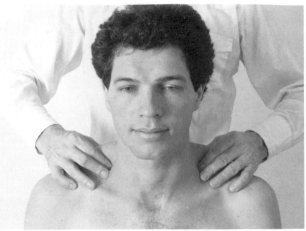

8.81

Insertion

Descending portion: the superior surface of the spine of the scapula, the acromioclavicular joint, and the posterosuperior margin of the lateral third of the clavicle (Fig. 8.**84a**).

Horizontal portion: the superior surface of the spine of the scapula from the base to the acromio-clavicular joint. At the spine of the scapula, this portion covers the insertion of the descending portion (important for palpation) (Fig. 8.**84b**).

Ascending portion: the inferior edge of the spine of the scapula, between the tuberosity and the lumbar triangle (Fig. 8.**84b**).

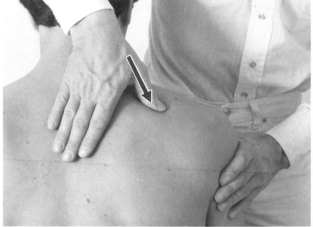

8.82

Course and Relations

The muscle bundles arising from the occipital bone run sharply inferiorly, whereas the fibers continuing below course away from the ligamentum nuchae at a sharp angle. The fibers from the most inferior portion of the cervical spine approximate the transverse direction (Fig. 8.**83**).

Innervation

The descending portion of the spinal accessory nerve and the rami of the cervical plexus C2−C4.

Function

Descending portion: elevation of the shoulder blade.

Horizontal portion: adduction of the scapula.

Ascending portion: pulling down of the scapula.

Palpatory Technique

Since the trapezius muscle is located subcutaneously, palpating it serves as good training for the beginner. All anatomic structures can be exactly located and easily reached. To gain an overview of whether myotendinotic changes are present, the muscle belly

of the descending portion is grasped halfway between the shoulder and the neck between the thumb and index finger, upon which the examiner moves up and down perpendicularly in the direction of the muscle fibers (Fig. 8.**81**). At the spinous processes, the spine of the scapula, and the clavicles, the tendinoses must be palpated in the direction of the incoming fibers (Figs. 8.**82**, 8.**84**). It should be noted that the descending and ascending portions are partially covered at the spine of the scapula by fibers of the horizontal portion.

SRS Correlation

The trapezius muscle is extremely important for routine diagnosis of the SRS. Seldom is the trapezius muscle responsible for the abnormal position of individual vertebrae. In contrast, individual myotenones result in painful pathological changes (myotendinosis) when problems in the region of the thoracic and lumbar vertebrae arise. When the muscle is palpated precisely, the spondylogenic pathology of the entire thoracic and lumbar spine can be deduced. The spondylogenic correlation of the myotenones is indicated for the descending portion in Figure 8.**84a** (myotenones), for the horizontal and ascending portions in Figure 8.**84b**.

Length Testing

Examination Procedure

The examiner stands behind the upright, seated patient. Using the forearm, the examiner stabilizes one of the patient's shoulders at the level of the acromio-clavicular joint. While cradling the patient's parietal region with the other hand, the examiner introduces sidebending and slight rotation to the opposite side (i. e. in the direction opposite to the location of the stabilized shoulder). The examiner evaluates muscle tension and the contour of the trapezius muscle, as well as the range of motion and endfeel at the barrier (Fig. 8.**85**). This examination can also be performed with the patient in the supine position (Fig. 8.**86**).

Possible Pathological Findings

Motion restriction with significant soft endfeel is an indication of muscle shortening and is usually accompanied by an insertion tendinosis at the spine of the scapula or the clavicle.

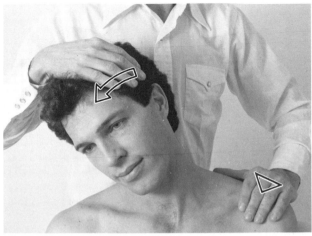

8.85

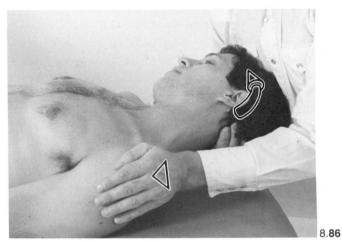

8.86

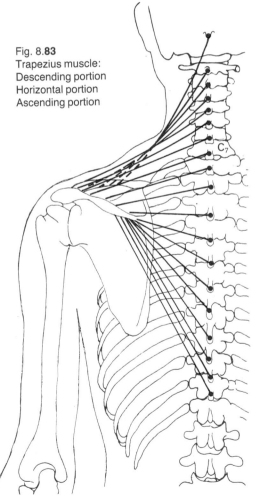

Fig. 8.**83**
Trapezius muscle:
Descending portion
Horizontal portion
Ascending portion

Fig. 8.**84**   Insertions of the myotendinoses at the spine of the scapula and the clavicle **a** Descending portion **b** Ascending and horizontal portion

8.18 Quadratus Lumborum Muscle

Anatomically as well as spondylogenically, this muscle consists of superficial (posterior) and deep (anterior) layers (Fig. 8.**90**).

Superficial (Posterior) Layer
(Fig. 8.**89**).

Origin

The origin of this muscle spreads over the horizontal portion of the internal lip of the iliac crest (about 6 cm long; partially from the iliolumbar ligament).

Insertion

The anterior side of the tips of the costal processes L1−L4; some of the fibers radiate to the iliolumbar ligament (L5). The most anterior fibers reach to the twelfth rib.

Palpatory Technique

Due to its position, it cannot be palpated easily. Confusion, especially with the longissimus lumborum muscle, is possible. The palpating finger must reach around the iliac crest superiorly in a hooklike manner in order to reach the painful tendinoses. The insertions at the tips of the costal processes are palpated lateroinferiorly (L4 can be palpated sometimes, whereas L5 is practically never palpated).

Deep (Anterior) Layer
(Fig. 8.**88**)

Origin

The inferior margin of the medial half of rib XII.

Insertion

The medial fibers insert at the anterior portion of the tips of the costal processes of L1−L5; the lateral fibers insert at the iliac crest, in about the same region as the superficial layer.

Course and Relations

The posterior surface of the quadratus lumborum muscle lies over the deep portion of the thoracolumbar fascia of the aponeurosis of the transverse abdominis and the internal abdominal oblique muscles. The anterior portion borders on the kidneys and the colon. The psoas major muscle slides over the medial margin, and the quadratus lumborum muscle is laterally covered by the thick mass of the deep back muscles. In the inferior quarter it is covered by the pelvic portion of the latissimus dorsi muscle.

Innervation

The subcostal nerve and ventral ramus (n. lumbalis) T12 and L1−L3.

Function

Bilateral contraction results in extension of the lumbar spine, and unilateral contraction results in lateral bending of the vertebral column to the side of the contracted muscle. In addition, the muscle fixes the twelfth rib. It therefore facilitates diaphragm contraction.

Palpatory Technique

The tendinoses at the twelfth rib, which often are painful, are palpated medioinferiorly, and the costal processes are palpated laterosuperiorly.

SRS Correlation

Spondylogenic changes can be observed with regional dysfunction of the lower thoracic spine.

Length Testing

Examination Procedure

Passive trunk sidebending is introduced to the standing patient. Both the overall range of motion and in particular the muscle contours in the lumbar area are evaluated. Asymmetric movement to one side (i. e., less excursion to one side) with the induced sidebending motion may indicate that the muscle is shortened. This muscle can also be evaluated with the patient in the side-lying position while resting on one elbow with normal lumbar spine lordosis. Again, the examiner observes for asymmetry in range of sidebending motion and the contour of the muscle (Fig. 8.**87**).

Possible Pathological Findings

Asymmetric contraction and movement in the lumbar spine with induced sidebending or even symmetric broad retraction in the flank may indicate shortening of the quadratus lumborum muscles.

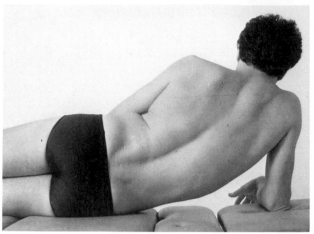

8.87

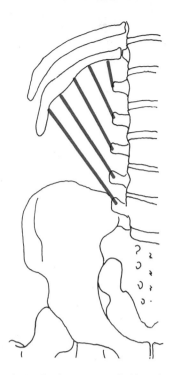

Fig. 8.88   Quadratus lumborum muscle (deep layer)

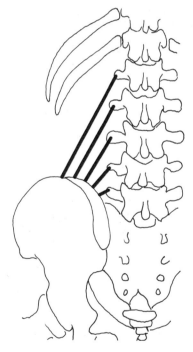

Fig. 8.89   Quadratus lumborum muscle (superficial layer)

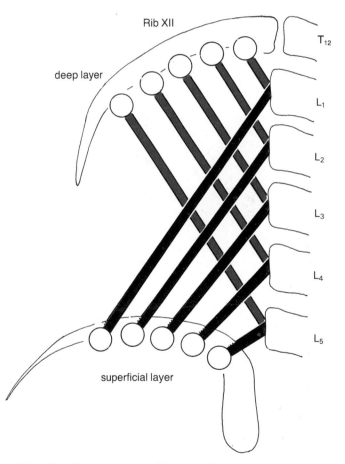

Fig. 8.90   The myotenones of the superficial and deep layers of the quadratus lumborum muscle (from posterior)

8.19 Psoas Major Muscle

Origin

It arises from the anteroinferior surfaces of the transverse processes L1–L5, not including the tips (where the quadratus lumborum muscle arises). The origin at L5 covers the complete anterior surface. Furthermore, the psoas major muscle arises from the lateral and lateroanterior circumference of the intervertebral discs of T12–L5 and their respective vertebral bodies of L1–L4 (Fig. 8.**93**).

Insertion

The anterior half of the lesser trochanter of the femur.

Course and Relations

The muscle runs downward, alongside the lumbar spine (psoas shadow on X-rays) into the true pelvis and, below the inguinal ligament, through the lacuna musculorum (ilium) to the lesser trochanter. Upon exit from the lacuna musculorum, the muscle lies directly on the anterior side of the hip joint.

Innervation

Rami of the lumbar plexus and the femoral nerve. The psoas major and minor muscles are segmentally innervated by L1–L3, sometimes by T12 and L4.

Function

Flexion of the thigh, possibly adduction and lateral rotation of the thigh. When the extremity is fixed, bilateral contraction causes the trunk to flex, whereas unilateral contraction of the muscle rotates the pelvis and trunk in opposite directions.

Palpatory Technique

With the patient supine, the origin is palpated through the abdominal wall, which should be completely relaxed. The promontory is located (correlating to L5). The fingers then follow the vertebral bodies laterally, reaching the lateral circumference and consequently move superior to L1 level (Fig. 8.**91**). The four fingers then move laterally along the vertebral bodies to the muscle belly, and the patient is asked to raise the leg straight up (when myotendinotic changes have occurred, painfulness normally increases) (Fig. 8.**92**).

The insertion at the lesser trochanter can also be palpated. Again the patient is supine, and the fingers search the lesser trochanter behind the adductors while the legs are flexed and abducted.

SRS Correlation

The psoas major muscle, which is important for maintaining body posture, tends to shorten and is very often involved in the spondylogenic event (it is possibly correlated with the upper cervical spine). Myotendinosis and muscle shortening can develop as a result of an anteriorly functionally abnormal position of the vertebra. This has to be taken into account when establishing diagnosis and therapy.

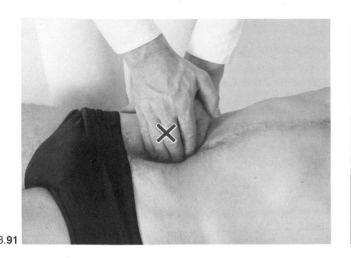

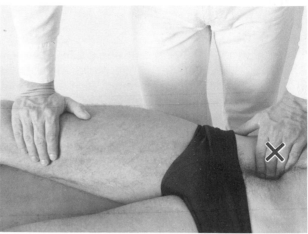

8.91

8.92

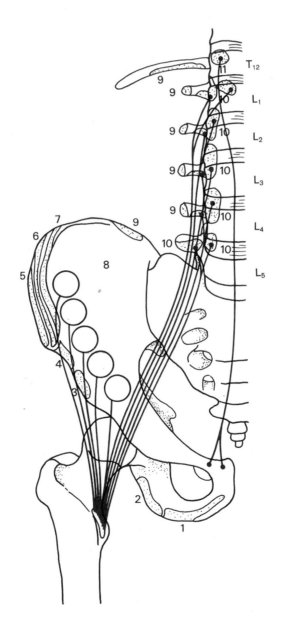

Fig. 8.93   Iliopsoas muscle

1   Adductor magnus m
2   Quadratus femoris m
3   Rectus femoris m
4   Sartorius m
5   External abdominal oblique m
6   Internal abdominal oblique m
7   Transversus abdominis m
8   Iliacus m
9   Quadratus lumborum m
10 Psoas major m
11 Psoas minor m

Length Testing

Examination Procedure

The patient is in the prone position. The examiner stabilizes the patient's pelvis by pressing one hand flat against the examination table. The other hand takes hold of the patient's thigh and slowly introduces extension the ipsilateral thigh. During this maneuver, the examiner observes the thoracolumbar junction (Fig. 8.**94**).

Possible Pathological Findings

1. Diminished (restricted) hip extension with soft end feel. This is most likely due to shortening in the psoas major muscle.
2. Diminished (restricted) hip extension with hard end feel. This may be due to degenerative changes within the joint itself, that is, at the hip joint or possibly the SIJ.
3. Prominent retraction of the thoracolumbar area during this maneuver. This may be an indication that there is psoas major shortening.

Variation

With the patient in the supine position, the length of the hip flexor muscles (iliopsoas m, rectus femoris m, tensor fasciae latae m) is evaluated. The height of the examination table is adjusted exactly to the height of the standing patient's ischium. The patient then actively flexes the hip and knee (Fig. 8.**95**). From this position, the patient then reclines onto the examination table and actively participates in stabilizing the pelvis by bringing the knee towards the chest until the lumbar lordosis is reversed. The leg that is being examined hangs freely off the table.

Possible Pathological Findings

1. The leg that is being examined rises above the horizontal plane and resists being pushed in the direction of the floor (Fig. 8.**96**). This indicates that there is shortening of the iliopsoas muscle.
2. If, in addition to shortening of the iliopsoas muscle, there is simultaneous shortening of the rectus femoris muscle, the knee will also be extended.

8.20 Psoas Minor Muscle

Origin

Vertebral bodies of T12 and L1 below the arcuate ligament of the diaphragm.

Insertion

At the pecten ossis pubis, the inguinal ligament (broad junction), and the iliopectineal line (iliopectineal eminence).

The psoas minor muscle is mentioned for the sake of completeness only. It is very difficult to palpate and is of no significance for SRS aspects.

8.21 Iliacus Muscle

Origin

Upper margin of the iliac fossa (Fig. 8.**93**).

Insertion

Lesser trochanter of femur.

Course and Relations

The muscle fibers converge toward the lacuna musculorum (ilium) where they attach to the lateral edge of the psoas major muscle to insert together at the lesser trochanter of the femur.

Innervation and Function

Same as the psoas major muscle.

Palpatory Technique

The iliac muscle can be palpated in the iliac fossa only with difficulty, and then incompletely. In order to relax the abdominal musculature, the patient is brought into a halfsitting position. The thumb reaches around the anterior-superior iliac spine and slides deep along the upper part of the illum (Fig. 8.**97**).

The iliac muscle can be followed along the iliac crest from the anterior iliac spine by going superior for about three finger widths and inferior by two finger widths, at the most. The remaining fibers at the origin cannot be followed distinctly due to their anatomic position and the overlying abdominal musculature.

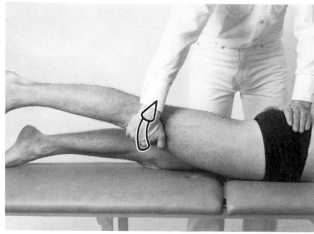

8.94

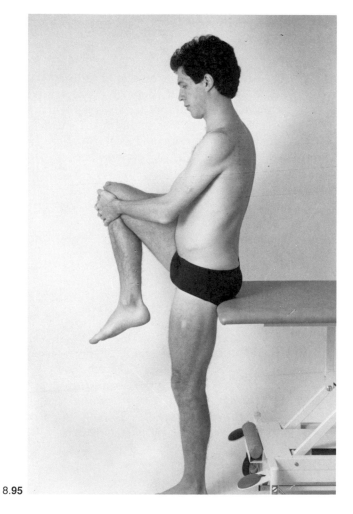

8.95

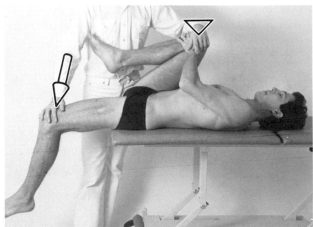

8.96

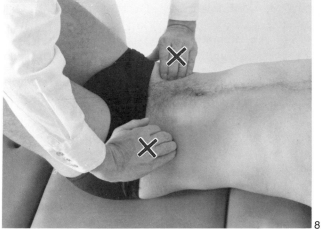

8.97

8.22 Abdominal Muscles

The abdominal wall, largely formed by the antero-lateral abdominal muscles, is confined superiorly by the infrasternal angle, and inferiorly by the iliac crest and the inguinal and pubic sulci. Due to their anatomic arrangement, the superficial abdominal muscles function very efficiently as a unit. The superficial abdominal muscles can be divided into two major groups, a lateral and medial group:

– *lateral group:* the external abdominal oblique, internal abdominal oblique, and transverse abdominal muscles.
– *medial group:* rectus abdominis muscle and the pyramidalis muscle.
  The broad tendons and aponeuroses of the more *lateral abdominal muscles* envelope the rectus abdominis muscle, forming the rectus sheath.

8.22.1 External Oblique Abdominal Muscle

Origin

This muscle arises by eight fleshy slips from the external surface of the eight lower ribs (ribs V–XII). In part, it inserts between the fifth and ninth rib together with the slips of the anterior serratus muscle, and between the tenth and twelfth rib together with slips of the latissimus dorsi muscle (Fig. 8.**98b**).

Insertion

The fibers that originate from the lowermost three ribs run almost vertically to the iliac crest and its external labrum (Fig. 8.**99**). The remainder of the fibers run obliquely from superior and lateral to inferior and medial in order to join the broad aponeurosis (Fig. 8.**98b**).

Course and Relations

As a rule, the muscle fibers run from superior, lateral, and posterior to inferior, medial, and anterior.

Innervation

Intercostal nerves (T5–T12).

Function

With a fixed pelvis, both external oblique abdominal muscles introduce forward flexion to the spine and pull the ribs in an inferior direction. Unilateral obliquus muscle contraction causes the thorax to be rotated into the direction opposite to that of the side of muscle contraction. It is also elicited with the Valsalva maneuver.

Palpatory Technique

The lateral portion of the superficial abdominal muscle can easily be palpated at its origin along the ribs where the fibers run obliquely. It is best to examine the patient in the side-lying position with the arm abducted. This also allows differentiation between the borders of the serratus anterior muscle, latissimus dorsi muscle, and the fibers of the external abdominal oblique muscle.

8.22.2 Internal Abdominal Oblique Muscle

Origin

This muscle originates at the intermediate line of the iliac crest, the thoracolumbar fascia, and the anterior superior iliac spine (ASIS) (Fig. 8.**99**).

Insertion

The superior portion of the muscle inserts at the inferior borders of the lower three ribs. The central portion of the muscle continues medially to become part of the aponeurosis, which is separated into two laminae, namely, an anterior and posterior one. In the male, the muscle continues below to become the cremasteric muscle along the spermatic cord (Fig. 8.**98a**).

Course and Relations

This fan-shaped muscle passes superiorly and medially, originating inferiorly at the iliac crest.

Innervation

Intercostal spinal nerves of T10–T12 and L1.

Function

Function is similar to that described for the external oblique muscle. With the pelvis fixed, muscle contraction will pull the ribs inferiorly and introduces flexion to the trunk. Unilateral contraction rotates the thorax to the same side as contraction. The muscle is also involved in the valsalva maneuver.

Palpatory Technique

It is best to palpate this muscle with the patient in the supine position. After the origin has been located at the iliac crest, the muscle fibers can be followed upwards along the lowermost rib, and then in the direction of the aponeurosis (medial).

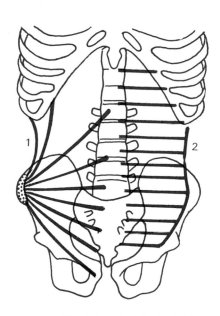

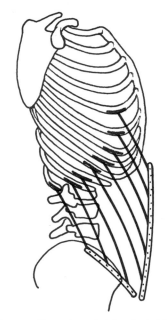

Fig. 8.**98a**   Course of the internal abdominal oblique muscle (1) and the transverse abdominal muscle (2)

Fig. 8.**98b**   Course of the external abdominal oblique muscle

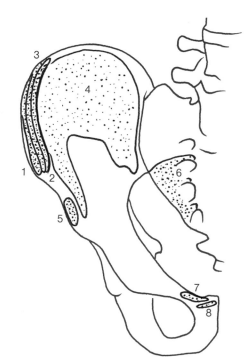

Fig. 8.**99**   Muscle insertions at the pelvis

1   External abdominal oblique m
2   Internal abdominal oblique m
3   Transverse abdominis m
4   Iliacus m
5   Rectus femoris m
6   Piriformis m
7   Rectus abdominis m
8   Pyramidalis m

8.22.3 Transverse Abdominis Muscle

Origin

This muscle originates via six slips from the internal aspects of the lower costal cartilage (ribs VII−XII), the deep lamina of the thoracolumbar fascia, the inner lip of the iliac crest, the ASIS, and the inguinal ligament (Figs. 8.**98a**, 8.**99**).

Insertion

At the abdominal aponeurosis.

Course and Relations

The fibers of the transverse abdominis muscle run obliquely and horizontally towards the median plane to end in the aponeurosis and thus, the linea alba (Fig. 8.**100**).

Innervation

Intercostal spinal nerves T7−T12, and L1.

Function

The superior segments of the muscle internally pull the ribs from which they originate. In addition, and similar to the typical action of the inferior muscle portion, muscle contraction causes the abdominal cavity to become smaller. This muscle is also involved in the valsalva maneuver.

Palpatory Technique

Starting medially, the muscle can be palpated perpendicular to the direction of its muscle fibers.

8.22.4 Rectus Abdominis Muscle

Origin

The muscle originates from outer surface of the fifth, sixth and seventh costal cartilage, the xiphoid process, and the ligaments connecting the xiphoid process and the ribs (Fig. 8.**101**).

Insertion

The superior surface of the crest of the pubis close to the symphysis pubis (Fig. 8.**99**).

Course and Relations

From its origin, the muscle courses straight down to its insertion. The fibers are interrupted by three fibrous bands, the so-called tendinous intersections (Fig. 8.**100**).

Innervation

Lower six or seven thoracic spinal nerves.

Function

With a fixed pelvis, contraction of this muscle pulls the thorax inferiorly and introduces flexion to the spine. With the thorax fixed, muscle contraction causes the pelvis to rise. This muscle plays a significant role in the Valsalva maneuver.

Effect of the Valsalva Maneuver

The combined action of the abdominal muscles is responsible for the Valsalva maneuver, where the abdominal cavity's space is reduced and increased pressure is exerted upon the viscera located in the abdomen and pelvis.

Palpatory Technique

With the patient in the supine position and the abdominal wall totally relaxed, this muscle can be followed from its origin to the insertion, palpating the muscle perpendicular to the fiber direction.

Strength and Endurance Testing of the Abdominal Muscles: Procedure

The patient is in the supine position and the legs are somewhat flexed both at the hip and the knee (to eliminate action of the psoas major muscle) (Fig. 8.**102**). The patient is requested to raise the arms and then to lift the head, upper thoracic spine, and shoulder blades off the table. The patient should then remain in this position for thirty seconds without having to alter respiration (Fig. 8.**103**).

Possible Pathological Findings

The patient may not be able to assume the above described position or maintain it for at least thirty seconds. Any of these two findings is indicative of weak abdominal muscles.

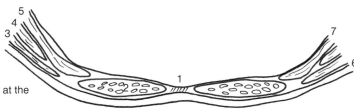

Fig. 8.**100** Transverse section through the abdominal wall at the level of the umbilicus

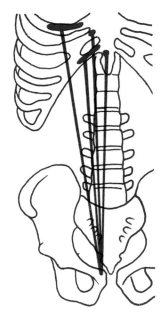

Fig. 8.**101** Course of the rectus abdominis muscle

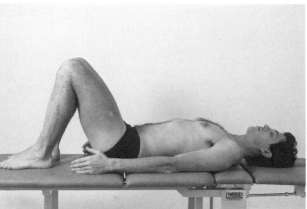

8.**102**

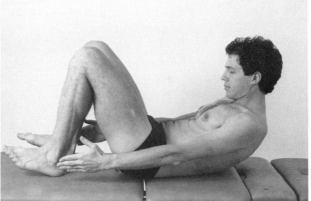

8.**103**

8.23 Sternocleidomastoid Muscle

This large, rounded muscle passes obliquely across the side of the neck, being twisted 90° around its longitudinal axis in a screwlike manner so that its inferior portion is directed anteriorly and its superior portion laterally. At the origin, the tendon of the sternocleidomastoid muscle is divided into a clavicular and a sternal portion. The muscle belly unites to form one strong insertion.

Origin

Sternal portion: The muscle arises as a rounded, strong tendon from the anterior surface of the manubrium of the sternum, immediately medial and somewhat inferior to the sternoclavicular joint (Fig. 8.**106**).

Clavicular portion: This portion is composed of both muscular and aponeurotic (tendon) fibers and arises from the superior surface and the posterior border of the sternal end of the clavicle. The origin extends laterally from the joint to the first third of the clavicle. The flat muscle belly slides under the inferior surface of the sternal portion and becomes enlarged superiorly.

Insertion

The muscle inserts into the outer surface of the mastoid process from its tip to its superior border and further to the center of the superior nuchal line (Figs. 8.**106**, 8.**107**).

Course and Relations

(See Fig. 7.**4**, the cross-section of the cervical spine). The sternocleidomastoid muscle is covered to a great extent by the platysma muscle. From its origin to its insertion, the muscle passes superficially and obliquely across the anterior side of the neck, thereby dividing the neck region in two: the anterior and lateral regions (Fig. 8.**104**). It would be beyond the scope of this book to cover the topographical importance of these two anatomical triangles in further detail (please refer to anatomy texts).

Innervation

The spinal accessory nerve and partially the cervical plexus (C2−C3).

Function

Bilateral contraction results in flexion of the head, and unilateral contraction results in lateral bending of the head to the side of the contracted muscle and rotation to the opposite side.

Palpatory Technique

The origin of the sternal portion at the manubrium of the sternum is palpated superolaterally. The examiner has to remain immediately medial to the sternoclavicular joints. When palpating the clavicular portion, the finger reaches around the posterior margin of the clavicle in a hooklike manner (Fig. 8.**105**). The homologous insertion tendinoses are palpated at the external surface of the mastoid process, going inferior from its apex to the superior nuchal line.

SRS Correlation

The sternocleidomastoid muscle consists of four myotenones, which are correlated with the vertebrae of the middle thoracic spine. Their arrangement can be seen in Figure 8.**106**.

Length Testing

Procedure

The patient is sitting. The examiner, who is standing behind the patient, fixates the shoulder with one hand and at the same time localizes the clavicular and sternal muscle insertions of the sternocleidomastoid muscle with the index finger. The patient's trunk rests against the examiner's thighs. Using the other hand, which is placed over the patient's parietal region, the examiner introduces first maximal flexion to the head and then maximal sidebending to the opposite side, with subsequent minimal rotation to the same side. During this maneuver, the examiner evaluates the tension of the muscle insertion at the sternum and clavicle (Fig. 8.**108**).

Possible Pathological Findings

1. Soft endfeel at the extreme (barrier) of motion, with prominent muscle contour and tenderness at the insertion. Functional shortening of the sternocleidomastoid muscle, often in association with increased use of the accessory respiratory musculature; may occasionally be observed in patients with pulmonary disorders.
2. Slowly progressive vertigo. This may be suspicious of circulatory compromise related to the vertebral artery. Further workup is necessary.
3. Vertigo which occurs immediately with this maneuver. This may be due to the cervical type of vertigo, but differentiation is difficult.

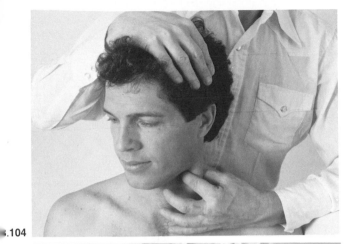

8.104

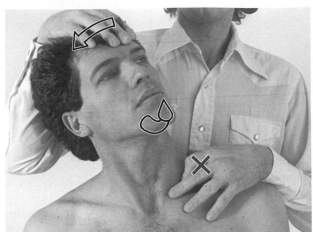

8.108

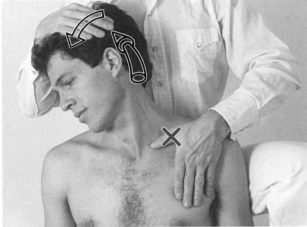

8.105

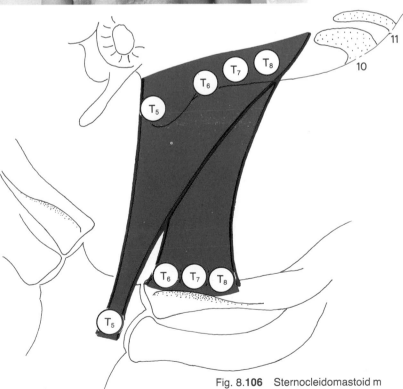

Fig. 8.106   Sternocleidomastoid m

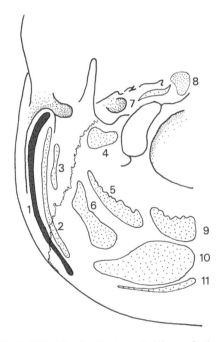

Fig. 8.107   Muscle attachment at the occiput

1   Sternocleidomastoid m
2   Splenius capitis m
3   Longissimus capitis m
4   Rectus capitis lateralis m
5   Rectus capitis posterior major m
6   Obliquus capitis superior m
7   Rectus capitis anterior m
8   Longus capitis m
9   Rectus capitis posterior minor m
10   Semispinalis capitis m
11   Trapezius m

8.24   Deltoid Muscle

Origin

Clavicular portion: lateral third of the clavicle.

Acromial portion: the acromion.

Scapular portion: from the spine of the scapula.

The most posterior fibers arise from the infra-spinatous fascia (Fig. 8.**111**).

Insertion

The muscle inserts at the deltoid tuberosity of the humerus. The relatively small area of insertion has the shape of an escutcheon (Fig. 8.**112**). It passes to the intermuscular septum of the lateral and medial arm.

Course and Relations

The broad deltoid muscle covers all muscles inserting at the proximal end of the humerus.

The broad origin (more than 20 cm), in contrast to the small area of insertion (15 × 15 mm), is responsible for the extensive convergence of the fibers.

Innervation

Suprascapularis nerve.

Function

The main function of the muscle is abduction in the shoulder joint, the acromial portion of the muscle being the main abductor.

The clavicular portion is synergistic to the pectoralis major muscle; the scapular portion is synergistic to the latissimus dorsi and teres major muscles.

Palpatory Technique

Similar to the gluteal musculature, the deltoid muscle can be palpated directly (Fig. 8.**109**). The origin tendinoses must be especially demarcated exactly in the direction of the converging fibers (Figs. 8.**110**, 8.**112**). The transitional tendinoses are located at the fibers most posterior, that is, at the transition into the infraspinous fascia. The insertion tendinoses can be defined only theoretically, according to their spondylogenic correlation. The intermuscular septum, however, which is often subject to pain, can be palpated practically to its insertion at the lateral epicondyle.

SRS Correlation

The SRS correlation, which can only be differentiated at the origin, is reproduced in Figure 8.**111**.

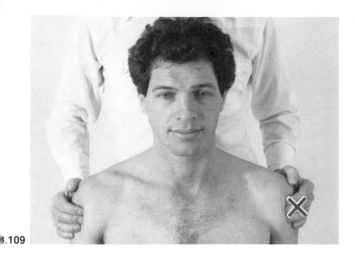

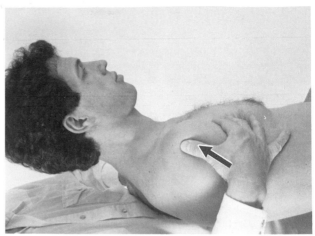

8.109

8.110

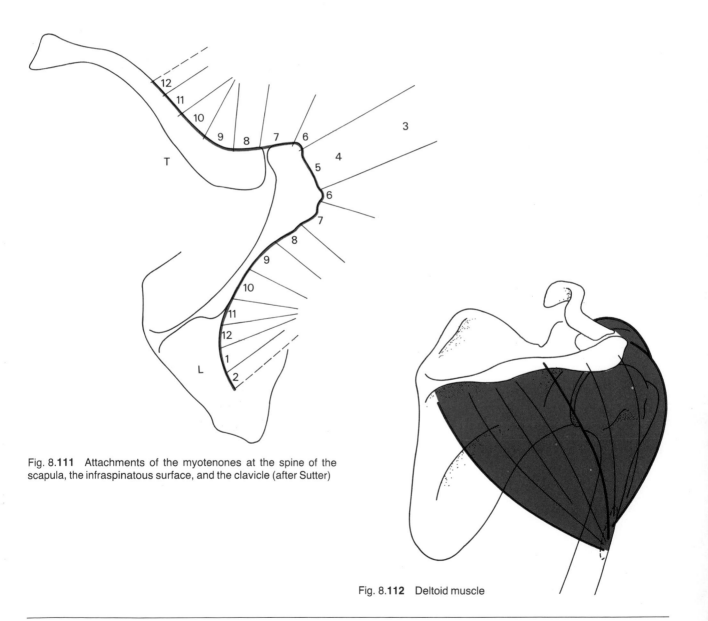

Fig. 8.111 Attachments of the myotenones at the spine of the scapula, the infraspinatous surface, and the clavicle (after Sutter)

Fig. 8.112 Deltoid muscle

8.25 Pectoralis Major Muscle

In general, the pectoralis major muscle is divided into the three parts, consisting of the clavicular, sternocostal, and abdominal portions.

Origin

The clavicular fibers arise from the anterior surface of the medial half of the clavicle. The sternal portion originates from the sternal membrane and the costal cartilage between the second and sixth ribs. The weakest part, the abdominal portion of this muscle, takes its origin from the anterior layer of the rectus sheath in the uppermost area (Fig. 8.**115**).

Insertion

Lateral lip of the intertubercular groove of the humerus. The muscle attaches via a tendon in which the fibers cross and form an anterior and posterior lamina. The fibers of the abdominal portion attach most proximally.

Course and Relations

The fibers of the abdominal portion run rather vertically from inferior to superior, whereas the fibers of the sternocostal and clavicular portions are arranged more horizontally (Fig. 8.**115**).

Innervation

Lateral and medial pectoral nerves (C5−T1).

Function

As a whole, the pectoralis major muscle is able to abduct and internally rotate the arm. The muscle also functions to assist deep inhalation.

Palpatory Technique

This superficial muscle can easily be palpated at the anterior surface of the thorax. The muscle is usually palpated by following it from its origin at the thorax to the insertion at the humerus in accordance with the fibers' direction.

Length Testing of the Pectoralis Major Muscle: Procedure

The supine patient flexes the legs slightly at the hip and knees. The patient's thorax is stabilized by the examiner's hand placed broadly over it (Fig. 8.**113**). With the other hand the examiner abducts the patient's arm, which should be able to be carried beyond the horizontal in the healthy person. The degree of range of motion for this movement is evaluated (Fig. 8.**114**).

Possible Pathological Findings

1. Decreased range of motion for abduction or extension at the shoulder with soft endfeel. This is probably due to a shortened pectoralis major muscle.
2. Decreased range of motion for abduction or extension with hard endfeel. This may be caused by structural changes at the joint, such as the result of a shrunken capsule.
3. Pain during the arc of movement or at the extreme (barrier) of movement. This requires further detailed examination to determine the cause of the pain.

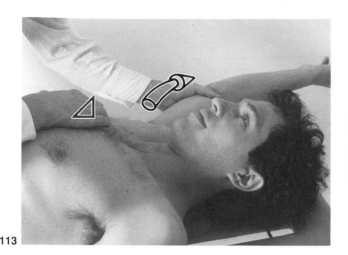

8.113

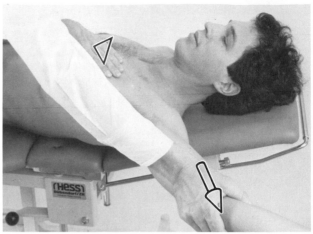

8.114

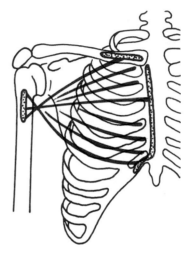

Fig. 8.115   Pectoralis major m

8.26 Gluteus Maximus Muscle

Origin

In the area of origin, the gluteus maximus muscle can be divided into two layers; this fact is of spondylogenic importance (see below).

Superficial layer (Fig. 8.**117a**):
– From the iliac crest
– From the posterior superior iliac spine
– From the thoracolumbar fascia
– From the lateral sacral line
– From the coccyx

Deep layer:
– From the broad, upper portion of the ilium, behind the posterior gluteal line
– From the sacrotuberous ligament
– From the fascia covering the gluteus medius (Fig. 8.**117b**).

Insertion

The superficial and the deep layers unite in their course. The superior portions pass into the iliotibial tract (tibial portion) at the level of the greater trochanter, and the inferior fibers insert at the gluteal tuberosity of the femur, being about 10 cm long (femoral portion): (see the diagram of the pelvis, Fig. 7.**27**).

Course and Relations

The fibers of the tibial portion pass obliquely in a lateroinferior direction. The strong aponeurotic transition into the iliotibial tract is located at the lateral margin of the greater trochanter (transitional tendinoses). The fibers of the femoral part also pass obliquely lateroinferior; thus, the inferior edge of the muscle crosses the horizontal gluteal sulcus.

Innervation

The inferior gluteal nerve L5, S1.

Function

Extension of the thigh, adduction and lateral rotation of the femur.

Palpatory Technique

See diagram of the pelvis, Fig. 7.**27**.

The origin tendinoses of the superficial layer can easily be reached, the palpatory direction being lateroinferior (Fig. 8.**116**). The pressure of palpation is exerted tangentially and is of specific importance at the lateral sacral line in order to avoid confusion with the sacral zones of irritation. Myotendinotic changes are palpated obliquely in the direction of the fibers from the origin to insertion, the aponeurotic transition. Even the less experienced examiner should be able to complete this procedure successfully. Thus, the gluteus maximus muscle is used for teaching and practice purposes. The sacral or lumbar zones of irritation, in contrast, serve for comparison and control. Palpation of the deep layer is performed in the same manner, the only difference being the greater palpatory depth which, however, requires the examiner to be more experienced.

SRS Correlation

With abnormal position of the sacral or lumbar vertebrae, the gluteus maximus muscle develops myotendinosis rapidly and consistently. The superior fibers (tibial portion) are correlated with the SIJ and L5, the inferior fibers (femoral portion) with the superficial layer of the lumbar spine. The fibers of the lower layer have a possible reflexogenic and spondylogenic relationship to the upper thoracic spine. The arrangement and correlation of individual myotendinoses are depicted clearly in Figure 8.**117a**.

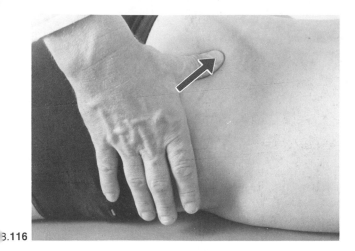

8.116

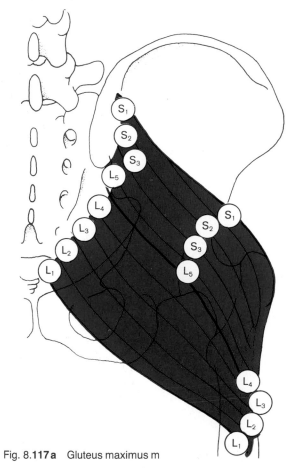

Fig. 8.**117a**   Gluteus maximus m

Fig. 8.**117b**   Muscle insertions at the lateral side of the ilium

1   Gluteus maximus m
2   Gluteus medius m
3   Gluteus minimus m
4   Rectus femoris m
5   Semimembranosus m
6   Biceps femoris muscle
7   Semitendinosus muscle

8.27 Gluteus Medius Muscle

Origin

The gluteus medius muscle arises from a triangle whose sides are formed by the anterior and posterior gluteal lines and the external lip of the iliac crest (Figs. 8.**117b**, 8.**120**).

Insertion

The muscle inserts in the outer surface of the greater trochanter (superior, lateroposterior quadrant).

Course and Relations

The gluteus medius muscle is fan-shaped with its fibers arranged like roof tile (Fig. 8.**120**). Due to this arrangement, a superficial and deep layer can be differentiated in the area of origin both anatomically and spondylogenically; these two layers are also separated from each other by loose connective tissue.

Innervation

Superior gluteal nerve L4–S1.

Function

The muscle as a whole unit serves for the abduction of the thigh; the anterior portion flexes and rotates the thigh medially; the posterior portion extends and rotates the thigh laterally.

Palpatory Technique

The tendinoses as well as the myotendinoses of the superficial layer can be found without difficulty; of importance is the differentiation from the gluteus maximus muscle. For precise palpation as well as to obtain clear information from the patient, the thumb must reach the insertion tendinoses just barely inferior to the iliac crest along the muscle fibers' direction (Figs. 8.**118**, 8.**120**). Myotendinotic changes can be followed to the insertion at the greater trochanter without any difficulty. The insertions of the deep layer are located at the anterior gluteal line.

SRS Correlation

The division of the gluteus medius muscle into two parts is also obvious from the spondylogenic correlation: with abnormal positions (segmental dysfunction) in the cervical spine, the deep layer shows myotendinosis, whereas the superior layer reacts upon segmental dysfunctions in the lumbar spine region (Fig. 8.**120**).

The myotenone L5 in the superficial layer arises from a characteristic location in a flat groove at the junction of the ascending portion and the horizontal portion of the iliac crest. This groove is not a bony formation, yet it can be palpated very easily. L1 arises directly medial from the iliac spine pointing in the anteroinferior direction, whereas T12 arises laterally. When the muscle is well developed, a further myotenone is present, which is correlated with T10.

Strength and Endurance Testing of the Gluteal Muscles

Procedure

The patient is in the prone position. The knee is flexed to 90° in order to eliminate the action of the hamstring muscles. The patient should be able to lift the thigh off the table and hold it there for at least 30 seconds (Fig. 8.**119**).

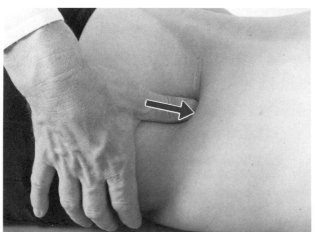

8.118

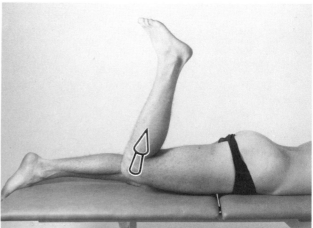

8.119

Possible Pathological Findings

The patient is unable to perform the above described maneuver at all or is able to hold the leg off the table only for a short period of time before it drops back. This is a sign of a functional weakness of the gluteal muscles.

Function

Abduction of the thigh in addition to the same functions as the gluteal medial muscle.

Palpatory Technique

In order to reach the origin of the gluteus minimus muscle, the examiner has to penetrate the gluteus medius and partially penetrate the gluteus maximus muscles. The myotendinoses of the origin are palpated along a convex line (pointing slightly superior) from the anterior margin of the ilium to the vicinity of the posterior inferior iliac spine. In practice, palpation is performed from the apex of the trochanter in the direction of the posterior iliac spine, whereby the finger during palpation presses deeply into the soft tissue of the buttocks at different angles.

SRS Correlation

The gluteus minimus muscle is correlated spondylogenically with the lower thoracic spine.

Strength and Endurance Testing

Cf. gluteus medius muscle, p. 308.

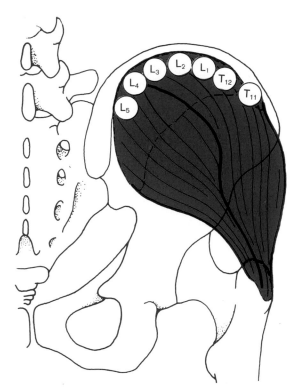

Fig. 8.120 Gluteus medius m

8.28 Gluteus Minimus Muscle

Origin

This fan-shaped muscle arises from the outer surface of the ilium, between the inferior and anterior gluteal lines. The posterior fibers arise from the greater sciatic notch (Figs. 8.117b, 8.121).

Insertion

Anterolateral and superior quadrant of the greater trochanter.

Course and Relations

This deep, flat muscle converges toward the greater trochanter and is totally covered by the gluteus medius muscle.

Innervation

Superior gluteal nerve L4−S1.

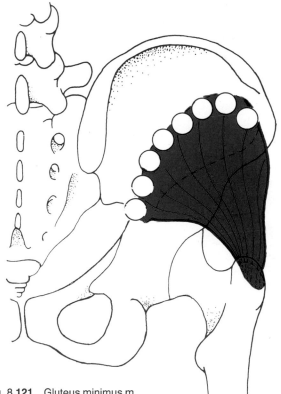

Fig. 8.121 Gluteus minimus m

8.29   Piriformis Muscle

Origin

The anterior surface of the pelvis between the sacral foramina II to IV (Fig. 8.**124**).

Insertion

The superomedial apex of the greater trochanter.

Course and relations

The piriformis muscle passes from the lateral surface of the sacrum to the greater sciatic foramen, thereby leaving the lesser pelvis to insert finally at the greater trochanter (Fig. 8.**125**).

Passing through the greater sciatic foramen, the piriformis muscle divides this foramen into superior and inferior portions. This is of great clinical importance, since the piriformis muscle is in close proximity to the sciatic nerve, the inferior gluteal nerve, the posterior cutaneous nerve of the thigh, and the pudendal nerve.

Innervation

Rami from the sacral plexus of S1.

Function

Lateral rotation of the thigh.

Palpatory Technique

The piriformis muscle can be palpated at one particular point in the gluteal region after its exit from the greater sciatic foramen. This point is the intersection of two lines that are constructed as follows: the first line is the connection between the superior posterior iliac spine and the greater trochanter; the other line runs from the anterior superior iliac spine and the lower pole of the coccyx (Figs. 8.**122**, 8.**125**). Myotendinosis of the piriformis muscle can be very painful. In order to eliminate doubt or for further verification, the origin must be examined rectally at the anterior surface of the sacrum.

SRS Correlation

The piriformis muscle represents one single myotenone that is correlated with L5. The piriformis muscle is important in posture, and it decidedly tends to shorten. Similar to the psoas major muscle, the piriformis muscle is often involved in the SRS event. Chronic myotendinosis in the piriformis muscle can even cause neurologic symptoms as a result of its anatomical proximity to the sciatic nerve. These symptoms are difficult to differentiate from a discogenic radicular condition.

Length Testing

Examination Procedure

The patient is in the supine position with the hip flexed to 90° on the side where the muscle is being examined. The examiner adducts the patient's thigh (passive adduction), while at the same time providing an axial pressure force to the femur in order to prevent the pelvis from lifting off the table (Fig. 8.**123**).

Possible Pathological Findings

Loss of range of motion with soft endfeel, accompanied by stretch pain, may be due to functional shortening of the piriformis muscle. This test, however, does not differentiate between shortening of the piriformis muscle and a painful iliolumbar ligament (Fig. 5.**84**).

Provocative Testing Using Pressure on the Piriformis Muscle

Examination Procedure

The patient is in the prone position, relaxing the gluteal muscles as much as possible. Two imaginary lines are constructed as follows: one that connects the anterior iliac spine and the ischium, and the other between the posterior iliac spine and the major trochanter. At the point of intersection of these two lines the examiner presses deeply with the palpating fingers, slowly and repetitively moving up and down from superior to inferior and back (Fig. 8.**122**).

Possible Pathological Findings

1. If a hard, cordlike muscle (oblique orientation) can be palpated in the deeper layers of the buttocks, it is most likely the shortened piriformis muscle. This diagnosis may be ascertained through improvement with a provisional treatment ("test treatment").
2. Localized pain during deep palpation. This is probably due to shortening of the piriformis muscle. At that location of palpation, this must be differentiated from a painful ischial tuberosity that lies beneath the sciatic nerve. This requires further detailed examination.
3. Radiating pain becomes apparent during deep palpation. The differentiation between pseudoradicular radiation or pain caused by pressure on the sciatic nerve is very difficult and calls for a more detailed examination, possibly including other diagnostic studies.

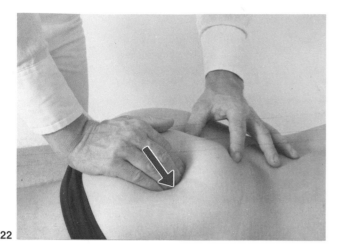

8.122

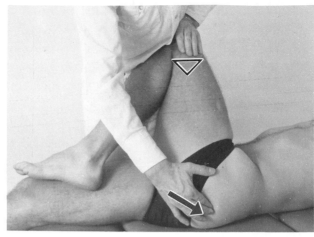

8.123

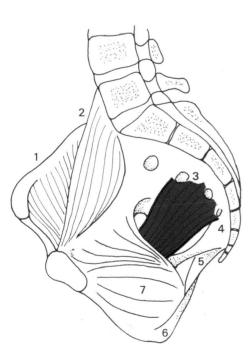

Fig. 8.124 Muscle attachments at the pelvis

1   Iliacus m
2   Psoas major m
3   Piriformis m
4   Sacrospinous ligament
5   Sacrotuberous ligament
6   Ischial tuberosity
7   Obturator fascia

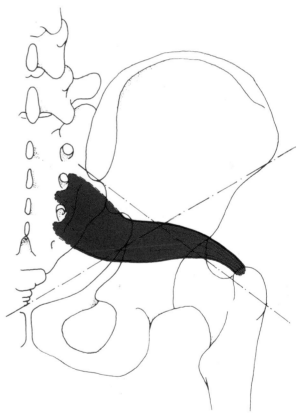

Fig. 8.125 Piriformis m

8.30 Biceps Femoris Muscle

The long head of this muscle crosses over two joints whereas the short head of the biceps femoris only crosses over one joint.

Origin

The long head arises from the ischial tuberosity together with the semitendinosus muscle. The short head arises from the central third of the lateral lip of the linea aspera and the lateral intermuscular septum of the femur (Fig. 8.**126**).

Insertion

The head of the fibula (Fig. 8.**127**).

Course and Relations

The long and short heads unite to form the biceps femoris muscle. A subtendinous bursa is located at the insertion at the fibular head between the muscle and the lateral collateral ligament of the knee.

Function

Flexes the leg at the knee and externally rotates the leg when the knee is flexed.

Innervation

Long head: tibial nerve (L5−S2).
Short head: common peroneal (S1−S2).

Palpatory Technique

The origin of the long head can be palpated at the ischial tuberosity through the gluteus maximus and partially through the gluteus medius. The short head can be palpated at the linea aspera of the femur between the long head and the vastus lateralis muscle.

8.31 Semitendinosus Muscle

Origin

The muscle arises at the upper part from the ischial tuberosity via a tendon shared by the long head of the biceps femoris muscle (Fig. 8.**126**).

Insertion

Medial body of the tibia where it unites at the superficial pes anserinus together with the gracilis and sartorius muscle (Fig. 8.**127**).

Course and Relations

Located between the surface of the tibia and the pes anserinus; there is a rather large bursa in front of the insertion.

Innervation

Tibial nerve (L5−S2).

Function

Since this muscle crosses two joints, it has two actions: extension of the thigh, and flexion and internal rotation of the leg.

Palpatory Technique

At its origin at the ischial tuberosity, this muscle can be palpated through the gluteus maximus muscle. At the insertion, the muscle can be palpated at the common tendon shared with the pes anserinus at the medial surface of the tibia.

8.32 Semimembranosus Muscle

Origin

Superolateral impression at the ischial tuberosity, lateral to the long head of the biceps femoris muscle (Fig. 8.**126**).

Insertion and Course

Below the medial collateral ligament, the insertion is actually divided into three parts. The first part is located anteriorly at the medial condyle of the tibia; the second component is confluent with the fascia of the popliteus muscle; and the third part enters the posterior wall of the capsule, forming the oblique popliteal ligament (Fig. 8.**127**).

Innervation

Tibial nerve (L5−S1).

Function

This muscle extends the thigh and flexes the leg at the knee together with internal rotation.

In the manual medicine and orthopedic literature, the biceps femoris and semitendinosus and semimembranosus muscles are often grouped together as what have become known as the *hamstring muscles*.

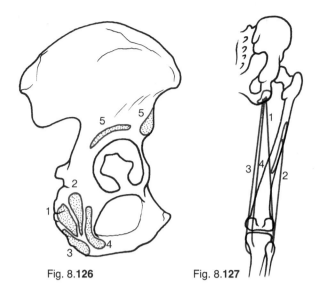

Fig. 8.**126**   Fig. 8.**127**

Fig. 8.**126**   Muscle insertions at the ischial tuberosity

1   Biceps femoris muscle, long head
2   Semimembranosus muscle
3   Semitendinosus muscle
4   Quadratus femoris muscle
5   Rectus femoris muscle

Fig. 8.**127**   Hamstring muscles

1   Biceps femoris muscle, long head
2   Biceps femoris muscle, short head
3   Semitendinosus muscle
4   Semimembranosus muscle

Possible Pathological Findings

1. Loss of flexion motion at the hip with knee extended; soft end feel. This is a clear indication that the hamstring muscles are shortened (Pseudo-Lasègue). This does not, however, rule out the possibility of a lumboradicular syndrome. Flexion can be improved stepwise with specific treatment up to a point where a lumbar root can be mechanically irritated by a herniated disk.

2. Loss of hip flexion with knee extended; hard end feel. A hard end feel elicited with this maneuver may be due to lumboradicular irritation secondary to a herniated disk. A hard end feel may also be due to degenerative processes at the hip joint. Hip mobility, however, does not improve when the knee is flexed simultaneously, whereas the Lasègue phenomenon with a hard (reflexive) end feel does tend to disappear when the knee is allowed to flex.

3. Loss of hip flexion with hard end feel and pain in the lumbar spine. Lumboradicular irritation secondary to a herniated disk may range between possible to probable, depending on the individual clinical situation.

4. Loss of flexion motion in the lumbar spine with low back pain, radiating in a dermatomal distribution; the knee remains extended during this maneuver. The likelihood of a lumboradicular irritation ranges between possible to probable.

8.33   **Length Testing of the Hamstring Muscles**

(Cf. sections 8.30−8.32)

Examination Procedure

The patient is in the supine position. With one hand placed flat over the patient's leg, the examiner introduces passive hip flexion. In order to be sure that the knee is not flexed, the examiner repositions the hands in a screwlike formation over the anterior part of the thigh (Fig. 8.**128**).

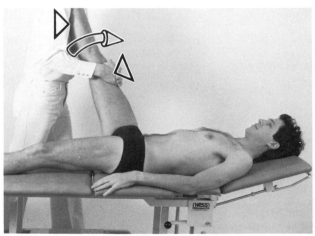

8.**128**

8.34　Rectus Femoris Muscle

Origin

This muscle arises from the anterior inferior iliac spine and the rim of the acetabulum of the hip joint (Fig. 8.**117b**).

Insertion

At the base of the patella, within the medial and lateral retinacula of the patella (Fig. 8.**129**).

Course and Relations

The rectus femoris muscle is part of the quadriceps femoris system. Together with the vastus medialis, vastus lateralis, and intermedius muscles, it inserts via a common tendon at the patella. Some of the fibers of the vastus medialis and rectus femoris muscles form the medial retinaculum of the patella, and the fibers of the vastus lateralis and portions of the rectus femoris muscles form the lateral retinaculum of the patella. These retinacula then attach at the tibial condyles, bypassing the patella.

Innervation

Femoral nerve (L2−L4).

Palpatory Technique

This muscle, being the most superior member of the quadriceps femoris group, should not be difficult to palpate at its origin at the anterior inferior iliac spine. In contrast, the fibers that become part of the common tendon and the retinaculum of the patella cannot be easily distinguished by palpation.

Length testing

Procedure

The pelvis of the patient in the prone position is stabilized by the examiner's hand pushing against the sacrum in direction of the table. With the other arm, the examiner then flexes the patient's knee (passive flexion) and evaluates movement at the pelvic girdle (Fig. 8.**130**).

Possible Pathological Findings

With progressive knee flexion, the patient's pelvis on the tested side starts to lift off the examination table as a result of hip flexion. This is highly indicative of pronounced rectus femoris muscle shortening. Differential-diagnostically, the possibility of lumboradicular irritation in the mid- or upper lumbar roots with a reverse Lasègue-phenomenon must be considered.

The length of the rectus femoris muscle can be tested at the same time the hip flexors are being examined (iliopsoas muscle, tensor fasciae latae muscle). The patient's starting position is the same as that described for the iliopsoas muscle (p. 294). After the examination of the iliopsoas muscle, the patient's knee is flexed further (passive flexion) (Fig. 8.**131**).

While knee flexion is being increased, the thigh continues to rise further above the horizontal line. When the rectus femoris muscle is shortened, flexion of the knee joint induces the hip to flex as well, in the form of a compsensatory movement.

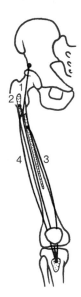

Fig. 8.**129**   Quadriceps muscle of thigh

1   Rectus femoris m
2   Vastus intermedius m
3   Vastus medialis m
4   Vastus lateralis m

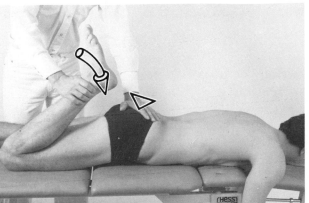

8.**130**

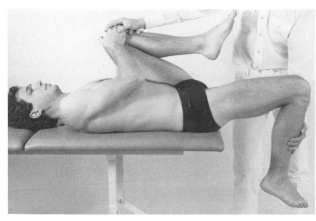

8.**131**

9　Radiologic Diagnosis

9.1　Functional Radiologic Examination of the Cervical Spine

In manual medicine, the standard anteroposterior and lateral views are usually sufficient in the routine evaluation of the midcervical and lower cervical spine. Evaluated are continuity and symmetry of the individual bony structures, as well as the patient's usual resting position. The right and left oblique views with the beam angled in the superior direction allow visualization of the anterior portion of the foramina, whereas the oblique view with the beam directed inferiorly (after Dorland) focuses more on the posterior parts of the foramina, especially the articular surfaces of the smaller facet joints.

When a functional disturbance is suspected, the lateral functional views according to Penning are indicated (Fig. 9.**1**). Clinical experience has shown that it is beneficial to guide and stabilize the head in flexion and extension, since movement is frequently decreased secondary to pain inhibition (Dvořák et al., 1988). Functional diagrams may graphically reveal the presence of segmental hypermobility or hypomobility (Fig. 9.**2**) (Dvořák et al. 1990a, b).

Both the lateral X-rays of the cervical spine in the neutral position and the functional views provide information about the possibility of spinal stenosis. Causes of spinal stenosis include hypoplasia of the lamina, transverse orientation of the pedicle, or vertebral body hypertrophy (Fig. 9.**3**). (Wackenheim and Dietemann, 1985). One of the potential complications of a cervical spine stenosis is cervical myelopathy.

Semioblique views in flexion and extension are useful in the evaluation of a patient complaining of post-traumatic neck and arm pain with radicular changes (cervicobrachialgia). This view may reveal foramen

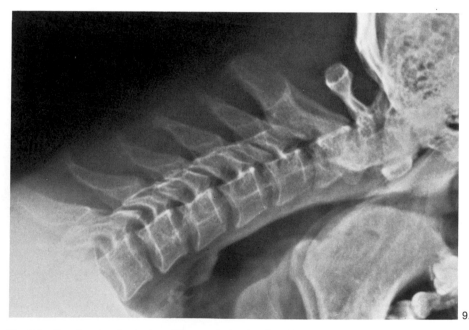

9.**1**a

Fig. 9.**1**　Functional radiographs of the cervical spine (head position held by examiner), **a** flexion and **b** extension views. The articular processes are projected over each other as a result of coupled rotation

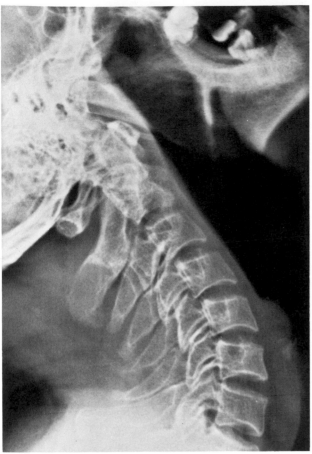

9.1 b

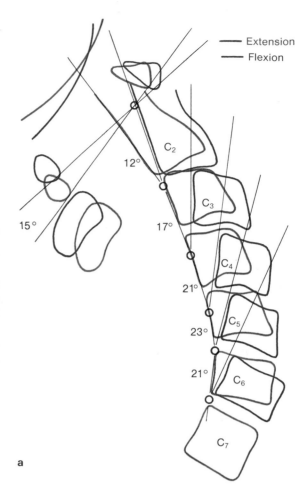

a

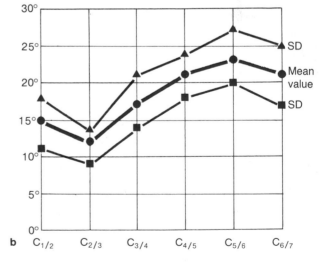

b

encroachment caused by fragments stemming from articular or uncinate processes, for instance (Fig. 9.**4**). The diagnosis of spinal stenosis, however, can more easily be ascertained through axial CT-scans. Since the interpretation of semioblique views is very difficult, especially in patients with cervical degenerative changes, reconstructive CT scans are the preferred technique for the evaluation of nerve root compression.

Fig. 9.**2** **a** Functional diagram for flexion and extension in the cervical spine (Dvořák et al. 1988, 1990 a)

b Functional analysis
SD = Standard deviation

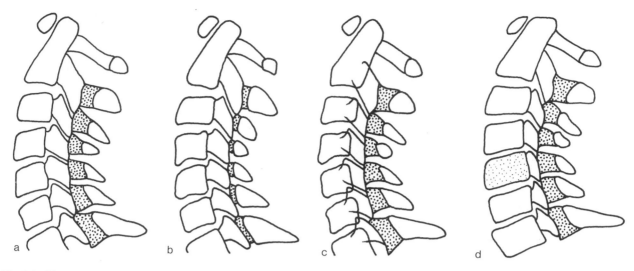

Fig. 9.3 The various forms of cervical spine stenosis in the lateral view

a Normal cervical spinal canal. The "safety zone," which correlates with the projection of the laminae, is bound by the posterior margin of the articular processes and the anterior margin of the spinous processes. The anteroposterior diameter measures approximately 4 mm

b Constitutional spinal stenosis due to hypoplasia of the laminae. The "safety zone" measures less than 2 mm and can be totally obliterated. This form is found most frequently, that is, in up to 90% of the cases of spinal stenosis

c Spinal stenosis due to the pedicles assuming too transverse of an orientation. The articular processes are displaced more anteriorly and are projected against the posterior quarter of the vertebral bodies. The "safety zone" is normal

d Spinal stenosis due to vertebral body hypertrophy. The latter reveals flattened vertebral bodies (platyspondylisis) with anteroposterior extension of the vertebral bodies and spinal stenosis (after Wackenheim and Dietemann)

9.2 Radiologic Examination of the Thoracic and Lumbar Spine

9.2.1 Thoracic Spine

Functional disturbances in the thoracic spine can rarely, and even less frequently than in the cervical spine, be demonstrated on static X-rays. Usually a straight anteroposterior and lateral view suffice.

The anteroposterior view (Fig. 9.5) clearly reveals the root of the arch and the spinous processes, but less so the joint processes or joint spaces. Typically, the head of the rib and its close anatomic relationship to the disk can be visualized in addition to the neck of the rib laterally and the tubercle of the rib. The costotransverse joint space, however, is not visible in the lower segments. In the midthoracic spine, the tip of a spinous process, due to its oblique and inferiorly directed arrangement, is projected over the next inferior vertebral body. Again, positional asymmetries should not be overinterpreted. Vertebral rotation should only be suspected when positional asymmetry is found in addition to an asymmetry in dis-

tance between the root of the arch and the outer margin of the vertebral body. In this instance, the root of the arch appears broader on the side to which it is rotated and narrower on the opposite side. Such isolated rotations are not rare, and in most cases rotation is in the direction of the convexity.

The lateral view (Fig. 9.6) clearly reveals the shape of the vertebrae and the intervertebral disks as well as the intervertebral foramina, the joint space, and articular processes. The ribs are frequently projected over the vertebral arch and the spinous process. When numbering the individual vertebral bodies, the position of the diaphragm in the anteroposterior view may be used as a guide. In special cases, a needle may need to be placed between specific vertebrae for exact localization. Abnormal posture, growth abnormalities (e. g., status post-Scheuermann's disease or juvenile kyphosis), and degenerative disk disease can be demonstrated on the lateral views. According to Lewit, unilateral changes of the intercostal space secondary to somatic dysfunctions of the joints at the rib can be detected in the anteroposterior view.

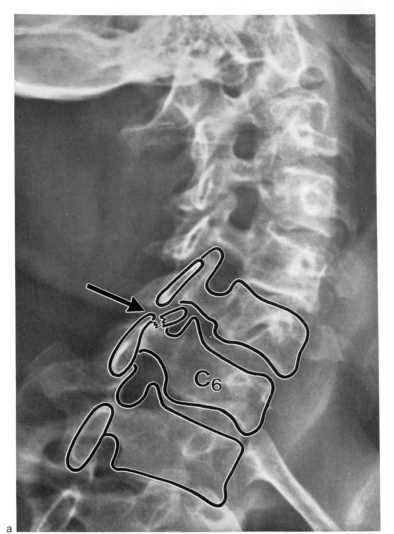

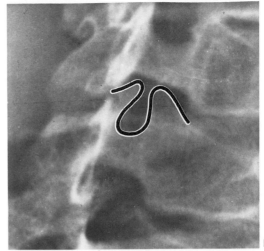

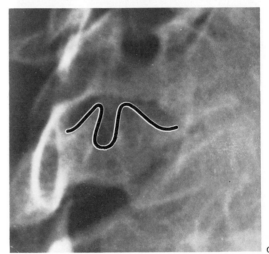

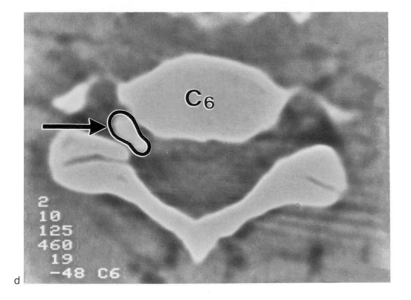

Fig. 9.4 44-year-old male patient after indirect cervical spine injury in motor vehicle accident. Left-sided neck and arm pain with deficits in the C7 distribution

a Semioblique view: the foramen at C5–C6 is significantly diminished in size due to a fractured/dislocated articular process
b Semioblique view in maximal flexion
c Extenison
d CT scan at the C6 level reveals obstruction of the foramen by the fractured/dislocated articular process

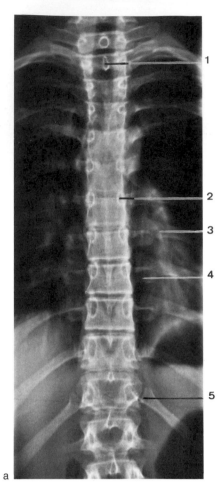 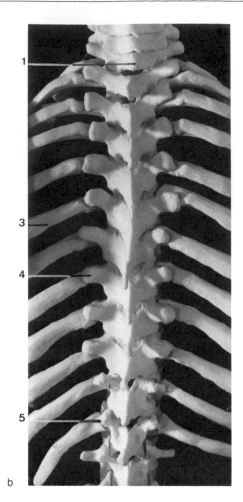

Fig. 9.**5a, b** Radiograph and skeletal model of the thoracic
spine, anteroposterior views (after Lewit)

1 Spinous process
2 Root of the arch
3 Rib
4 Transverse process
5 Costotransverse joint

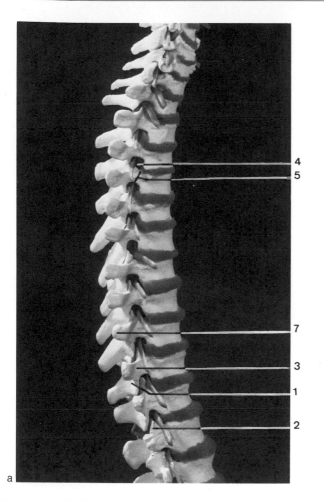 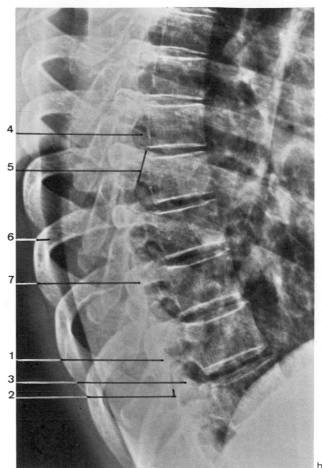

Fig. 9.**6a, b** Radiographic skeletal model of the thoracic spine, lateral view (after Lewit)

1 Inferior articular process
2 Joint space
3 Superior articular process
4 Intervertebral foramen
5 Vertebral arch
6 Rib
7 Transverse process

9.2.2 Lumbar Spine with Pelvis

The plate size commonly used for thorax exposures (35 mm × 43 mm) is actually well suited to provide an anteroposterior view of both the entire lumbar spine and pelvis, including the symphysis pubis and femoral heads (Fig. 9.**7**). This view, taken with the patient in the standing position, provides more meaningful information than the narrow view of the spine alone or a pelvic view with the patient in the supine position. Again, the examiner is cautioned against

the temptation of overinterpretation, since minor asymmetries may simply be the result of uneven patient positioning. Yet, pelvic torsions that may cause a functional disturbance in the SIJ can be recognized if both halves of the pelvis appear asymmetric on the radiograph (Fig. 9.**8**). In this view, the examiner evaluates whether or not the symphysis pubis is level (unilateral elevation of symphysis), if there is asymmetry of the obturator foramina, and unilateral hiking of the pelvic crest with the ilium

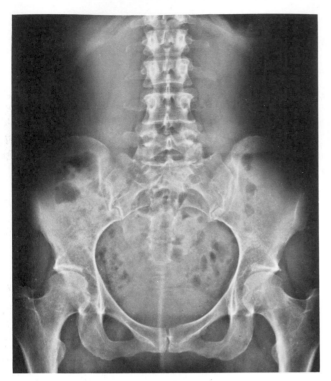

Fig. 9.7 Lumbar spine and pelvis, anteroposterior view. Facet joints at L4—L5 and L5—S1 lie in frontal plane on the right and in sagittal plane on the left

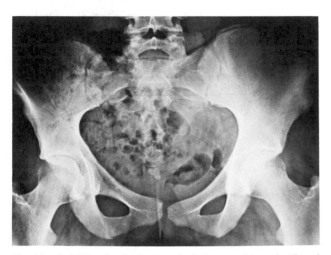

Fig. 9.8 Pelvic torsion (patient supine). Asymmetric projection of the pelvic halves, superior symphysis, and asymmetric obturator foramen

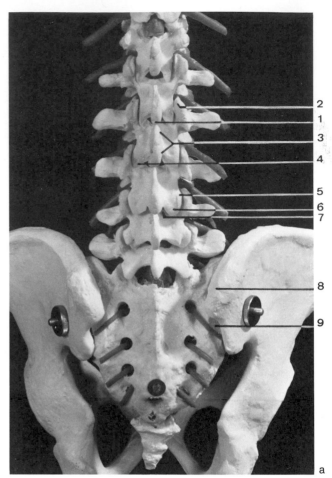

Fig. 9.9a—c Skeletal model and anteroposterior view of the lumbar spine (after Lewit)

1	Spinous process	8	Posterior iliac spine
2	Superior articular Surface	9	Sacroiliac joint
3	Vertebral arch	10	Intervertebral disk
4	Interarticular space	11	Transverse process
5	Joint space	12	Vertebral body
6	Inferior articular Surface	13	Vertebral arch
7	Spinal canal	14	Sacroiliac joint

being narrower on the same side when compared to the other (Cramer, 1965). This view also allows preliminary interpretation of the hip joint, especially the relationship between femoral head and neck, as well as the hip socket and leg length. Respective asymmetries can cause the sacrum to become uneven

and thus be the cause of scoliosis formation. Whether, and to what extent, a leg length difference causes changes in the lumbar spine is in part dependent on the position of the lumbar facet joints. Between L1 and L3, the facet joints, due to their orientation being more in the sagittal plane, can be well visualized on the anteroposterior projection. In contrast, asymmetries of the facet joints at the L4—L5 level, and in particular the L5—S1 level, are frequent, and on radiographs these joints appear oriented more in the frontal plane unilaterally. Such changes may then alter the relationship of the loading forces, leading to abnormal movement patterns and

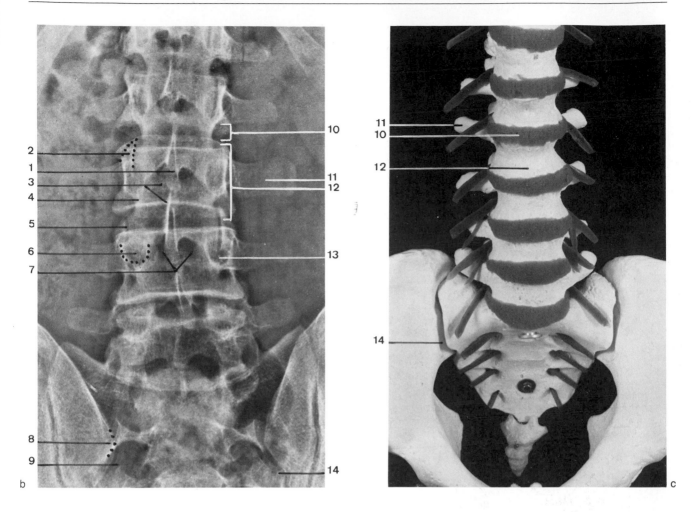

thus contributing to asymmetric degenerative changes.

In the lumbar spine (Fig. 9.9), shape and positional relationships of the vertebral bodies, the intervertebral disks, and the roots of the vertebral arch are specifically evaluated. The latter usually conceal the joints in the lumbar spine. The spinous processes may occasionally make contact with each other (Baastrup syndrome). The lowermost lumbar vertebra has the greatest tendency to reveal an anomaly: spina bifida occulta, the incomplete union of both laminae to form the spinous process, is usually of less significance than those unilateral junctional abnormalities, for instance, in which the transverse processes have become unfittingly large. In the latter case, these huge transverse processes may make actual contact with the lateral mass of the sacrum, leading to irritations in that area and subsequently causing sclerosis in the adjoining bony components. In this sense, the term nearthrosis, that is, the formation of a false joint, may be applied. Of less significance for

the practitioner of manual medicine than for the surgeon is the decision of whether the transitional vertebra has sacralized or lumbarized. Occasionally, the presence of stub ribs or architectural changes of the transverse processes are helpful in this determination. These altered transverse processes reveal a very broad costal process at the L3 vertebra, while that of L4 and L5 may be distinguished by the extent to which they point upwards in the superior direction (L5 significantly more so than L4).

Again, it is important for the examiner to remember that an isolated finding of an asymmetric spinous process should not be overinterpreted. According to Lewit (1984), however, signs on the radiograph that speak for vertebral rotation include a broader root of the arch on the side to which the vertebra has rotated, clearly visible joint space, and a transverse process that appears shorter and narrower. More important than radiologic evaluation is adequate palpation, which determines the direction and extent of the mobilizing therapeutic technique.

The lateral view (Fig. 9.**10**), which should, if possible, always include the femoral heads, may demonstrate a pelvic torsion. In the latter case, the pelvic crests are not congruent but rather intersect at the level of the facet joints (Fig. 9.**11**).

The degree of the spinal curvatures in the sagittal plane (i. e., exaggerated versus reversed lordotic curvature in the lumbar spine), along with variations in sacral base inclination have been used to define three pelvic types: the arched type (or high-assimilation pelvis), the normal pelvis ("block pelvis"), and the flat type (Gutmann, 1985). It is also possible to statically differentiate between a real spondylolisthesis with a bony break in the interarticular portion from an anterior or posterior pseudolisthesis with spondyloarthrosis and osteochondrosis. For manual therapy, the differentiation between instability and osteophytic reaction is more important than pelvic type, junctional anomalies, or spondylolisthesis. According to Macnab (1977), instability can be detected on a radiograph by so-called traction marks that are due to overstretching of the outermost fibers of the anulus (Figs. 9.**12**, 9.**13**). On the radiograph, these appear as horizontal ossifications of up to 1 mm from the edge of the vertebral body. This is in contrast to the marginal osteophytes that grow towards each other and restrict movement, but do not usually cause a segmental dysfunction. Hypermobile spinal segments, on the other hand, are frequently the nidus for segmental dysfunction and require very specific therapy. Functional views in

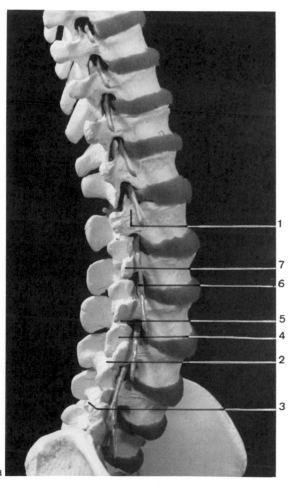

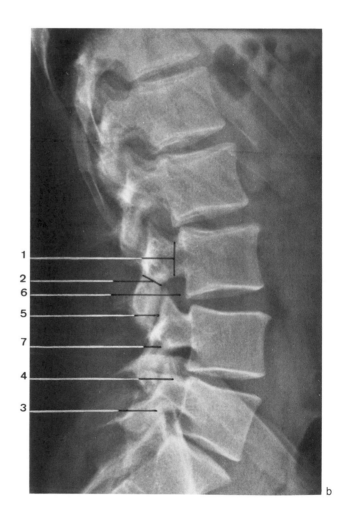

Fig. 9.**10a, b**   Lateral view of the lumbar spine. Skeletal model and X-ray (after Lewit)

1	Vertebral arch	5	Joint space
2	Interarticular space	6	Intervertebral foramen
3	Inferior articular surface	7	Transverse process
4	Superior articular surface		

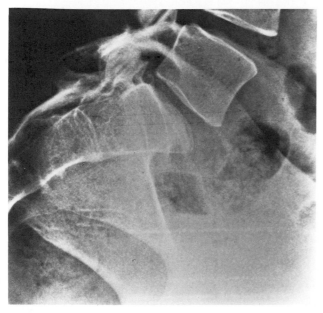

Fig. 9.11 Lateral view of the lumbosacral junction that may reveal pelvic torsion when the pelvic crests intersect at the level of the facet joints

extension and flexion may occasionally reveal excessive hypermobility, but due to the great normal variation it is difficult to set abnormal values (Dvořák et al., 1989). Typically, there is greater mobility at L4 than at L5. In some cases, and with appropriate studies, the lateral views may provide information about the presence of hypermobility or hypomobility.

On the lateral view, the interspinous nearthrosis associated with the Baastrup syndrome is visualized. In the Baastrup syndrome, with exaggerated lordosis, the spinous processes of the lower vertebrae run into each other and by friction cause a false joint with marginal osteophytic changes. This is often accompanied by pain.

In summary, the radiologic evaluation of the thoracic and lumbar spine and the pelvis concentrates primarily on static abnormalities and helps in the exclusion of potential contraindications. Radiologic studies are useful in manual medicine to the extent that they assist in the evaluation of pelvic torsions and segmental instability.

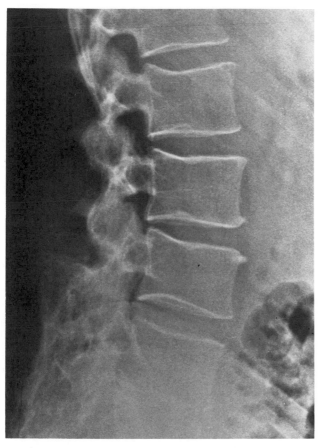

Fig. 9.12 Lateral view of the lumbar spine with traction marks at the L3−L4 segment

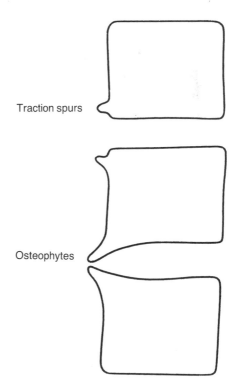

Traction spurs

Osteophytes

Fig. 9.13 Instability results in overstretch of the outermost fibers of the anulus fibrosus leading to horizontal traction marks. Osteophytes grow towards each other, leading to less mobility and greater stabilization where they grow together

10 Individual Spondylogenic Reflex Syndromes

The development of a spondylogenic reflex syndrome begins with segmental dysfunction in particular motion segments (clinical finding: Zone of irritation). This causes myogelosis as a reflex response in the corresponding myotendinoses.

Only the most important myotendinoses of isolated SRS are represented. Depending upon the extent of the SRS, the muscles represented can take part in the complete appearance of SRS, but do not necessarily have to do so. In practice, we most often find a mixture of two, three, or more SRSs, causing certain diagnostic difficulties at the beginning of treatment.

This is due to the fact that reflexogenically initiated myotendinosis of a myotenone can bring those vertebrae into abnormal position at which it inserts. This abnormal position, in turn, can cause another myotendinosis of those myotenones which are spondylogenically related to it.

All abnormal positions (segmental dysfunctions) that have been elicited must be treated. After two or three treatments, the original problem is less obscure and is represented as mixed myotendinoses.

Selected examples of spondylogenic reflex syndromes are given in the illustrations on the following pages.

C₁

**Myotendinoses
(= Myotenones) in the:**

1	Anterior cervical intertransverse m
2	Thoracic intertransverse m
1	Interspinous ligament
2	Supraspinous ligament
1	Levator costae brevis m
	Rotatores muscles
2	Multifidus m
	Semispinalis lumborum m
	Psoas major m
	Gluteus medius m (deep layer)
	Latissimus dorsi m
*****	Zone of irritation

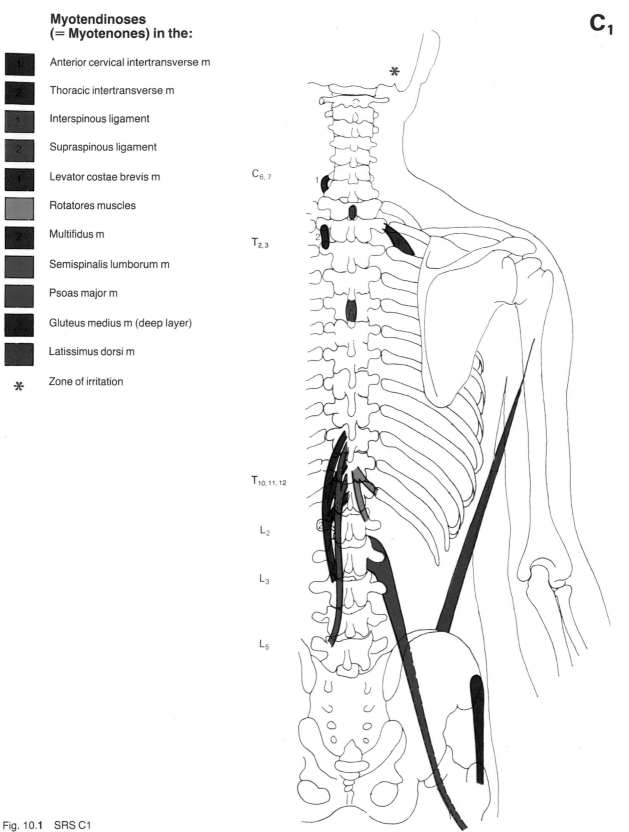

C₆,₇

T₂,₃

T₁₀,₁₁,₁₂

L₂

L₃

L₅

Fig. 10.**1** SRS C1

Myotendinoses (= Myotenones) in the:

C_4

Anterior cervical intertransverse m

Thoracic intertransverse ligament

Interspinous ligament

Supraspinous ligament

Levator costae brevis m

Rhomboid minor m

Rotatores muscles

Multifidus m

Semispinalis lumborum m

Psoas major m

Gluteus medius m (superficial layer)

Latissimus dorsi m

✳ Zone of irritation

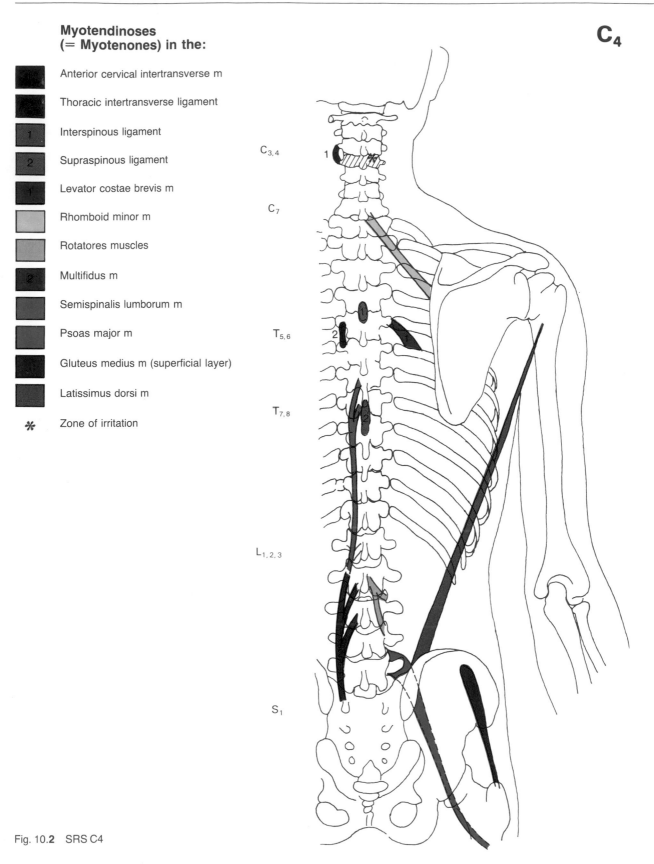

Fig. 10.2 SRS C4

**Myotendinoses
(= Myotenones) in the:**

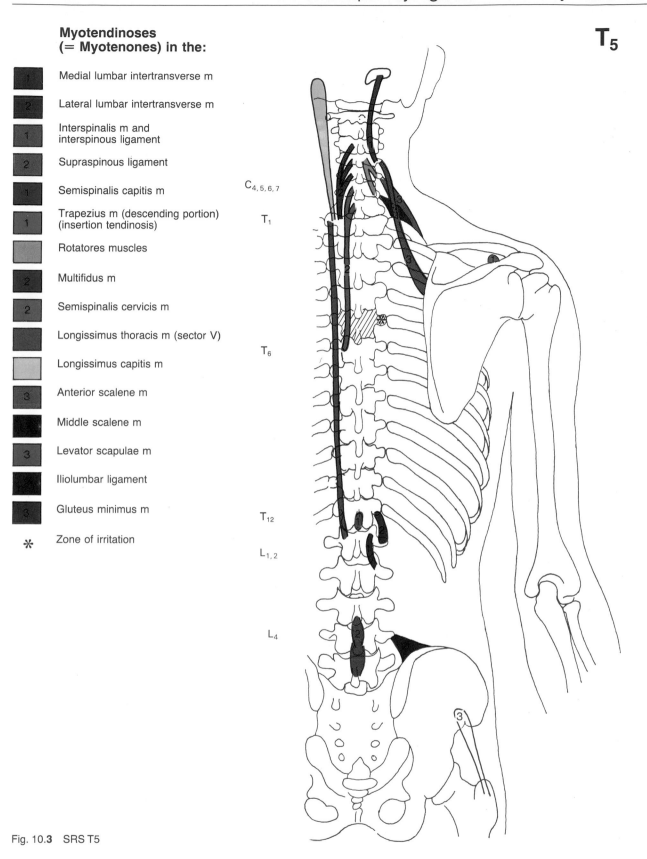

T$_5$

1 Medial lumbar intertransverse m

2 Lateral lumbar intertransverse m

1 Interspinalis m and interspinous ligament

2 Supraspinous ligament

1 Semispinalis capitis m

1 Trapezius m (descending portion) (insertion tendinosis)

Rotatores muscles

2 Multifidus m

2 Semispinalis cervicis m

Longissimus thoracis m (sector V)

Longissimus capitis m

3 Anterior scalene m

Middle scalene m

3 Levator scapulae m

Iliolumbar ligament

3 Gluteus minimus m

✳ Zone of irritation

C$_{4, 5, 6, 7}$

T$_1$

T$_6$

T$_{12}$

L$_{1, 2}$

L$_4$

Fig. 10.**3**   SRS T5

Myotendinoses (= Myotenones) in the:

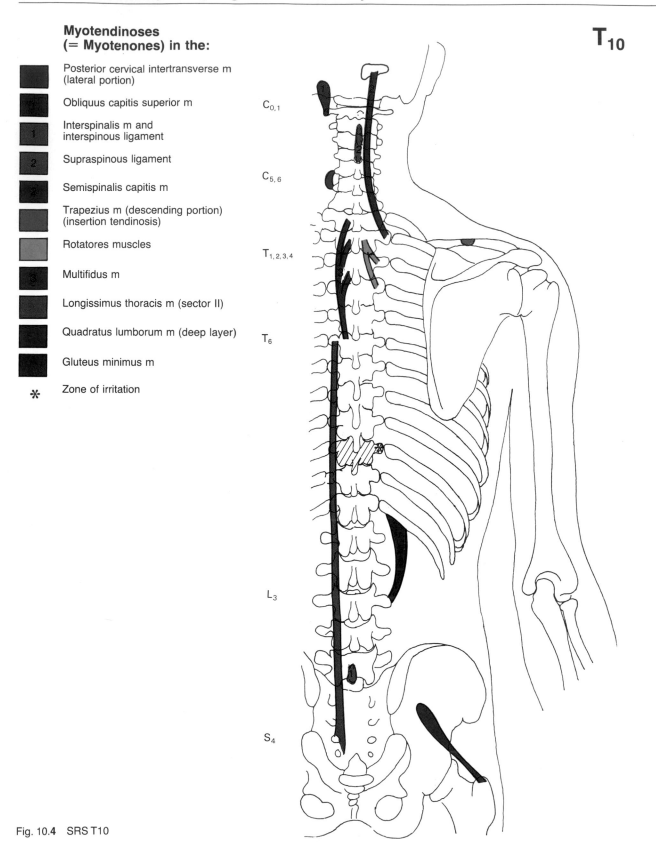

Posterior cervical intertransverse m (lateral portion)

Obliquus capitis superior m

Interspinalis m and interspinous ligament

Supraspinous ligament

Semispinalis capitis m

Trapezius m (descending portion) (insertion tendinosis)

Rotatores muscles

Multifidus m

Longissimus thoracis m (sector II)

Quadratus lumborum m (deep layer)

Gluteus minimus m

∗ Zone of irritation

T_{10}

$C_{0,1}$

$C_{5,6}$

$T_{1,2,3,4}$

T_6

L_3

S_4

Fig. 10.4 SRS T10

**Myotendinoses
(= Myotenones) in the:**

L_3

Rectus capitis lateralis m

Posterior cervical intertransverse m $C_{0,1}$

Interspinales muscles

Semispinalis capitis m $C_{4,5}$

Trapezius m (ascending portion)

Rotatores muscles

Multifidus m

Spinalis thoracis m

Longissimus thoracis m (sector I)

Longissimus thoracis m (sector III)

Gluteus medius m (superficial layer) $T_{6,7,8}$

Gluteus maximus m (femoral portion)

* Zone of irritation

T_{10}

T_{11}

L_5, S_1

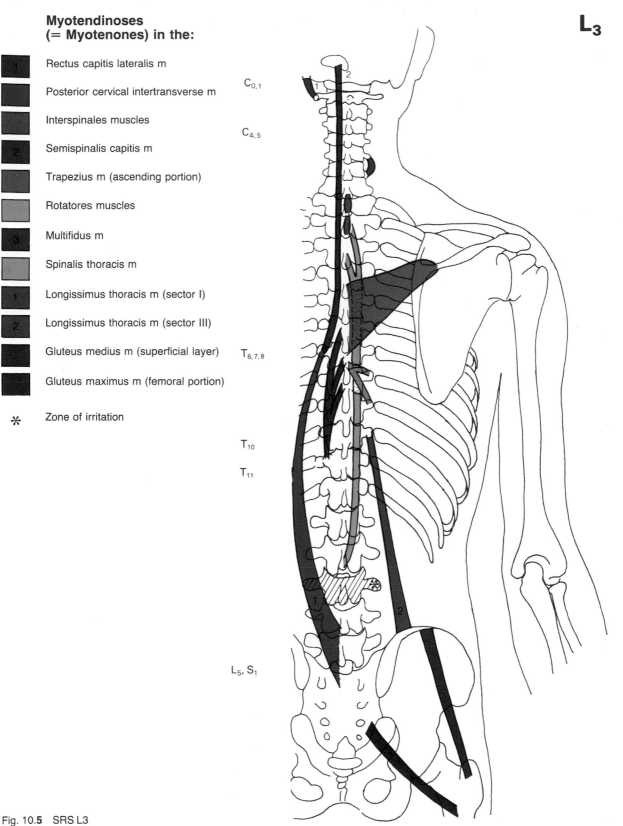

Fig. 10.**5** SRS L3

**Myotendinoses
(= Myotenones) in the:**

L$_5$

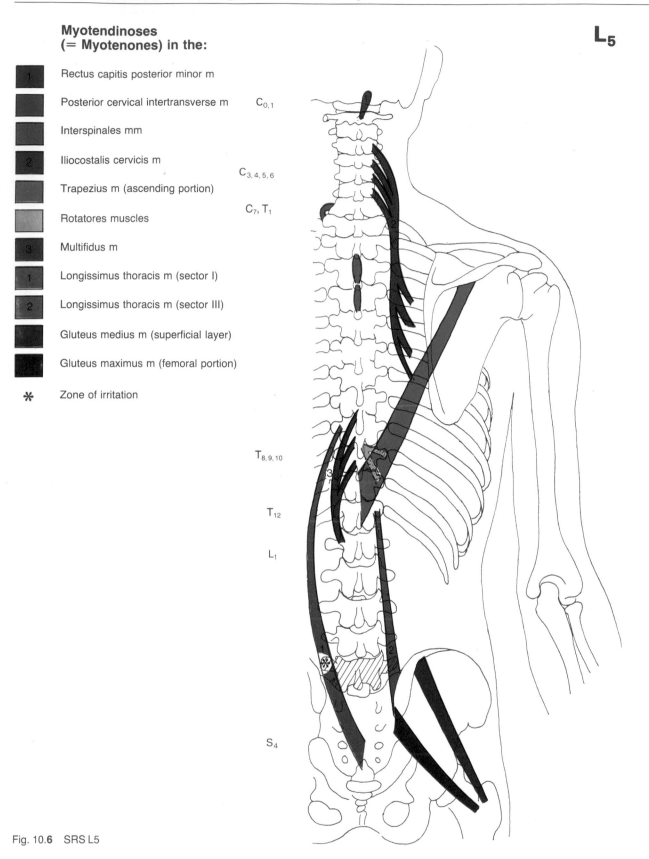

Rectus capitis posterior minor m

Posterior cervical intertransverse m   C$_{0,1}$

Interspinales mm

Iliocostalis cervicis m

Trapezius m (ascending portion)   C$_{3,4,5,6}$

Rotatores muscles   C$_7$, T$_1$

Multifidus m

Longissimus thoracis m (sector I)

Longissimus thoracis m (sector III)

Gluteus medius m (superficial layer)

Gluteus maximus m (femoral portion)

✳   Zone of irritation

T$_{8,9,10}$

T$_{12}$

L$_1$

S$_4$

Fig. 10.**6**   SRS L5

**Myotendinoses
(= Myotenones) in the:**

1 Longissimus thoracis m (sector IV)

2 Longissimus lumborum m (lateral head)

Gluteus maximus m (tibial portion)

Obliquus capitis inferior m

✳ Zone of irritation

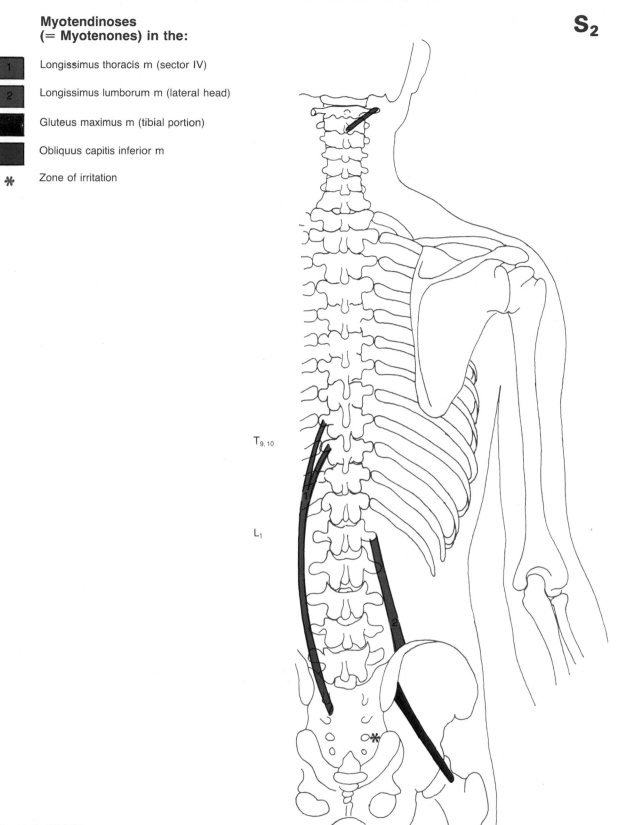

T₉,₁₀

L₁

Fig. 10.**7** SRS S2

References

Arlen, A.: Die „paradoxe Kippbewegung des Atlas" in der Funktionsdiagnostik der Halswirbelsäule. Manuelle Med. 15 (1977) 16–22

Arnold, F.: Handbuch der Anatomie, Bd. I, 1845

Andriacchi, L. P., A. B. Schulz, T. B. Betrytsko, I. O. Galente: A model for studies of mechanical interactions between the thoracic spine and rib cage, J. Biomech. 7 (1974) 497

Auteroche, P.: Innervation of the zygapophyseal joints of the lumbar spine. Anat. Clin. 5 (1983) 17–28

Baker, A. S., R. G. Ojemann, M. N. Swartz, E. P. Richardson jr.: Spinal epidural abscess. New. Engl. J. Med. 293 (1975) 463–468

Beal, M.: Palpatory testing for somatic dysfunction in patients with cardiovascular disease. J. Amer. osteopath. Ass. (1984)

Beal, M. C.: The sacro-iliac problem revies of anatomy, mechanics and diagnosis. J. AOA 81 (1982) 10

Beal, M., J. Dvořák: Palpatory examination of the spine: a comparison of the results of two methods. Relationship of segmental (somatic) dysfunction to visceral disease. J. Manual Med. 2 (1984)

Benett, G. J., M. A. Ruda, S. Gobel, R. Dubner: Enkephalin immunoreactive stalked cells and lamina II b islet cells in cat substantia gelatinosa. Brain Res. 240 (1982) 162–166

Benini, A.: Claudicatio intermittens der Cauda equina. Praxis 12 (1981) 504–510

Bernhard, W.: Kraniometrische Untersuchung zur funktionellen Morphologie des oberen Kopfgelenkes beim Menschen. Gegenbaurs morph. Jb. 122 (1976) 497

Biemond, A., J. de Jong: In cervical nystagmus and related disorders. Brain 92 (1969) 437

Blau, J. N., V. Loque: The natural history of intermittent claudication of the cauda equina. Brain 101 (1978) 211–222

Bonica, J. J., D. Albe-Fessard: Advances in Pain Research and Therapy. Raven, New York 1980

Borovansky, L.: Soustavna Anatomie Cloveka, 3. Aufl. SZN, Praha 1967

Bowen, V., J. D. Cassidy: Macroscopic and microscopic anatomy of the sacroiliac joint from embryonic life until the eight decade. Spine 6 (1981) 820–827

Brodal, A.: Neurological Anatomy in Relation to Clinical Medicine, 3rd ed. Oxford University Press, Oxford 1981

Brown, M. G., G. M. Goodwin, P. B. G. Matthews: The persistence of stable bonds between actin and myosin filaments of intrafusal muscle fibers following their activation. J. Physiol. Lond. 210 (1970) 9–10

Brügger, A.: Über die Tendomyose. Dtsch. med. Wschr. 83 (1958) 1048

Brügger, A.: Vertebrale Syndrome. Acta rheum. 18 (1960) 1

Brügger, A.: Pseudoradikuläre Syndrome. Acta rheum. 19 (1962) 1

Brügger, A.: Pseudoradikuläre Syndrome des Stammes. Huber, Bern 1965

Brügger, A.: Die Erkrankungen des Bewegungsapparates und seines Nervensystems. Fischer, Stuttgart 1977

Buerger, A. A.: Experimental neuromuscular models of spinal manipulative techniques. Manual Medicine 1 (1983) 10–17

Burger, P. C., F. S. Vogel: Surgical pathology of the nervous system, 2. Aufl. Wiley, New York 1982

Cashion, E. L., W. J. Lynch: Personality factors and results of lumbar disc surgery. Neurosurgery 4 (1979) 141–145

Caviezel, H.: Beitrag zur Kenntnis der Rippenläsionen. Manuelle Med. 5 (1974) 110

Caviezel, H.: Klinische Diagnostik der Funktionsstörung an den Kopfgelenken. Schweiz. Rundsch. Med. Praxis 65 (1976) 1037

Clark, F. J.: Information signaled by sensory fibers in medial articular nerve. J. Neurophysiol. 38 (1975) 1464–1472

Clark, F. J., P. R. Burgess: Slowly adapting receptors in cat knee joint: Can the signal joint angle? J. Neurophysiol. 38 (1975) 1448–1463

Colachis, S. C., et al.: Movements of the sacroiliac joint in the adult male. A preliminary report. Arch. phys. med. Rehab. 44 (1963) 490

Cooper, S., P. M. Daniel: Muscle spindles in man, their morphology in the lumbricals and the deep muscles of the neck. Brain 86 (1963) 563–586

Cramer, A.: Iliosakralmechanik. Asklepios 6 (1965) 261–262

Crisco III, J. J., M. M. Panjabi, J. Dvořák: A model of the alar ligaments of the upper cervical spine in axial rotation. J. Biomech. (1990) (submitted)

Dejung, B.: Iliosacralblockierung – eine Verlaufsstudie. Manuelle Med. 23 (1985) 109–115

Delmas, A.: Fonction sacroiliaque et statique du corps. Rev. Rhumatisme 9 (1950) 475–481

Depreux, R., H. Mestdagh: Anatomie fonctionelle de l'articulation sousoccipitale. Lille méd. 19 (1974) 122

Dimnet, J.: Cervical spine motion in the sagittal place. Kinematic and geometric parameters. J. Biomech. 15 (1982) 959–964

Dubs, R.: Beitrag zur Anatomie der lumbosakralen Region unter besonderer Berücksichtigung der Discushernie. Fortschr. Neurol. Psychiat. 18 (1950) 69

Duckworth, J. W. A.: The anatomy and movements of the sacroiliac joint. In: Manuelle Medizin und ihre wissenschaftlichen Grundlagen. Verlag für physikalische Medizin, Heidelberg 1970

Dul, J.: Bewegungen und Kräfte im oberen Kopfgelenk beim Vorbeugen der Halswirbelsäule. Manuelle Med. 20 (1982) 51–58

Dunbar, H., B. Ray: Chronic atlantoaxial dislocation with late neurologic manifestation. Surg. Gynec. Obstet. 113 (1961) 757

Dvořák, J.: Rippenfrakturen. Diss. Zürich 1976

Dvořák, J.: Manuelle Medizin in USA in 1981. Manuelle Med. 20 (1982) 1

Dvořák, J., F. v. Orelli: Das Verhältnis der Komplikationen zu durchgeführten Manipulationen in der Schweiz. Schweiz. Rundsch. Med. Praxis 71 (1982) 64

Dvořák, J., M. M. Panjabi: The functional anatomy of the alar ligaments. Spine 12 (1987) 183–189

Dvořák, J., V. Dvořák, W. Schneider: Manuelle Medizin 1984. Springer, Heidelberg 1984

Dvořák, J., M. Gauchat, L. Valach: The outcome of surgery for lumbar disc herniation. Part I: a 4–17 years' follow-up with emphasis on somatic aspects. Spine 13 (1988) 1418–1422

Dvořák, J., J. Hayek, R. Zehnder: CT-functional diagnostics of the rotatory instability of upper cervical spine. II. An evaluation on healthy adults and patients with suspected instability. Spine 12 (1987) 726–731

Dvořák, J., M. M. Panjabi, J. E. Novotny: In vito kinematics of the normal cervical spine. J. orthop. Res. (1990) (submitted)

Dvořák, J., M. M. Panjabi, J. E. Novotny: Clinical validation of functional flexion/extension X-rays of the lumbar spine. Spine (1990) (in print)

Dvořák, J., L. Valach, S. Schmid: Verletzungen der Halswirbelsäule in der Schweiz. Orthopäde 16 (1987) 2–12

Dvořák, J., M. M. Panjabi, M. Gerber, W. Wichmann: CT-functional diagnostics of the rotatory instability of upper cervical spine. I. An experimental study on cadavers. Spine 12 (1987) 195–205

Dvořák, J., L. Valach, P. Fuhrimann, E. Heim: The outcome of surgery for lumbar disc herniation. Part II: a 4–17 years' follow-up with emphasis on psychosocial aspects. Spine 13 (1988) 1423–1427

Dvořák, J., E. Schneider, P. Saldinger, B. Rahn: Biomechanics of the cranio-cervical region: the alar and transverse ligaments. J. orthop. Res. 6 (1988) 452–461

Dvořák, J., D. Fröhlich, L. Penning, H. Baumgartner, M. M. Panjabi: Functional X-ray diagnostic of the cervical spine: flexion/extension. Spine 13 (1988) 748–755

Dvořák, J., M. M. Panjabi, D. Chang, R. Theiler, D. Grob: Functional radiographic diagnosis of the lumbar spine: flexion/extension and lateral bending. Spine (1990) (in print)

Dvořák, J., L. Penning, J. Hayek, M. M. Panjabi, D. Grob, R. Zehnder: Functional diagnostics of the cervical spine by using computertomography. Neuroradiology 30 (1988) 132–137

Egund, N., T. H. Olsson, H. Schmid, G. Selvik: Movements in the sacroiliac joints demonstrated with Roentgen stereophotogrammetry. Acta Radiol. Diagn. 19 (1978) 5

Eisler, P.: Die Muskeln des Stammes. Fischer, Jena 1912

Eldred, E., R. S. Huttow, J. C. Smith: Nature of the presisting changes in afferent discharge from muscle following its contraction. Progr. Brain Res. 44 (1976) 157–170

Fassbender, H. G.: Der rheumatische Schmerz, Med. Welt 36 (1980) 1263

Fassbender, H. G., K. Wegner: Morphologie und Pathogenese des Weichteilrheumatismus. Rheumaforschung 32 (1973) 355

Feinstein, B., J. N. K. Langton, R. M. Jameson, F. Schitter: Experiments on pain referred from deep somatic tissues. J. Bone Jt Surg. 36-A (1954) 981

Fielding, J. W.: Cineroentgenography of the normal cervical spine. J. Bone Jt Surg. 39-A (1957) 1280

Fielding, J. W.: Spine fusion for atlanto axial instability. J. Bone Jt Surg. 58-A (1976) 400

Fielding, J. W., G. V. B. Cochron, J. F. Lansing III, M. Hohl: Tears of the transverse ligament of the atlas. J. Bone Jt Surg. 56-A (1974) 8

Fielding, J. W., R. J. Hawkins, R. N. Hensinger, W. R. Francis: Deformities, Orthop. Clin. N. Amer. 9 (1978) 955

Foo, D., A. B. Rossier: Preoperative neurological status in predicting surgical outcome of spinal epidural hematomas. Surg. Neurol. 15 (1981) 389–401

Fredrikson, J. M., D. Schwarz, H. H. Kornhuber: Convergence and interaction of vestibular and deep somatic afferents upon neurons in the vestibular nuclei of the cat. Acta oto-laryng. (Stockh.) 61 (1965) 168–188

Freeman, M. A. R., B. D. Wyke: The innervation of the knee joint. An anatomical and histological study in the cat. J. anat. (Lond.) 101 (1967) 505

Frigerio, N. A., et al.: Movements of the sacroiliac joint. Clin. Orthop. rel. Res. 100 (1970) 370

Frigerio, N.: Movement of the sacroiliac joints. Clin. Orthop. 100 (1974) 370

Frisch, H.: Programmierte Untersuchung des Bewegungsapparates, 4. Aufl. Springer, Berlin 1990

Fryette, M.: Principles of Osteophatic Technique. Academy of Applied Osteopathy, Carmel/Cal. 1954

Gerstenbrand, F., H. Tilscher, M. Berger: Radikuläre und pseudoradikuläre Symptome der mittleren und unteren Halswirbelsäule. Münch. med. Wschr. 121 (1979) 1173

Gibson, R. W.: The evolution of chiropractic. In Haldeman, S.: Modern Developments in the Principles and Practice of Chiropractic. Appleton Century Crafts, New York 1980

Glen, W. V., M. L. Rhodes, E. M. Altschuler, L. L. Wiltse, Ch. Kostanek, Y. M. Kuo: Multi planar display computerized body tomography applications in the lumbar spine. Spine 4 (1979) 108

Goldstein, M.: The research status of spinal manipulative therapy. 1975 National Institute of Neurological and Communicative Disorders and Stroke, Monograph, No. 15, US. Department of Health, Education, and Welfare Publication No. (National Institutes of Health 76–998)

Granit, R.: Receptors and Sensory perception. Yale University Press, New Haven 1955

Granit, R.: The functional role of the muscle spindles – facts and hypotheses. Brain 98 (1975) 531–556

Granit, R., O. Pompeiano: Reflex control of posture and movement. Progr. Brain Res. 50 (1979) 1

Greenman, Ph.: Wirbelbewegung. Manuelle Medizin, 22 (1984) 13

Greenman, P., A. A. Buerger: Empirical Approaches to the Validation of Manual Medicine. Thomas, Springfield/Ill. 1984

Grice, A.: Mechanics of walking. Development and clinical significance. J. Canad. Chiropractiv Ass.

Grigg, P., B. J. Greenspan: Response of primate joint afferent neurons to mechanical stimulation of knee joint. J. Neurophysiol. 40 (1977) 1–8

Guillain-Barré-Syndrome. Ann. Neurol. 1981 (suppl. to vol. 9)

Gutmann, G.: Die Halswirbelsäule. Die funktionsanalytische Röntgendiagnostik der Halswirbelsäule und der Kopfgelenke, Band I/1. Fischer, Stuttgart 1981

Gutmann, G.: Die funktionsanalytische Röntgenuntersuchung der Wirbelsäule und ihre tatsächliche klinische Bedeutung. In: H. Frisch (Hrsg.): Manuelle Medizin heute. Springer, Berlin 1985

Gutzeit, K.: Der vertebrale Faktor im Krankheitsgeschehen. In Junghanss, H.: Röntgenkunde und Klinik vertebragener Krankheiten. Hippokrates, Stuttgart 1955

Gutzeit, K.: Der vertebrale Faktor im Krankheitsgeschehen. Manuelle Medizin 19 (1981) 66

Harner, R. N., M. A. Wienir: Differential diagnosis of spinal disorders. In: R. H. Rothman, F. A. Simeone (ed.): The spine, 2nd ed. Saunders, Philadelphia 1982

Hassler, R.: Neuronale Grundlagen der spastischen Tonussteigerung. In Bauer, H. J., W. P. Koella, A. Struppler: Therapie der Spastik. Verlag für angewandte Wissenschaften, München 1981

Herron, L. D., J. Turner: Patient selection for lumbar laminectomy and dissectomy with a revised objective rating system. Clin. Orthop. 199 (1985) 145–152

Hess, K.: Lage- und Lagerungsnystagmus aus neurologischer Sicht. Akt. Neurol. 10 (1983) 113–117

Hikosaka, O., M. Maeda: Cervical effect on abducens motoneurones and their interaction with the vestibulo-ocular reflex. Exp. Brain Res. 18 (1973) 512

Hnik, P., N. Kruz, J. Vyskocil: Work-induced potassium changes in muscle venous effluent blood measured by ionspecific electrodes. Pflügers Arch. 338 (1973) 177–181

Hockaday, J. M., C. W. M. Whitty: Patterns of referred pain in normal subject. Brain 90 (1967) 481

Hohermuth, H. J.: Spondylogene Kniebeschwerden. Vortrag anläßlich der 4. Deutsch-Schweizerischen Fortbildungstagung für Angiologie und Rheumatologie. Rheinfelden, Mai 1981

Hohl, M., H. Baker: The atlanto-axial joint. J. Bone Jt Surg. 46-A (1964) 1739

References

Hohmann, D., B. Kügelgen, K. Liebig, M. Schirmer (Hrsg.): Neuroorthopädie. 2. Lendenwirbelsäulenerkrankungen mit Beteiligung des Nervensystems. Springer, Berlin 1984

Hoover, H. V.: Functional technic. Yearbook, Academy of Applied Osteopathy, Carmel/Cal. 1958 (S. 47)

Howald, H.: Training induced morphological and functional changes in sceletal muscle. Int. J. Sport Med. 3 (1982) 1–12

Huguenin, F.: Der intrakanalikuläre Bandapparat des zerviko-okzipitalen Überganges. Manuelle Medizin 22 (1984) 25

Hülse, M.: Die Gleichgewichtsstörung bei der funktionellen Kopfgelenksstörung. Manuelle Med. 19 (1981) 92–98

Hülse, M.: Die differentialdiagnostische Auswertung des Zervikalnystagmus. HNO 30 (1982) 192–197

Hülse, M.: Die zervikalen Gleichgewichtsstörungen. Springer, Berlin 1983

Igarashi, M., H. Miyata, B. R. Alford, W. K. Wright: Nystagmus after experimental cervical laesion. Laryngoscope (St. Louis) 82 (1972) 1609

Illi, F.: The vertebral column lifeline of the body. Nat. Coll. Chiropractic, Chicago 1951

Ingelmark, B. E.: Über den craniocervicalen Übergang beim Menschen. Acta anat. (Basel), Suppl. 6 (1947) 1

Janda, V.: Muskelfunktionsdiagnostik. Fischer, Leuven 1979

Jayson, M. I. V.: The Limbar Spine and Back Pain, 2nd Ed. Pitman, London 1980

Jirout, J.: Changes in the atlas-axis relations on lateral flexion of the head and neck. Neuroradiology 6 (1973) 215

Jörg, J.: Therapie des akuten „Bandscheibenvorfalls". Dtsch. med. Wschr. 107 (1982) 465–567

Jones, L. M.: Spontaneous release by positioning. Doctor of Osteopathy 4 (1964) 109

Jones, L. M.: Strain and Counterstrain. The American Academy of Osteopathy, Colorado Springs 1981

De Jong, P. T. V. M., J. M. B. Vianney, B. Cochen, L. B. W. Jongkees: Ataxia and nystagmus induced by injection of local anaesthetics in the neck. Ann. Neurol 1 (1977) 240

Jowett, R. L., M. W. Fidler: Histochemical changes in the multifidus in mechanical derangements of the spine. Orthop. Clin. N. Amer. 6 (1975) 145–161

Kapandji, A.: The physiology of joints: the trunc and the vertebral column, vol. 3. Churchill-Livingston, London 1974

Kaufman, D. M., J. G. Kaplan, N. Litman: Infectious agents in spinal epidural abscess. Neurology 30 (1980) 844–850

Keller, H. M., W. E. Meier, D. A. Kumpe: Noninvasive angiography for the diagnosis of vertebral artery disease using Doppler-ultrasound. Stroke 7 (1976) 364

Kellgren, J. H.: Observation of referred pain arising from muscles. Clin. Sci. 3 (1938) 175

Kellgren, J. H.: On the distribution of pain arising from deep somatic structures with charts of segmental pain areas. Clin. Sci. 4 (1939) 35

Kennedy, J. C., R. J. Hawkins, R. B. Willis, K. D. Danylchuck: Tension studies of human knee ligaments. J. Bone Jt Surg. 58-A (1976) 350

Knese, K.: Kopfgelenk, Kopfhaltung und Kopfbewegung des Menschen. Z. Anat. Entwickl.-Gesch. 114 (1947/50) 67

Kornhuber, H. H.: Handbook of Sensory Physiology, Vol. IV/1. Vestibular System. Springer, Berlin 1974

Korr, I. M.: Proprioceptors and somatic dysfunction. J. Amer. Osteopath. Ass. 74 (1975) 638

v. Lanz, T., W. Wachsmuth: Praktische Anatomie, Bd. I, Teil 1, Kopf. Springer, Berlin 1979

Larson, J. N.: Summary of side and occurrence of paraspinal soft tissue changes of patients in the intensive care unit. Amer. osteopath. Ass. 75 (1976) 840–842

Lewis, T., J. H. Kellgren: Observations relating to referred pain viscero-motor reflexes and other associated phenomena. Clin. Sci. 4 (1939) 47

Lewit, K.: Möglichkeiten der Prävention vertebragener Störungen. Arch. physik. Ther. 1 (1968) 103–116

Lewit, K.: Blockierung von Atlas-Axis und Atlas-Occiput im Rö-Bild und Klinik. Z. Orthopädie 108 (1970) 43

Lewit, K.: Manuelle Therapie im Rahmen der ärztlichen Rehabilitation. Barth, Leipzig 1973

Lewit, K.: Muskelfazilitations- und Inhibitionstechniken in der Manuellen Medizin. Manuelle Med. 19 (1981) 12

Lewit, K.: Manuelle Medizin im Rahmen der medizinischen Rehabilitation, 4. Aufl. Urban & Schwarzenberg, München 1984

Löffel, N. B., L. N. Rossi, M. Mumenthaler, J. Lütschg, H. P. Ludin: The Landry-Guillain-Barré syndrome. Complications, prognosis and natural history in 123 cases. J. neurol. Sci. 33 (1977) 71–79

Ludwig, K.: Über das Lig. alare dentis. Z. Anat. Entwickl.-Gesch. 116 (1952) 442

Lumsden, R. M., J. M. Morris: An in vivo study of axial rotation and immobilization at the lumbosacral joint. J. Bone Jt Surg. 50-A (1968) 1591

Lysell, E.: Motion in the cervical spine. Acta orthop. scand., Suppl. 123 (1969) 1

Macalister, A.: Notes on the development and variations of the atlas. J. Anat. Physiol. 27 (1893) 518

MacDonald, G. R., T. E. Hunt: Sacroiliac joints. Observations on the gross and histological changes in the various age groups. Canad. med. Ass. J. 66 (1952) 157–173

MacNab, J.: Backache. Williams, Baltimore 1977

Maeda, M.: Neck influences on the vestibulo-ocular reflex arc and the vestibulo-cerebellum. Progr. Brain Res. 50 (1979) 551–559

Maigne, R.: Wirbelsäulenbedingte Schmerzen. Hippokrates, Stuttgart 1970

Mattle, H.: Zur Diagnose und Differentialdiagnose des Rückenschmerzes aus neurologischer Sicht. Schweiz. med. Wschr. 116 (1986) 1550–1560

Mattle, H., J. P. Sieb, M. Rohner, M. Mumenthaler: Nontraumatic spinal epidural and subdural hematomas. Neurology 37 (1987) 1351–1356

Mattle, H., A. Jaspert, M. Forsting, J. P. Sieb, P. Hänny, U. Ebeling: Der akute spinale Epiduralabszeß. Dtsch. med. Wschr. (1986)

Melzack, R.: Phantom body pain in paraplegics: evidence for central „pattern generating mechanism" for pain. Pain 4 (1978) 195

Melzack, R.: Myofascial trigger points: relation to acupuncture and mechanism of pain. Arch. phys. Med. 62 (1981) 114

Memorandum der Deutschen Gesellschaft für Manuelle Medizin: Zur Verhütung der Zwischenfälle bei gezielter Handgriff-Therapie an der HWS. Manuelle Med. 17 (1979) 53

Mense, S.: Nervous outflow from sceletal muscle following chemical noxious stimulation. J. Physiol. (Lond.) 267 (1977) 75–88

Miles, M., W. E. Sullivan: Lateral bending at the lumbar and lumbosacral joints. Anat. Rec. 139 (1961) 387

Mitchell, F. L., P. S. Moran, N. A. Pruzzo: An Evaluation and Treatment Manual of Osteopathic Muscle Energy Procedures, Mitchell, Moran, Pruzzo, Valley Park/Mo. 1979

Mixter, W. J., J. S. Barr: Rupture of intervertebral disc with involvement of spinal canal. New Engl. J. Med. 211 (1934) 210

Molina, F., J. E. Ramcharan, B. D. Wyke: Structure and function of articular receptor system in the cervical spine. J. Bone Jt Surg. 58-B (1976) 255

Moll, J. M., V. Wright: Normal range of spinal mobility. Ann. rheum. Dis. 30 (1971) 387

Mumenthaler, M.: Der Schulter-Arm-Schmerz. Huber, Bern 1981

Mumenthaler, M.: Zosterinfektionen des Nervensystems. Klinik und Therapie. Akt. Neurol. 12 (1985) 145–152

Mumenthaler, M., H. Schliack: Läsion der peripheren Nerven, 3. Aufl. Thieme, Stuttgart 1977

Niethard, F. U.: Die Form-Funktionsproblematik des lumbosakralen Überganges. Die Wirbelsäule in Forschung und Praxis, Bd. 90. Hippokrates, Stuttgart 1981

Northup, G. W.: Osteopathic Medicine: An American Reformation, edited by American Osteopathic Association, Chicago 1966

Oppenheim, H.: Lehrbuch der Nervenkrankheiten. 6. Aufl. Karger, Berlin 1913

Pacher, A. R., A. C. Steere: The triad of neurologic manifestations of Lyme-disease: Meningitis, cranial neuritis and radiculoneuritis. Neurology 35 (1985) 47–53

Panjabi, M. M., J. Hausfeld, A. White: Experimental determination of thoracic spine stability. Presented at the 24th annual meeting of Orthopaedic Research Society. Dallas 1978

Panjabi, M. M., J. Dvořák, J. Duranceau, M. Gerber, I. Yamamoto: Threedimensional movements of the upper cervical spine. Spine (im Druck)

Panjabi, M. M., D. Tech, J. Dvořák, J. Crisco III, T. Oda: The role of alar ligaments in the three-dimensional stability of the upper cervical spine. Part I: axial rotation. J. orthop. Res. (1990) (submitted)

Panjabi, M. M., J. Dvořák, J. Crisco III, T. Oda, A. Hilibrand, D. Grob: The role of alar ligaments in the three-dimensional stability of the upper cervical spine. Part II: flexion, extension and lateral bending. J. orthop. Res. (1990) (submitted)

Penning, L.: Functional pathology of the cervical spine. Excerpta Medica Foundation, Amsterdam 1968

Perl, E.: Pain, spinal and peripheral nerve factors. 1975 National Institute of Neurological and Communicative Disorders and Stroke. Monograph 173–185, 1975

Pfaltz, C. R.: Der vestibuläre Spontannystagmus. Akt. Neurol. 10 (1983) 110–112

Pitkin, H. C., H. C. Pheasant: Sacroarthrogenic Telalgia. A study of referred pain. J. Bone Jt Surgery 18 (1936) 111–133

Putschar, W.: Entwicklung der Beckenverbindungen des Menschen. Fischer, Jena 1931

Reich, Ch., J. Dvořák: Diagnostik der atlanto-axialen Instabilität mittels transbukalen Röntgenaufnahmen. Man. Med. 24 (1986) 123

Rethelyi, M., J. Szentagothai: Distribution and connections of afferent fibers in the spinal cord. In Handbook of Sensory Physiology, Vol. 1. Springer, Berlin 1973

Reynolds, M. D.: Myofascial trigger point syndromes in the practice of rheumatology. Arch. phys. Med. 62 (1981) 111

Richmond, F. J., V. C. Abrahams: What are the proprioceptors of the neck? Progr. Brain Res. 50 (1979) 245

Rolander, S. D.: Motion of the lumbar spine with special reference to the stabilizing effect of posterior fusion. Acta orthop. scand., Suppl. 1966

Rubin, D.: Myofascial trigger point syndromes: an approach to management. Arch. phys. Med. 62 (1981) 107

Rudolf, T., D. Benecke: Zur Problematik des Iliosakralgelenkssyndroms. Manuelle Therapie beim ISG-Syndrom: Eine Pilotstudie. Diss., Bern 1985

Saldinger, P., J. Dvořák, B. A. Rahn, S. M. Perren: The histology of alar and transverse ligaments. Spine 15 (1990) 257–261

Sandoz, R. W.: Structural and functional pathologies of the pelvic ring. Annals 7 (1981) 101–160

Sato, A.: The somato-sympathetic reflexes: their physiological and clinical significance. 1975 National Institute of Neurological and Communicative Disorders and Stroke. Monograph No. 15, 163–172

Schirmer, M.: Indikation zur Nachoperation nach lumbalen Bandscheibenoperationen. Dtsch. med. Wschr. 106 (1981) 373

Schmid, H.: Das Iliosacralgelenk in einer Untersuchung mit Röntgenstereophotogrammetrie und einer klinischen Studie. Akt. Rheumatol. 5 (1980) 163

Schmidt, R., R. Ackermann: Durch Zecken übertragene Meningo-Polyneuritis (Garin-Bujadoux-Bannwarth). Erythema-chronicum-migrans-Krankheit des Nervensystems. Fortschr. Neurol. Psychiat. 53 (1985) 145–153

Schmidt, R. F., K. D. Kniffki, E. D. Schomburg: Der Einfluß kleinkalibriger Muskelafferenzen auf den Muskeltonus. In Bauer, H. J., W. P. Koella, A. Struppler: Therapie der Spastik. Verlag für angewandte Wissenschaften, München 1981

Schmorl, G., H. Junghanns: Die gesunde und die kranke Wirbelsäule in Röntgenbild und Klinik, 5. Aufl. Thieme, Stuttgart 1968

Schneider, W., T. Trischler: Testung und Dehnung der verkürzten tonischen Muskulatur. Dokumentation der orthopädischen Universitätsklinik Balgrist, Zürich 1981

Schoultz, T. W., J. E. Swett: The fine structure of the Golgi tendon organ. J. Neurocytol. 1 (1972) 1–26

Schulz, A. B., D. Benson, O. Hirsch: Force deformation properties of human ribs. J. Biomech. 7 (1974) 303

Schulz, A. B., D. Benson, O. Hirsch: Force deformation properties of human costosternal and costovertebral articulations. J. Biomech. 7 (1974) 311

Schunke, G. B.: The anatomy and development of the sacro-iliac joint in man. Anat. Record 72 (1938) 313–331

Schwarz, E.: Manuelle Medizin und innere Medizin. Schweiz. Rundsch. Med. (Praxis) 63 (1974) 837

Sell, K.: Spezielle manuelle Segment-Technik als Mittel zur Abklärung spondylogener Zusammenhangsfragen. Manuelle Med. 7 (1969) 99

Selvik, G.: A Roentgen stereophotogrammetric method for the study of the kinematics of the sceletal system. AV-Centralen, Lund 1974

Simons, D. G.: Electrogenic nature of palpable bands and local twitch response associated with myofascial trigger points. In Bonica, J. J., D. Albe-Fessard: Advances in Pain Research and Therapy, Vol. I. Raven Press, New York 1976

Simons, D. G.: Muscle pain syndromes. Amer. phys. Med. 54 (1975) 289 und 55 (1976) 15

Sinclair, D. C., W. H. Feindel, G. Weddell, M. A. Falconer: The intervertebral ligaments as a source of segmental pain. J. Bone Jt Surg. 30-B (1948) 515

Southwick, S. M., A. A. White: The use of psychological tests in the evaluation of low back pain. J. Jt. Bone Surg. 65-A (1983) 560–565

Steel, H.: Anatomical and mechanical consideration of the atlanto-axial articulation. J. Bone Jt Surg. 50-A (1968) 1481

Steere, A. C., G. J. Hutchinson, D. W. Rahn, L. H. Sigal, J. E. Craft, E. T. DeSanna, S. E. Malawista: Treatment of early manifestations of Lyme-disease. Ann. intern. Med. 99 (1983) 22–26

Stoff, E.: Zur Morphometrie der Gelenkflächen des oberen Kopfgelenkes. Verh. anat. Ges. (Jena) 70 (1976) 575

Stoobey, J. R.: Motion testing of the cervical spine. J. Amer. osteopath. Ass. 66 (1967) 381

Sutter, M.: Versuch einer Wesensbestimmung pseudoradikulärer Syndrome. Schweiz. Rundsch. Med. Praxis 63 (1974) 842

Sutter, M.: Wesen, Klinik und Bedeutung spondylogener Reflexsyndrome. Schweiz. Rundsch. Med. Praxis 64 (1975) 42

Sutter, M.: Rücken-, Kreuz- und Beinschmerzen bei funktionell instabilen Becken. Ther. Umsch. 34 (1977) 452

Sutter, M., R. Fröhlich: Spondylogene Zusammenhänge im Bereiche der oberen Thorax-Apparatur. Vortrag auf der Jahresversammlung der Schweiz. Ärztegesellschaft für Manuelle Medizin 1981

Travell, J.: Myofascial trigger points: clinical view. In Bonica, J. J., D. G. Albe-Fessard: Advances in Pain Research and Therapy, Vol. I. Raven Press, New York 1976 (S. 199)

Travell, J.: Identification of myofascial trigger point syndromes: a case of atypical facial neuralgia. Arch. phys. Med. 62 (1981) 100

Travell, J., S. H. Rinzler: The myofascial genesis of pain. Postgrad. Med. 2 (1952) 425

Travell, J. G., G. D. Simons: Myofascial Pain and Dysfunction. The Trigger Point Manual. Williams & Wilkins, Baltimore 1983

Verner, E. F., D. M. Musher: Spinal epidural abscess. Med. Clin. N. Amer. 69 (1985) 375–384

Vrettos, X. C., B. Wyke: Articular reflexogenic systems in the costovertebral joints. J. Bone Jt Surg. 56-B (1979) 382

Wackenheim, A., J. L. Dietemann: Die Kanalstenose der Halswirbelsäule. Orthopäde 14 (1985) 93–100

Waller, U.: Pathogenese des spondylogenen Reflexsyndroms. Schweiz. Rundsch. Med. Praxis 64 (1975) 42

Walther, D. S.: Applied Kinesiology. SDC System, Pueblo/Col. 1981

Ward, R. C., S. Sprafka: Glossary of osteopathic terminology. J. Amer. osteopath. Ass. 80 (1981) 552–566

Wardwell, W. I.: The present and future role of the chiropractor. In Haldeman, S.: Modern Developments in the Principals and Practice of Chiropractic. Appleton, New York 1980

Weisl, H.: The articular surfaces of the sacro-iliac joint and their relation to the movements of the sacrum. Acta anat. 22 (1954) 1–14

Werne, S.: Studies in spontaneous atlas dislocation. Acta orthop. scand., Suppl. 23 (1957) 1

White, A., M. M. Panjabi: The basic kinematics of the human spine. Spine 3 (1978a) 13

White, A., M. M. Panjabi: Clinical Biomechanics of the Spine. Lippincott, Philadelphia 1978b

White, A. A., R. M. Johnson, M. M. Panjabi: Biomechanical analysis of clinical stability in the cervical spine. Clin. Orthop. 10 (1975) 85

Wolf-Heidegger, G.: Atlas der systematischen Anatomie des Menschen. Karger, Basel 1961

Wyke, B. D.: The neurological basis of thoracic spinal pain. Rheum. phys. Med. 10 (1967) 356

Wyke, B. D.: Morphological and functional features of the innervation of the costovertebral joints. Folia morph. 23 (1975) 296

Wyke, B. D.: Clinical significance of articular receptor system in the limbs and spine. Proc. of the 5th Int. Congress of Manual Medicine, Copenhagen 1977

Wyke, B. D.: Neurological mechanisms in the experience of pain. Acupuncture and Electro-Ther. Res. 4 (1979a) 27

Wyke, B. D.: Neurology of the cervical spinal joints. Physiotherapy 65 (1979b) 72

Wyke, B. D.: Perspectives in physiotherapy. Physiotherapy 32 (1980) 261

Wyke, B. D., P. Polacek: Structural and functional characteristics of the joint receptor apparatus. Acta Chir. orthop. Traum. Čech. 40 (1973) 489

Wyke, B. D., P. Polacek: Articular neurology – the present position. J. Bone Jt Surg. 57-B (1975) 401

Yoshimura, M., A. North: Substantia gelatinosa neurones hyperpolarized in vitro by enkephalin. Nature (Lond.) 305 (1983) 529–530

Index

Index

Index

Index

Index